Pediatric Procedural Adaptations for Low-Resource Settings

Tina M. Slusher • Ashley R. Bjorklund
Stephanie M. Lauden
Editors

Pediatric Procedural Adaptations for Low-Resource Settings

A Case-Based Guide

Emily Danich
Copyeditor

Springer

Editors
Tina M. Slusher
Department of Pediatrics
University of Minnesota
Minneapolis, MN, USA

Department of Pediatrics
Hennepin Healthcare
Minneapolis, MN, USA

Ashley R. Bjorklund
Department of Pediatrics
University of Minnesota
Minneapolis, MN, USA

Department of Pediatrics
Hennepin Healthcare
Minneapolis, MN, USA

Stephanie M. Lauden
Nationwide Children's Hospital
The Ohio State University
Columbus, OH, USA

ISBN 978-3-030-99954-4 ISBN 978-3-030-99955-1 (eBook)
https://doi.org/10.1007/978-3-030-99955-1

This Springer imprint is published by the registered company Springer Nature Switzerland AG
The registered company address is: Gewerbestrasse 11, 6330 Cham, Switzerland

To the Stop Kernicterus In Northern Nigeria Collaboration; to Professors Angela Okolo, William Ogala, and Joshua Owa, and all the pediatricians and healthcare team members who have taught me to care for children around the world; to the Global Pediatrics Program at the University of Minnesota; to my colleagues at Hennepin Healthcare as well as my friends and family who have made it possible for me to travel; and, finally, to all the children God has blessed me to care for over these past 34 plus years.

Tina M. Slusher

Foreword

Manufactured equipment for pediatric procedures and medical devices are typically very costly, often prohibitively so, in low- and middle-income countries (LMICs). For over three decades, Professor Tina M. Slusher, senior editor of this book, has spent her career dedicated to advancing the care of children across the globe. Through inter- national multi-disciplinary team collaboration, she has studied common pediatric procedures and device designs, in order to modify, teach, and implement adaptations for common pediatric procedures in LMICs.

Prof. Slusher has practiced in settings across the spectrum of resources, learning from her LMIC partners, and working together with them collaboratively, to build strong equitable partnerships in pediatric and neonatal care. Always seeking to practice the best medicine possible in each locale, she has gathered ideas about innovations and adaptions from anyone willing to spend time thinking about how to make more out of less.

Most of these effective "innovations" are resourceful modifications and adaptations that simplify the device design toward the blueprint and the basic concepts behind the design. A few of these adaptations are original with Prof. Slusher, though they would not have come to fruition without the countless collaborators from around the world being willing to share their secrets and brainstorm about the challenges of doing a procedure without a commercial kit or high-cost supplies and equipment.

As a skillful teacher, Prof. Slusher has helped to share the adaptations she has learned from global colleagues and then co-taught with these colleagues in limited resource settings. She has dedicated her career to sharing knowledge of these procedures, teaching countless residents, students, nurses, and other healthcare providers, at the bedside, in conferences and hands-on workshops, and digitally (including free online material), and the content of her teachings have been well received – both in the United States and around the world.

This unique book is the first to package this content in a user-friendly, highly adaptable, pocket size format that is likely to find wide usage around the globe. It uniquely supports different learner preferences, with opportunities to learn via cases, reading, videos, and visual diagrams. This is very welcome given the variable needs and situations of learners, from limited access to Internet in some places, to visual learners, and those who need an on-the-go resource. Furthermore, having the content in this easily usable format will enable practitioners especially in LMICs to care for children in a cost-effective, evidence-based, and safe way – despite resource limitations.

I congratulate Prof. Tina M. Slusher and her team of co-editors and authors for compiling this very resourceful book, and highly recommend it to practitioners especially in low resource settings, and those (including students) preparing to practice in those settings.

Professor Fidelia Bode Thomas
Department of Paediatrics,
University of Jos & Jos University Teaching Hospital,
Jos, Nigeria

Acknowledgments

The editors would like to acknowledge and thank Emily Danich the Global Pediatrics Program Coordinator at the University of Minnesota, for her extensive work and dedication to the completion of this book as copy editor. She has served as our copy editor for this project, and without her tireless efforts, this book would not be possible.

We would also like to thank the chapter authors; the Pediatric Innovation Device Consortium at the University of Minnesota; Earl Bakken Medical Device Center; the Interdisciplinary Simulation Education Center at Hennepin Healthcare, with special thanks to Mr. Russ Siekman for his help with homemade models.

We would like to thank Dr. Jessica Jantzer, PharmD at Hennepin Healthcare Pharmacy, for her extensive help with the chapter on "Mixing Intravenous Fluids in a Low-Resource Setting". The editors/authors also thank Dr. Kristina Krohn and Mrs. Mary Greer for their substantial help in editing pictures and figures.

Contents

Editors and Contributors

About the Editors

Tina M. Slusher, MD, FAAP completed her undergraduate studies at Eastern Kentucky University and then medical school at the University of Kentucky. She completed her pediatric residency at Oklahoma University in Oklahoma City, OK. She practiced medicine in Pikeville, KY, for 7 years during which time she made her first trip to Nigeria. This trip led her to leave private practice and do a fellowship in pediatric critical care at the University of Texas Southwestern, Dallas, TX. She did her research year of her fellowship split between Nigeria and Kenya where she worked clinically covering busy neonatal and pediatric services. During that time, she has spent part of each year working on pediatric global health and often in Nigeria and other countries in sub-Saharan Africa with short stints in Asia, Europe, and Central America. She has had several funded pediatric global health research projects (NIH, Thrasher, USAID, etc.) most focused on severe neonatal hyperbilirubinemia/jaundice but on other subjects as well including breast milk use in low birth weight and sick neonates and respiratory support beyond the neonate. She is currently a pediatric intensivist at Hennepin Healthcare and Professor of Pediatrics at the University of Minnesota in the Division of Critical Care, and is the research director for the Global Pediatrics Program. She is active in the leadership of the Global Pediatric Program and continues to network striving for equitable partnerships with colleagues around the globe in research, teaching, and clinical care.

Ashley R. Bjorklund, MD, FAAP completed undergraduate at North Park University, and then medical school at Rush Medical College at Rush University in Chicago, IL. She went on to complete internal medicine and pediatric residency as well as pediatric critical care fellowship at the University of Minnesota. In residency, she completed both the internal medicine and pediatric global heath program tracks and gained experience training in international partner sites. In fellowship, she was awarded a Thrasher Early Career Award to be the lead investigator with a team of researchers in the USA and Uganda developing and studying a modification to a low cost bubble continuous positive airway pressure (BCPAP) device for use in children with respiratory distress in limited resource settings. She served as a pediatrician in the United States Navy Medical Corps. In 2019, she joined the Department of Pediatrics at Hennepin Healthcare in Minneapolis, MN, where she is currently the Medical Director of the Pediatric Intensive Care Unit and as an Assistant Professor at the University of Minnesota; she is the Program Director for the Pediatric Critical Care fellowship. As faculty of the University of Minnesota Global Pediatrics Program, she volunteers as co-director of the Global Research Program and she continues to work in partnership with an array of researchers and clinicians on development of low cost respiratory support device modifications and pediatric critical care training for limited resource settings.

Stephanie M. Lauden, MD, CTropMed®, FAAP completed dual-undergraduate degrees at the University of Rochester, and then medical school at the Boonshoft School of Medicine at Wright State University in Dayton, Ohio. She went on to complete pediatric residency at the University of Minnesota. In Minnesota, she served as a Pediatric Global Health Chief Resident, which allowed her to teach and conduct research in the USA, Cameroon, and Thailand, and earn a certificate in tropical medicine through the American Society of Tropical Medicine and Hygiene. Dr. Lauden joined Nationwide Children's Hospital in September 2017, initially in the division of Pediatric Emergency Medicine, and then transitioned to Pediatric Hospital Medicine in 2018. Dr. Lauden joined Nationwide Children's Hospital in 2017. There, she served as co-director for both the ethics and global health residency advanced competencies and Hospital Pediatrics Medical Director at the Behavioral Health Pavilion. In 2022, she was appointed as a Visiting Associate Professor at the University of Colorado and took on a new role as the Program Director for Pediatric and Psychiatric Integrative Services at Children's Hospital Colorado. She continues to be actively engaged in both local and national academic collaboratives with a focus on under-resource populations, communication with patients with limited-English proficiency, and global health education.

Contributors

Isa Abdulkadir, MBBS, PGDE, MPH, FMCPaed Department of Paediatrics, Division of Neonatology, Ahmadu Bello University, Zaria, Nigeria

Olumide T. Adeleke, MB, BS Department of Family Medicine, Bowen University Teaching Hospital, Ogbomoso, Nigeria

Michael A. Alao, MBBS, PMCPaed Department of Paediatrics, University College Hospital, Ibadan, Nigeria

Yaw Asamoa-Bonsu, MD Department of Pediatrics, Division of Pediatric Critical Care Medicine, University of Wisconsin, Madison, WI, USA

Kayode Bamigbola, MBBS, FWACS Department of Surgery, Federal Medical Centre, Ondo, Nigeria

Rachel Bensman, MD MPH Cincinnati Children's Hospital, Department of Pediatrics, Division of Emergency Medicine, University of Cincinnati, Cincinnati, OH, USA

Ashley R. Bjorklund, MD Department of Pediatrics, Division of Critical Care, Global Pediatric Program, University of Minnesota, Minneapolis, MN, USA

Department of Pediatrics, Division of Critical Care, Hennepin Healthcare, Minneapolis, MN, USA

Nathalie Charpak, MD Kangaroo Mother Care Program of the San Ignacio University Hospital Senior researcher and Director of the "Fundacion Canguro" in Bogotá, Bogotá, Colombia

Lindsey Cooper, MD (ABP) Centre Medicale Evangelique-Nyankunde, Democratic Republic of Congo, Department of Pediatrics, Nyankunde, Democratic Republic of Congo

Beverly Ann Curtis, DNP, PPCNP-BC, PMHS, IBCLC Keystone Pediatrics, Chambersburg, PA, USA

Louise Tina Day, MA, MBBS, MRCPCH, MRCOG London School Hygiene & Tropical Medicine Maternal and Newborn Group, London, UK

Brinda Desai, MD Division of Pulmonary, Critical Care, and Sleep Medicine, University of California San Diego, San Diego, CA, USA

Udochukwu M. Diala, MBBS, FMCPaed Department of Paediatrics, University of Jos, Jos, Nigeria

Chinyere Ezeaka, MBBS, FMC(Paed), FWACP(Paed) Department of Paediatrics, Division of Neonatology, University of Lagos, Lagos, Nigeria

Beatrice Ezenwa, BSc, MBBS, MPH, MSc, FMCPaed Department of Paediatrics, Lagos University Teaching Hospital (LUTH), Lagos, Nigeria

Iretiola Bamikeolu Fajolu, FMC(Paed), MSc.Neonatology, MBBS Department of Paediatrics, Lagos University Teaching Hospital (LUTH), Lagos, Nigeria

Colleen Fant, MD MPH Feinberg School of Medicine, Northwestern University, Chicago, IL, USA

Zubaida Farouk, MBBS, FWACP(Paed) Department of Paediatrics, Bayero University, Kano, Nigeria

Shady Fayik, MD Harpur Memorial Hospital, Menoufia, Egypt

Daniel A. Gbadero, MBBS, FWACP(Paed), FMC(Paed) Department of Paediatrics, Bowen University, Ogbomoso, Nigeria

Kristin Van Genderen, MD Feinberg School of Medicine, Northwestern University, Chicago, IL, USA

Scott Hagen, MD Department of Pediatrics, Division of Pediatric Critical Care Medicine, University of Wisconsin School of Medicine and Public Health, Madison, WI, USA

Cynthia Howard, MD, MPHTM Division of Hospital Medicine, University of Minnesota, Minneapolis, MN, USA

Olayinka R. Ibrahim, MBBS, MSc, FMC(Paed) Department of Paediatrics, Federal Medical Centre, Katsina, Nigeria

Caroline E. Jasada, MD Department of Paediatrics, Jos University, Jos, Nigeria

Andrew W. Kiragu, MD, FAAP, FCCM Department of Pediatrics, University of Minnesota, Minneapolis, MN, USA

Children's Hospital of Minnesota, Critical Care, Minneapolis, MN, USA

Department of Pediatrics, Division of Critical Care, Hennepin Healthcare, Minneapolis, MN, USA

Stephanie M. Lauden, MD, CTropMed® Department of Pediatrics, Division of Hospital Medicine, University of Colorado, Denver, CO, USA

Viviane Leuche, MD Department of Pediatrics, Division of Emergency Medicine, Global Pediatrics Program, University of Minnesota, Minneapolis, MN, USA

Justin Y. Lim Harpur Memorial Hospital, Menoufia, Egypt

Paul K. Lim, MD Harpur Memorial Hospital, Menoufia, Egypt

Department of Surgery, University of Minnesota, Minneapolis, MN, USA

Risha Moskalewicz, MD Department of Pediatrics, Division of Pediatric Emergency Medicine, University of Minnesota, Minneapolis, MN, USA

Gatwiri Murithi, BSc Center for Public Health and Development, Center for Experiential Learning, Safe Anesthesia and Surgery Advocate Project Manager, HRH Specialist, Kisumu, Kenya

Ndidiamaka L. Musa, MD, FCCM Department of Pediatrics, Division of Critical Care, University of Washington, Seattle, WA, USA

Victor Musiime, MBChB, MMed(Paed), PhD Makerere University, Department of Paediatrics and Child Health, Kampala, Uganda

Joint Clinical Research Centre, Kampala, Uganda

Margaret Nakakeeto-Kijjambu, MBChB, MMed Pediatrics, MUK Ministry of Health and Government Consultant on Neonatal Health Care, Kampala, Uganda

Biplab Nandi, MBBChir Kamuzu Central Hospital, Lilongwe, Malawi

Norah Ndi Nyah Njini, MD Baptist Institute of Health Sciences, Mbingo Baptist Hospital, Bamenda, Cameroon

Loma Linda University, Loma Linda, CA, USA

Agneta Odera, MBChB Tenwek Hospital, Bomet, Kenya

Beatrice Odongkara, MBChB, MMed, ESPE/PETCA, PhD Department of Paediatrics and Child Health Gulu, Gulu University, Gulu, Uganda

Akinyemi O. D. Ofakunrin, MBBS, FMC(Paed) Department of Paediatrics, Jos University, Jos, Nigeria

Stephen Oguche, BmBch, FMC(Paed) Department of Paediatrics, University of Jos, Jos, Nigeria

Alaba Ogunsiji, MBBS Intensive Treatment Unit, Epsom and St. Heller University Hospital, NHS Trust, Carshalton, UK

Ifelayo Ojo, MBBS, MPH Department of Pediatrics, Global Pediatrics Program, University of Minnesota, Minneapolis, MN, USA

Department of Pediatrics, Hennepin Healthcare, Minneapolis, MN, USA

Venice Omona, MBChB, MMed(Paed) Department of Paediatrics and Child Health, Gulu University, Gulu, Uganda

Department of Paediatrics and Child Health, St Mary's Hospital Lacor, Gulu, Uganda

Dennis Palmer, MD Baptist Institute of Health Sciences, Mbingo Baptist Hospital, Bamenda, Cameroon

Michael B. Pitt, MD Department of Pediatrics, Division of Hospital Medicine, University of Minnesota, Minneapolis, MN, USA

Mark Ralston, MD Department of Pediatrics, Uniformed Services University of the Health Sciences, Bethesda, MD, USA

Bhupinder Reel, MD Department of Pediatrics and Child Health, and Paediatric Emergency and Critical Care, University of Nairobi, Nairobi, Kenya

Amy R. L. Rule, MD, MPH Cincinnati Children's Hospital Medical Center, Neonatal and Pediatric Hospitalist, Perinatal Institute | Hospital Medicine | Global Health Center, Cincinnati, OH, USA

Katherine Satrom, MD Department of Pediatrics, Division of Neonatology, University of Minnesota, Minneapolis, MN, USA

Zubin Shah, MD Division of Neonatology, Nationwide Children's Hospital, Columbus, OH, USA

David Shwe, MBBS, FMC(Paed) Department of Paediatrics, University of Jos, Jos, Nigeria

Clark Sleeth, MD Tenwek Mission Hospital, Department of Pediatrics, Tenwek Mission Hospital, Bomet, Kenya

Departments of Internal Medicine and Pediatrics Lexington, University of Kentucky, Lexington, KY, USA

Tina M. Slusher, MD Department of Pediatrics, Division of Critical Care, Global Pediatric Program, University of Minnesota, Minneapolis, MN, USA

Department of Pediatrics, Division of Critical Care, Hennepin Healthcare, Minneapolis, MN, USA

Demet Sulemanji, MD MP Shah Hospital, Critical Care, Nairobi, Kenya

Bose O. Toma, MBBS, FWACP(Paed) Department of Paediatrics, Jos University, Jos, Nigeria

Fatima Usman, MBBS, FWACP(Paed) Department of Paediatrics, Bayero University, Kano, Nigeria

Yvonne E. Vaucher, MD, MPH Department of Pediatrics, Division of Neonatology, University of California San Diego, San Diego, CA, USA

Anne White, MD Department of Pediatrics, Division of Neonatology, University of Minnesota, Minneapolis, MN, USA

Andrew Wu, MD, MPH, CTropMed® Boston Children's Hospital, Boston, MA, USA

Background

Stephanie M. Lauden, Ashley R. Bjorklund, and Tina M. Slusher

Necessity is the mother of innovation

–Original source unknown

Abbreviations

HIC	High-income country
LMIC	Low- and middle-income country
SDG	Sustainable Development Goal
WHO	World Health Organization

Through robust international collaboration efforts, global partners have seen the under-five mortality rate drop of 61% since 1990, largely due to a decline in infectious diseases. Despite this significant progress, 5.2 million children died in 2019, mostly from preventable and treatable causes [1]. Per the World Health Organization (WHO), two regions accounted for more than 80% of the 5.2 million deaths in 2019—Sub-Saharan Africa and Central Asia. The third Sustainable Development Goal (SDG) [2] includes targets to "end preventable deaths of newborns and children under five years by 2030" and to "reduce newborn mortality to <12 per 1,000

S. M. Lauden
Department of Pediatrics, Division of Hospital Medicine, University of Colorado, Denver, CO, USA
e-mail: stephanie.lauden@childrenscolorado.org

A. R. Bjorklund (✉) · T. M. Slusher
Department of Pediatrics, Division of Critical Care, Global Pediatric Program, University of Minnesota, Minneapolis, MN, USA

Department of Pediatrics, Division of Critical Care, Hennepin Healthcare, Minneapolis, MN, USA
e-mail: bals0064@umn.edu

T. M. Slusher et al. (eds.), *Pediatric Procedural Adaptations for Low-Resource Settings*, https://doi.org/10.1007/978-3-030-99955-1_1

live births in every country." SDGs also strive to reduce under-five mortality to <25 per 1000 live births in every country. Meeting the SDG 3 target would reduce the number of under-five deaths by 11 million between 2017 and 2030, yet at least 60 countries would require accelerated progress to meet these goals [3, 4]; thus, we have a lot of work to do.

Pediatric and neonatal care continue to advance with the development of new technology and improvements in care delivery methods. However, these advancements are often not affordable, feasible, or available in resource-limited settings. This leads to significant discrepancies in what devices, equipment, monitoring, and therapeutics are available in low- and middle-income countries (LMICs) compared to what becomes standard of care in high-income countries (HICs). Inequalities in resource distribution and availability create significant barriers to providing evidence-based and equitable care for all people [5]. There are increasing calls to "empower frontline innovations" as a way to address these gaps and procure needed medical supplies [5].

Great Need Has Led to Significant Innovation and International Partnerships The first of its kind, we developed this book to compile a series of high yield procedural and device innovations for those working in limited-resource settings. Many of these adaptations are rooted in well-studied evidence, while others are the result of decades of clinical success and experience. It is intended to equip healthcare providers working in low-resource settings with (1) background for how, when, and why an adaptation may be useful, (2) evidence to support use of the adaptation, (3) indications and contraindications for different settings, (4) step-by-step instructions, and (5) advice for troubleshooting and monitoring for possible complications. Importantly, this book is not intended to teach novice providers *how* to perform invasive procedures, as this is beyond the scope of the book. Rather the case studies and topics are written to provide *skilled proceduralists* with alternative, creative, and evidence-based options when faced with patients who require procedural interventions not available in their resource-limited settings.

This collection of adaptations is the result of countless global collaborators in pediatric care who have generously shared their successes, failures, and ideas about ways to overcome the challenges encountered while providing care with limited resources. Each chapter is written by authors born in or working largely in a LMIC in collaboration with authors from a HIC with significant experience working in resource-limited settings. Where known, we have given credit to the team who originally adapted the procedure. However, the majority of these procedural adaptations are the result of many individuals and teams working together; therefore, who to credit is simply unknown to us.

By sharing these innovations and adaptations, we, the editors and authors, strive to join with all our global partners in reaching children who are the most vulnerable. We aspire to play a small part in decreasing the morbidity and mortality faced by those struggling to meet the SDG 3 goals through safe, efficacious, affordable, and locally available adaptations. We commit to providing high-quality, evidenced-based care, wherever we care for children, with what we have available. Additionally, we hope this book will inspire others to dream big, develop new and better adaptations, and share those innovations with the global community. Focusing on innovations does not minimize the importance of addressing larger systemic questions of affordability and ethics surrounding inequitable access to the newest technologies. We applaud those engaged in this work. However, focusing on what we can do right now, with what we have, for the patient in front of us, is a critical first step in improving care in low-resource settings.

References

1. WHO. Children: improving survival and well-being. 8 Sept 2020, [cited 11/11/2021]; Available from: https://www.who.int/news-room/fact-sheets/detail/children-reducing-mortality.
2. UNICEF. Sustainable development goal 3: ensure healthy lives and promote well-being for all at all ages. 2021, [cited 11/11/2021]; Available from: https://unric.org/en/sdg-3/.
3. McArthur JW, Rasmussen K, Yamey G. How many lives are at stake? Assessing 2030 sustainable development goal trajectories for maternal and child health. BMJ. 2018;360:k373.
4. UNICEF. Child survival and the SDGs. Sept 2020, [11/12/2021]; Available from: https://data.unicef.org/topic/child-survival/child-survival-sdgs/.
5. White AM, et al. Get me a mask! The challenge of equipment supply chains. Pediatrics. 2021;148(3):e2020044305.

Procedural Adaptation and Device Modification Concepts in a Low-Resource Setting

Ashley R. Bjorklund, Stephanie M. Lauden, and Tina M. Slusher

Abbreviations

BCPAP	Bubble continuous positive airway pressure
HIC	High-income countries
LMICs	Low- and middle-income countries

1 Background

A team of experienced practitioners from both high-income countries (HIC) and low-and middle-income countries (LMICs) collaborated to develop a collection of procedural and device modifications which have been used safely and successfully in limited-resource settings by experienced practitioners with advanced understanding of pediatric care. They sought to share lessons learned with individuals practicing in low-resource settings. This book reviews this series of "Procedural Adaptations" and "Device Modifications." The descriptions are intended to help those practicing in limited resource settings when they need to do a procedure (that they have been trained to perform) but do not have the standard supplies and

A. R. Bjorklund (✉) · T. M. Slusher
Department of Pediatrics, Division of Critical Care, Global Pediatric Program, University of Minnesota, Minneapolis, MN, USA

Department of Pediatrics, Division of Critical Care, Hennepin Healthcare, Minneapolis, MN, USA
e-mail: bals0064@umn.edu

S. M. Lauden
Department of Pediatrics, Division of Hospital Medicine, University of Colorado, Denver, CO, USA
e-mail: stephanie.lauden@childrenscolorado.org

T. M. Slusher et al. (eds.), *Pediatric Procedural Adaptations for Low-Resource Settings*, https://doi.org/10.1007/978-3-030-99955-1_2

equipment typically available in a higher resource setting. Our hope is that this resource will prevent practitioners from having to "reinvent the wheel." Each possible substitutions or adaptation is covered using case-based scenarios. For this textbook, terms such as under-resourced, resource-denied, underserved and resource-limited are used, though we recognize that these terms have limitations and must be considered in terms of a particular context. For a variety of complex reasons outside the scope of this textbook, the reality is that some patients have access to high-quality healthcare, and others do not. Regardless of origin, local resources, socioeconomic status, or demographics, all individuals are worthy of having access to and receiving high-quality, evidence-based, whole-person care.

2 Ethical Framework

For centuries, healthcare providers have been asked to adhere to the core tenant of the Hippocratic Oath – "First do no harm." Providers must consider the unique vulnerabilities faced by both children and individuals living in low-resource settings, and exercise discernment when weighing the risks and benefits of interventions. The recognition of the intrinsic value of all humans is essential.

Healthcare providers bring their own perspectives, biases, and experiences to clinical encounters. For example, some providers may incorrectly justify the delivery of substandard medical care in settings where resources are limited or denied. However, with the recognition of the intrinsic value of all persons, we argue that medicine practiced in any setting should be high in quality. This book uniquely provides practitioners with the tools to both recognize real resource limitations and provide high-quality medical care using available resources.

As providers consider what procedural adaptations and device modifications might be appropriate in a given setting, we must draw a distinction between merely *trying something* and *conducting research*. All the principles which guide ethical research in high-resource settings apply directly to studying adaptations and modifications in low-resource settings. Experimentation should only be done in the context of *research* with appropriate regulatory controls, research review board evaluation, consent, ethics committee approval, etc. Research conducted in low-resource or resource-denied settings must be both supported and desired by the local community. Ideally, the local healthcare providers lead or co-lead any research and are included in any publications.

Evidence-based medicine should be practiced in all settings, to the best of our ability, regardless of resource availability. All of the device modifications and procedural adaptations discussed in this book have been safely utilized in clinical practice by experienced practitioners. Clinical care should continue to be provided in a manner that is with a "best possible option/outcome" mindset in all populations, which sometimes includes "outside of the box" treatments in emergent or urgent situations. There is a growing body of evidence supporting many of the modifications and adaptations outlined in this book. When available, this evidence will be cited alongside each procedure.

Key Concepts in Procedures and Procedural Adaptations There are several key principles which must be understood by readers before attempting procedural adaptations in any setting:

1. *Weighing risks and benefits:* As is true with any procedure, attention should be given to weighing the risks and benefits of any proposed intervention. Complications for the individual patient and their families may carry an even more significant burden in LMIC settings due to resource limitations and fee-for-service models. Risks should be considered carefully prior to proceeding with any invasive procedure, especially if elective. In addition, careful consideration should be given as to which patients are most likely to benefit from aggressive or invasive interventions. In settings with fee-for-service models, the cost of care becomes another key consideration in deciding the extent or level of care pursued in order to avoid additional hardship or financial burdens for families. The ethics surrounding resource distribution and extent of care are outside the context of this textbook, though awareness of these factors is critical to whole-person care. Parents may be choosing between the medical intervention you recommended and funding education for their other three children.
2. *Informed consent:* Providers have an ethical obligation to make sure patients and their guardians understand the indications for the procedure, alternative options, and potential complications. Except in extreme circumstances, consent must be obtained using the patient's native language with consideration for patient's level of literacy. Generally, adaptations that have low to no risk, or have been demonstrated to be safe and efficacious over time, do not require an additional consent process specifically related to the adaptation. An example of this would be using a feeding tube as a safe alternative for an umbilical venous catheter. In contrast, new or unstudied adaptations with beyond minimal risk warrant additional discussion of potential unknowns and complications related specifically to the adaptation. This discussion should occur in addition to the usual procedure discussion and consent. Lack of a policy that specifies need for written consent should not negate families being involved in, at a minimum, a discussion of risks, benefits, and alternatives. Informed consent is guided by ethical and moral principles.
3. *Procedural skills:* Understanding the rationale underlying procedurals steps and specific equipment used in a procedure may allow the proceduralist to understand what can be modified safely. If a modification to an established procedure is to be performed, the proceduralist should rehearse the steps until they feel confident with the proposed adaptation and have all available supplies on-hand. Any provider, including those coming from a HIC, who has not been trained to perform a procedure should not be performing the procedure without the appropriate supervision and guidance. For many of the procedures described in this book, the most experienced providers (i.e., teachers) are the providers living and working in the low-resource setting.

4. *Emergent situations:* Although it would be of ethical and moral concern for a provider without proper training to perform one of the adaptations outlined in this book, there may be extremely rare, life-threatening situations where no other provider is available. In these emergent situations, where it would be impossible to wait for another provider or transfer the patient elsewhere, it may be more harmful to do nothing rather than attempt an emergent procedure. In any setting, when an emergency arises, the most skilled clinician should be identified with the goal of providing every child the highest quality of care available.

Key Concepts in Device Modifications and Innovations

Equipment is often donated to LMICs by well-intentioned HIC partners with the hope of overcoming financial burdens or material resource needs. While some of this equipment can be utilized appropriately, it is not uncommon to have "graveyards" of unused or broken equipment. Even small repair-parts may be unavailable in low-resource settings or too expensive to purchase. Without appropriate training, staff to monitor and implement use, bioengineering support to repair broken equipment, and access to commercialized specialized replacement pieces, donated supplies become unused supplies. It is out of this recognition that device modifications have become an important bridge to the disparities in technology available.

"Blueprint" Model of Device Design Appropriate device modification requires an understanding of the physics of the design and the pathophysiology associated with use of the device. Without this foundational understanding, it is possible to create a device that is dangerous and can do more harm than good. Many helpful "device innovations" are created by reviewing the basic blueprint or original product design that was created prior to commercialization. Examples of this "blueprint" innovation concept are bubble continuous positive airway pressure (BCPAP) and the chest drainage system described in this book – the designs shown/discussed in this text are simply the setup that was created prior to commercialization.

Bioengineers Adding biomedical engineers to any device innovation team should be encouraged. Projects often involve collaboration between engineers from both high- and low-resource sites as they design, troubleshoot, and test device safety. There are many examples of device innovations coming from innovators in LMICs. Input from LMIC engineers, practitioners, and healthcare workers is essential if the innovation is to be sustainable and maximally impactful [1, 2]. Without including engineers from low-resource settings, even the most effective and well-designed innovations will become useless if no one is able to maintain the equipment in its local home.

Local Resource Use Sustainability is critical. As healthcare providers and engineers consider potential modifications to commercialized devices or high-resource procedures, it is critical to consider what local supplies are currently available and how these supplies will continue to be sourced long-term. The use of local supplies for devices must not be so expansive that those supplies become unavailable for other common uses. For example, if all the Foley catheters are used for chest tubes, then a local site may run out of Foleys for urinary retention.

Chest tube placement is relatively rare compared to Foley placement. Similarly, if the nasal cannula supply is diminished as they are utilized for making BCPAP circuits, what happens when a patient needs a simple nasal cannula for low flow oxygen? Relying on supplies shipped from other countries or donated by volunteers creates significant barriers to sustainability and should be avoided if possible. Additionally, ideal devices do not rely on resources that can be unreliable (e.g., electricity or Internet).

Reproducible Device modifications should be easy to build and easy to reproduce. Design simplicity is key. As with any process, the more complicated and numerous the steps required, the more likely that error may be introduced.

Durability In environments with limited bioengineering support, lack of temperature control, and heavy patient loads in crowded conditions, the long-term durability of a device modification must be factored into the design. Examples of these factors include limited air conditioning, lack of reliable electricity, and dust storms (Harmattan in sub-Saharan African). In addition, fragile, temperature-sensitive devices may work well in a high-resource setting, but mechanically fail in a low-resource setting, even with well-trained and dedicated staff. Even the most highly trained staff cannot overcome a brownout, extreme weather, etc.

Cost-Effective "Low cost" is a relative term depending on the reach of the innovation and the efficacy of the device. The impact on resource allocation (nursing, electricity, bed space, families, communities, etc.) should be considered.

Safety It is essential to ensure safety as we design device modifications. As the device is designed, attention should be paid to how each modification might affect the safety. For example, before trialing a device which makes contact with a patient's skin, it is appropriate to question if this device has been tested on the skin previously. Is there a risk of skin irritation, pressure ulcers, etc.? Anyone using a modified device should understand potential complications or what could happen if that device were to malfunction. For example, with the chest tube/pleuro-drainage system, if this malfunctions or is set up inappropriately, it could cause a tension pneumothorax. Safety and risk considerations are balanced with patient acuity and overall harm vs benefit calculation.

Efficacy Finally, it is essential to evaluate device efficacy. Every effort should be made to promote clinical trials of modified devices, especially those that have not been used extensively in the past, prior to widespread adaptation. Several device modifications have successfully been studied and used in multiple low-resource settings without additional known complications. An example of this is using a using a home-made spacer for bronchodilator therapy [3]. This is both effective and without additional risk. Other procedural or device modifications have only been tested in certain populations or specific clinical contexts. For example, BCPAP is well-established as a safe alternative to conventional CPAP in the neonatal population, but additional studies are required to understand safety in efficacy in more acutely ill children [4].

Clinicians designing new low-cost adaptations should be encouraged to incorporate clinical trials into their design. Grant committees should be made aware of the value of funding research focused on evaluating the safety, efficacy, and implementation of these modifications.

3 Using This Book

Understanding the foundational concepts behind procedural adaptations and device modifications is required before utilizing the information contained in each chapter of this book. These chapters have been written in a format that outlines (1) the need for the innovation or adaptation, (2) the evidence behind the innovation or adaptation described, (3) step-by-step instructions, and (4) complications that should be understood prior to proceeding with the procedure or using the modified device. In addition to providing the device modifications and procedural adaptations that are currently available, we hope that understanding these concepts will help guide future innovators to advance pediatric care in limited resource settings with ethically responsible, sustainable, and effective innovations. Should this book lead to further questions, please do not hesitate to contact our corresponding author.

References

1. Ibitoye MO, Raji AO, Nafiu SO. Inexpensive automated medication dispenser for persons with neurodegenerative illnesses in low resource settings. J Med Eng Technol. 2019;43(8):451–6.
2. Gilligan MM, et al. From toy to tool: using water beads for insulin storage in Haiti. Pediatr Diabetes. 2021;22(5):729–33.
3. Zar HJ, et al. Home-made spacers for bronchodilator therapy in children with acute asthma: a randomised trial. Lancet. 1999;354(9183):979–82.
4. Kawaza K, et al. Efficacy of a low-cost bubble CPAP system in treatment of respiratory distress in a neonatal ward in Malawi. PLoS One. 2014;9(1):e86327.

Basics of Pediatric Intensive Care, Neonatal Intensive Care, and Pediatric Emergency Medicine in a Low-Resource Setting

Yvonne E. Vaucher, Yaw Asamoa-Bonsu, Risha Moskalewicz, and Scott Hagen

Abbreviations

BUN	Blood urea nitrogen
CBC	Complete blood count
CO2	Carbon dioxide
CPAP	Continuous positive airway pressure
CR	Cardiorespiratory
CSF	Cerebral spinal fluid
CT	Computed tomography
CVP	Central venous pressure
ED	Emergency department
EMR	Electronic medical records
ETCO2	End-tidal carbon dioxide
HAAs	High acuity areas
Hct	Hematocrit

Y. E. Vaucher (✉)
Department of Pediatrics, Division of Neonatology, University of California San Diego, San Diego, CA, USA
e-mail: yvaucher@ucsd.edu

Y. Asamoa-Bonsu
Department of Pediatrics, Division of Pediatric Critical Care Medicine, University of Wisconsin, Madison, WI, USA

R. Moskalewicz
Department of Pediatrics, Division of Pediatric Emergency Medicine, University of Minnesota, Minneapolis, MN, USA

S. Hagen
Department of Pediatrics, Division of Pediatric Critical Care Medicine, University of Wisconsin School of Medicine and Public Health, Madison, WI, USA

T. M. Slusher et al. (eds.), *Pediatric Procedural Adaptations for Low-Resource Settings*, https://doi.org/10.1007/978-3-030-99955-1_3

Hgb	Hemoglobin
IV	Intravenous
IVF	Intravenous fluid
LBW	Low birth weight
MD	Medical doctor
MOH	Ministry of Health
MRI	Magnetic resonance imaging
NG	Nasogastric
NICU	Neonatal intensive care unit
NIPVV	Noninvasive positive pressure ventilation
NPO	Nothing per os
NSAID	Nonsteroidal anti-inflammatory drugs
OR	Operating room
PCV	Packed cell volume
PED	Pediatric emergency department
PICU	Pediatric intensive care unit
PO	Per os
POC	Point of care
QI	Quality improvement
RN	Registered nurse
RT	Respiratory therapist
T&C	Type and cross
VLBW	Very low birth weight

1 Background

Many procedures described in this book are performed in high acuity areas such as the pediatric intensive care unit (PICU), neonatal intensive care unit (NICU), and pediatric emergency department (PED). The purpose of this chapter is to provide a basic outline for the development and sustainability of a PICU, NICU, or PED, subsequently referred to as high acuity areas (HAAs), in limited resource settings in order to provide good clinical care, thereby reducing morbidity and mortality. These general guidelines are intended to be adapted for specific local, regional, and countrywide circumstances and cultural considerations.

1.1 Administration

Essential to the successful development and maintenance of an HAA is not only the commitment from the local hospital administration and leadership but also commitment from all involved levels of government including district/regional administrators and the Ministry of Health (MOH). Establishing and maintaining good relationships with referral sources is essential. Bidirectional communication between and integration with regional healthcare sites (e.g., regional hospital, district hospital, health centers) is needed to assure provision of appropriate levels of care, consultation, referral, and transfer of patients between sites. The MOH and hospital administration, in consultation with the HAA team, should develop guidelines for referrals between HAA facilities and all associated healthcare sites to enable appropriate escalation or de-escalation of care. The care for critically ill neonates and children at each site should be performed according to protocols and treatment guidelines that meet the national standards.

The setting up and maintaining of an HAA in developing countries requires a long-term administrative and financial commitment. Sustaining a functional PED, PICU, or NICU may be more challenging than establishing one. The decision to develop and support an HAA should be congruent with overall hospital goals and objectives, and be independent of individual changes in hospital administrative positions or board membership. Sufficient, ongoing financial and administrative commitment from the hospital, government, and/or MOH is essential to prevent the collapse of the HAA. Annual MOH and hospital budgets need to be sufficient for the support of personnel; for procurement, maintenance, and repair of necessary capital equipment (e.g., ventilators, warmers, suction machines, and IV pumps); for replacement of associated disposables (e.g., IV tubing, ventilator/continuous positive airway pressure (CPAP) circuits, nasal cannula); and for other essential supplies (e.g., gloves, needles, syringes, feeding tubes, alcohol wipes). MOH funding and health insurance reimbursement should be sufficient to cover the level, type, and volume of care provided by the HAA rather than being based only on hospital location or designation. MOH funding and health insurance reimbursements need to be prompt; delays result in difficulty paying suppliers and staff salaries, adversely affecting the quality of patient care.

1.2 Levels of Care

Local experts, regional health leadership, and the MOH should develop standards for all levels of care associated with HAAs. Definitions of "levels of care" in the PICU, NICU, and PED may vary depending upon resources available or as determined by individual country standards and guidelines. There is no system that will fit the needs of every region or resource-limited setting. Defining tiered approaches to care should be considered by all administrative levels of healthcare (i.e., country, region, institution). An example of care levels is shown for NICUs in Table 1.

1.3 Personnel

Personnel are essential to the function of any unit. Hospital staffing or personnel is often provided through the cooperation between government and individual institutions. Personnel for an HAA include registered nurses (RN), medical doctors (MD),

Table 1 Examples of tiered levels of neonatal care

Level of care	Description
Basic	Provide emergency bag and mask resuscitation at delivery of a newborn; bulb suction or other suction device, intermittent vital sign monitoring (heart rate, respiratory rate, temperature); routine postnatal care for the healthy, physiologically stable term (≥38 weeks' gestation) and late preterm (35–37 weeks' gestation) newborns; enteral nutritional support, cup feeding, initial fluid resuscitation; administration of antimicrobials
Intermediate (basic plus the following)	Care for moderately preterm (32–34 weeks' gestation) and LBW (<2500–1500 g) newborns; vital sign monitoring (heart rate, respiratory rate, temperature, oxygen saturation); respiratory support including supplemental oxygen and CPAP; nutritional support with NG tube feeding; intravenous fluids and antibiotics; phototherapy, transfusion, surgical and medical subspecialty consults available; basic radiographic and laboratory support
Advanced (intermediate plus the following)	Comprehensive care for VLBW (<1500 g), very preterm (<32 weeks' gestation) neonates and sustained life support for any critically ill newborn; respiratory support including invasive mechanical ventilation; intravenous vasoactive support and parenteral nutrition; emergent surgical and medical specialty consultation; readily available radiographic and ultrasonic imaging; wide range of laboratory support

and mid-level providers such as clinical officers, respiratory therapists (RT), pharmacists, biomedical engineers, and environmental service workers. Commitment to provide sufficient annual funding for HAA personnel is essential. Nurses often provide the majority of patient care in the HAA. It is essential to recruit and retain a sufficient number of experienced, well-trained nursing staff in order to provide quality patient care. There should be a commitment to adequate initial training, ongoing medical education, as well as engagement of nursing at all levels in quality improvement initiatives.

The availability of personnel to fulfill specific roles involved in providing care for critically ill children is important. The training level of the personnel available to fulfill these roles may vary between institutions. In high-resource settings, individual specialists are responsible for performing specific functions such as overseeing respiratory care, medication management to assure proper drug selection and dosing, and equipment maintenance. Where staffing is limited, individual doctors and nurses can assume these specialized roles. On-call or standby staffing allows for some flexibility when patient census changes. Personnel assigned to perform duties other than direct patient care in the HAA may be able to provide patient care when census changes during surges. Having specifically designated staff to regularly clean all equipment and the physical environment is very important to reduce the risk of transmission of potentially deadly pathogenic organisms to the staff and from one patient to another.

Managing critically ill patients requires a team approach to care. The team includes all those providing patient care: physicians, nurses, and ancillary staff. Each team member should be aware of their individual responsibilities on the team. Respect for each other and open communication between team members are critical for a well-functioning team and optimal patient care. For instance, during resuscitation it is important to have a team leader – most often a physician – who oversees the resuscitation and coordinates care efforts among the team.

Staff burnout, low salaries, and the intensity of the work all threaten the integrity of HAAs. In addition to the initial training, regular education including in vivo simulation in the HAA or simulation mock codes reinforces familiarity with procedures, teaches team-building strategies, and encourages team cohesion. Once trained to provide care in an HAA, staff should be allowed to remain in such areas to maintain high levels of clinical competency. Every effort should be made to retain experienced staff who choose to work in the HAA and who find working there rewarding. Transfer into the HAA and/or retention of staff who are either disinterested or who have difficulty personally tolerating the stressful intensive care environment can be detrimental to patient care.

Initial and recurrent training of personnel, providing levels of staff certification, remuneration for subspecialty or advanced training and competitive salaries to encourage experienced staff to work in the unit, maintaining an adequate annual budget, establishing sources of funding commensurate with the goals of the unit, and a safe and robust system for addressing staff concerns without retribution will all help sustain a successful ED, NICU, and PICU.

2 Physical Resources and Spaces

The establishment and maintenance of an HAA in a resource-limited setting is contingent upon the availability of sufficient space for patient care and the healthcare workers. A reliable supply of electric power (including a backup generator if needed), oxygen (with backup tanks or concentrators as needed), and clean water is critical in any HAA to support the use of lifesaving equipment such as ventilators and infusion pumps and for the prevention of hospital-acquired infection by encouraging effective handwashing and environmental cleanliness.

Adequate physical space in which HAAs are located is essential. Depending on the source of admissions to the PICU, proximity to the emergency department (ED), operating room, or both may be important; the NICU should be located close to the labor and delivery areas and accessible to postpartum mothers; and the ED should be readily accessible to the public or an ambulance arriving to the hospital. The size of the area designated for each patient may be determined by governments or standards of care in a country, but ideally each patient area will have enough space for the patient bed, equipment, and medical personnel and for the presence of family. The area should have adequate lighting and temperature control, a dependable electrical supply, and a clean, potable water supply.

In addition to direct patient care areas, the PED and ICUs will require identified space for nursing and physician staff to perform charting, medication preparation, as well as cleaning equipment. The nurses' station should be located in a position to easily visualize patient care areas with the ability to readily identify changes in patient acuity and the recruit help when needed. Space should be designated for storage of durable and reusable equipment, readily available resuscitation equipment including a code cart, a procedural area, a family consultation room, as well as storage of medication and nutritional supplies. An area to express breast milk is important, especially in the NICU.

One of the most important advancements in medical care was the recognition of handwashing to prevent the spread of infectious disease. Designated wash stations with soap and clean water, emphasizing good handwashing technique, as well as provision of a hand-sanitizing gel for staff and family members are the most effective ways to prevent infection in the hospital setting.

3 Essential Durable Medical Equipment and Disposable Medical Supplies

High acuity medical care provided in areas such as a PED, NICU, and PICU requires equipment not necessarily found in general care units. The need for invasive and noninvasive monitoring, as well as providing respiratory, cardiovascular, and neurologic support, requires equipment and supplies specifically designed for use in HAAs. The type of equipment needed is dependent on the answer to two questions: (1) what resources are available, including equipment, personnel, and financial and (2) what are the most common life-threatening medical conditions patients will present with to the hospital? The answers to these questions will determine which equipment should be emphasized and procured. In general, the intended goal is to provide noninvasive care whenever possible, thus avoiding the complications, and advanced monitoring, training, and resources required to perform invasive procedures. There are, however, some basic equipment needs for any high acuity area (see Tables 2 and 3).

The method of procuring durable medical equipment is a decision that should include all the medical and institutional stakeholders. The discussion includes weighing benefits and disadvantages of accepting donated or previously used medical equipment versus purchasing new equipment. While accepting donated or previously used equipment may be attractive due to reduced cost, there are many limitations. Donated equipment may not fill the need of the unit; be more complex than what is needed; require unavailable expertise to maintain, troubleshoot, and repair; require disposables that are unavailable and/or unaffordable; and have incompatible electrical, gas, or water requirements. All these issues potentially limit the functionality and longevity of the donated equipment. Donated equipment may also result in a variety of brand and models, each with their own specific maintenance and repair requirements. Purchasing new equipment can provide uniformity and match the type and complexity of equipment to the specific needs and level of care of the unit. In addition, new equipment is easier to maintain, often including a warranty and/or a repair contract. Ideally, a unit should have equipment that fulfills basic clinical needs (e.g., monitoring, ventilation, IV fluids, oxygen saturation

Table 2 Examples of essential tiered resources and supplies for neonatal and pediatric care in resource-limited settings

	Basic	Intermediate (IM): basic resources plus	Advanced: IM resources plus
Vital sign, cardiorespiratory (CR) monitoring	Digital thermometer, stethoscope, blood pressure cuff (with at least infant, child, and adult cuff sizes)	Basic plus continuous noninvasive CR monitoring capabilities	Invasive CR monitoring such as umbilical, arterial, lines, CVP, ETCO2, CO2 detector, capnography
Nutrition	Oral nutritional support: Syringes, bottles, or cups	Nasogastric and nasojejunal feeding tubes, feeding pumps	Parenteral nutrition
Fluid and medications (see medication section)	Oral rehydration and maintenance fluids, enteral medications (liquid and tablet forms) for common life-threatening conditions	Intravenous isotonic and maintenance fluids, IV medications for common life-threatening conditions, IV tubing sets with volume chamber	Custom IV and enteral fluids, IV; enteral medications for less common life-threatening conditions, infusion pumps
Diagnostic resources	POC glucose	Complete blood counts, basic chemistry panel, urinalysis, microbiology (cultures), radiographs	POC laboratory, blood gas, advanced chemistries, genetic testing, POC ultrasound, CT, MRI
Other resources	Blankets, gloves, gowns, bulb suction	Radiant warmers, incubators, portable suction	Wall suction Refrigeration for medication, blood storage

monitoring), is simple to operate, can be maintained and repaired locally, and has readily available and affordable disposable parts. The decision to purchase and maintain equipment from local or in-country providers reduces cost and may improve responsiveness for maintenance and repair. When purchasing new equipment in-country, it is essential to look carefully at the quality of the equipment. High-quality equipment often costs more at the onset but ultimately saves money if it is more dependable and durable. Most durable medical equipment also includes disposable parts, such as ventilator circuits and IV tubing which require funding for regular replacement. Personnel with the responsibility and authority to maintain, repair, and replace medical equipment should be identified whenever equipment is first purchased. Developing a system to routinely track equipment purchases, maintenance, and repair, having a sufficient budget for maintaining and replacing equipment, and establishing a close working relationship with available biomedical engineers are all important.

As noted previously, an area to store the equipment is necessary, but may be shared between the HAAs and the hospital operating rooms (ORs)/theaters as long as the equipment is readily accessible to all HAAs.

Table 3 Equipment and supplies necessary for respiratory support for neonatal and pediatric care in resource-limited settings

PED, NICU, and PICU	Oxygen, with flowmeter	Nasal cannula and mask	Oxygen blender	Pulse oximeter	Ventilator	CPAP/ NIPPV	Blood gas	Surfactant	Resuscitation equipment[a]
Basic	x	x							x
Intermediate	x	x	x	x		x			x
Advanced	x	x	x	x	x	x	x	x	x

[a] As appropriate for level-dependent care: self-inflating resuscitation bag, face masks of all sizes, suction bulb/device, laryngeal mask, endotracheal tubes, laryngoscope blades, and handles

4 Essential Drugs

HAAs use medications including those in vasoactive, anti-infective, and sedative categories. The specific categories and specific medications available to an institution for procurement may be contingent on the national formulary as determined by national policy and/or the MOH. Medication procurement from independent sources may need to be approved by the hospital administration, MOH, or regional stores.

Accurate records of available medications and a reliable supply chain are essential to avoid critically low levels or outright absence of specific drugs. Accurate record keeping also allows for monitoring of drug usage, prevents wastage, and identifies medications that are close to expiring, all of which reduces cost to the institution.

Medications needed for emergencies, including those required for resuscitation, status epilepticus, treatment of sepsis, acute management of raised intracranial pressures, respiratory failure, and intubation, should be immediately available on-site. When ordering IVFs, check the electrolyte concentrations of the available solutions to verify the amounts of basic ingredients including sodium, potassium, glucose, and base. Double checks and dual signatures for drugs with high lethality such as potassium, calcium, and chemotherapeutics should be encouraged. The hospital administration and unit director need to maintain ongoing discussions with the MOH to assure that all drugs necessary for lifesaving care in the HAAs are immediately available on-site, reducing the time and cost of procurement from an outside source. Other medications and fluids should be obtained readily through the institution's pharmacy or other delivery system.

Due to the concern for opioid and other substance abuse, including among healthcare workers, a secure system of monitoring, storage, and dispensing of drugs of abuse (e.g., limited drug volume, lock box system with key, logbook, or a system requiring dual signatures) is necessary. Additionally, in very remote areas, where supplies of these medications may be extremely low, keeping them in a secure location with limited access may help reserve the supplies for patients that most need them.

Specific drugs will vary based upon availability from the national formulary, local availability, and HAA type, location, and level of care. A non-exhaustive list of examples of commonly used medication classes for critically ill pediatric and neonatal patients include:

- *Antibiotics/antivirals/antiparasitic/antifungal (*IV, PO, ointments, and creams): dependent on local community and nosocomial flora and sensitivities
- *IV fluids*: NS, LR, or similar solutions like Hartman's, dextrose (5%, 10%, 50%), electrolyte additives, parenteral nutrition
- *Cardiovascular*: diuretics, vasoactive medications (pressors, inotropes, vasodilators, antihypertensive), antiarrhythmic
- *Respiratory*: inhaled/systemic bronchodilators, oral steroids, surfactant
- *Anticonvulsants*

- *Sedation/analgesia*: opioids, nonsteroidal anti-inflammatory drugs (NSAID), sedatives/hypnotics, amnestic agents
- *Muscle relaxants/paralytics*
- *Prophylaxis*: vitamin K (if possible, vitamin K1), ophthalmologic prophylaxis for newborns
- *Other*: systemic steroids, prostaglandin inhibitors

5 Essential Laboratory Tests

Many healthcare centers around the world provide the most essential components of lifesaving critical care using excellent clinical skills (i.e., history and physical examination) despite limited or no access to laboratory tests. However, the availability of laboratory tests impacts the ability to diagnose, facilitate medical decision-making, and improve the efficacy of interventions and treatments. Laboratory tests needed for a given HAA will depend on the patient population it serves, laboratory facilities available, and the administrative and financial support from the institution and the MOH. Laboratory testing may be point of care (POC) or centralized, depending on the complexity of the test, training of bedside personnel, and test supplies available. Examples of essential laboratory tests are shown in Table 4.

Table 4 Essential laboratory tests for neonatal and pediatric care in resource-limited settings

	Basic	Intermediate	Advanced
Hgb/Hct[a], CBC, differential/malaria screening	x	X	x
Coagulation			x
Transfusion services (T&C, Coombs, antibody testing)		X	x
Bilirubin (total and direct)	x	X	x
Basic electrolytes[b]		X	x
Glucose	x	X	x
BUN[c]/creatinine		X	x
Liver function tests		X	x
Urinalysis with microscopy[a]		X	x
Cultures (blood, urine, CSF[d])		X	x
Blood gas[e]			x

[a] May be point of careHgb/Hct/PCV: hemoglobin/hematocrit/packed cell volumeCBC: complete blood countT&C: type and cross
[b] Basic electrolytes: Na, K, CL, CO2
[c] BUN: blood urea nitrogen
[d] CSF: cerebral spinal fluid
[e] Blood gas: pH, pCO2, pO2, BE

6 Clinical Care Protocols: Policies

Standardized, written clinical care protocols improve the quality of care for critically ill neonatal and pediatric patients. Perhaps the most important to prevent death is a triage protocol with a standardized plan for assessing and recognizing very ill children as early as possible so that stabilizing measures and critical interventions can be immediately initiated. Such a triage protocol is implemented upon presentation, and can be a guideline thereafter for reassessing the patient over time during their initial hospital course. The World Health Organization has produced a free training program and manual, *Emergency Triage Assessment and Treatment* [1], which provides guidelines and protocols for identifying children in critical condition and providing initial interventions [2]. The *Helping Babies Breath* protocol is another excellent example of a worldwide, standardized protocol enabling birth attendants to recognize an effectively resuscitate infants demonstrating signs of neonatal asphyxia and to reprocess or clean that equipment after use (Fig. 1a and b) [3].

Examples of PICU/NICU/PED clinical scenarios that benefit from standardized protocols include shock, sepsis, neonatal jaundice, seizures, severe anemia, dehydration, malnutrition, respiratory failure, neonatal asphyxia, and informed consent for procedures. Detailed protocols should be provided for all procedures as well as for sterilization and cleaning of equipment.

7 Infection Control

Nosocomial infection, the greatest invisible threat in critical care units, substantially increases morbidity and mortality. All invasive procedures such as umbilical catheter, central line, and chest tube placement must be performed under sterile conditions.

Infective organisms are transferred to patients from hands, equipment, unit surfaces, and water collections. Handwashing or use of alcohol-/antiseptic-based preparations before and after touching each patient is essential. Antiseptic solutions placed at each bedside are the most effective way to assure adequate hand hygiene, even when soap and water are readily available. Frequent, thorough environmental cleaning of all unit surfaces including the floor is important. To reduce the risk of nosocomial infection, a system must be in place for disinfection for all durable equipment (e.g., respiratory equipment, radiant warmers, incubators, cots, monitors, oximeters, stethoscopes) by designated staff using task-specific protocols between patient use. Any reused disposable equipment with direct patient contact (e.g., respiratory circuits and resuscitation devices) must be adequately cleaned and sterilized prior to each reuse.

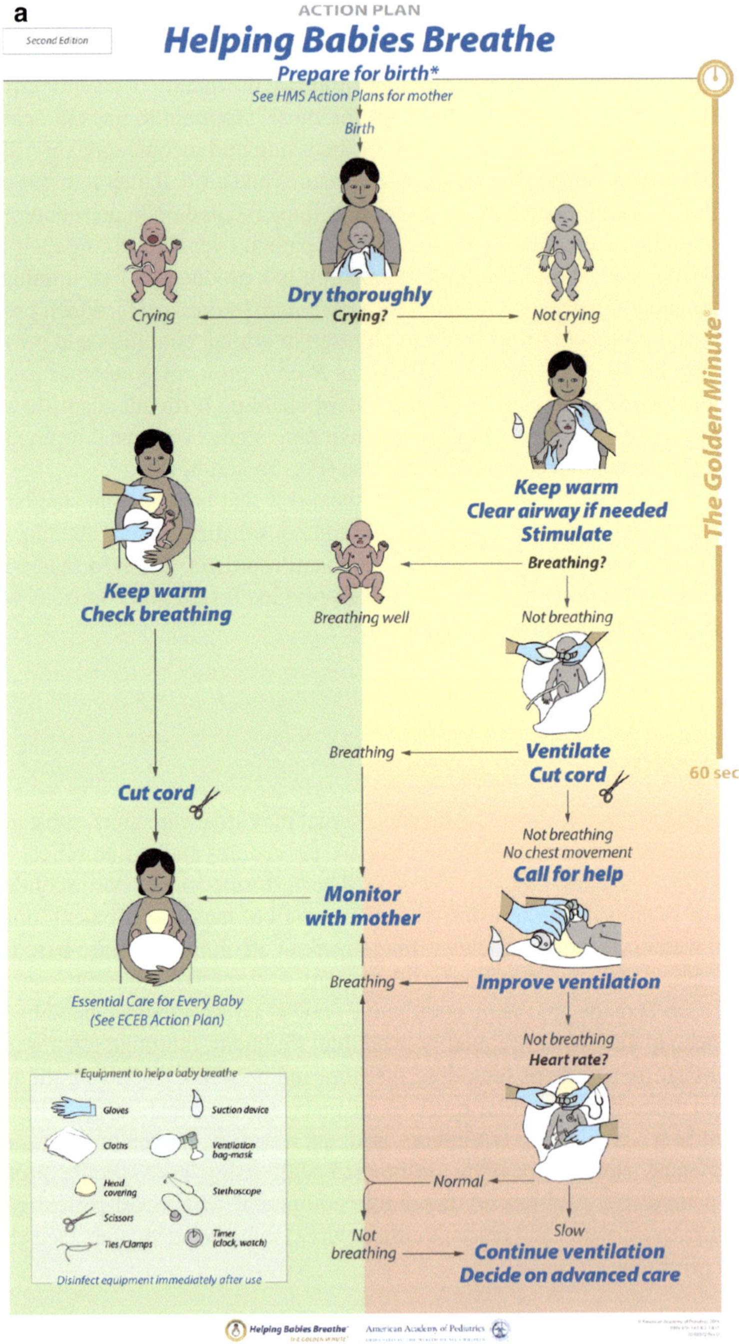

Fig. 1 (**a**) Helping Babies Breath Flowchart. (**b**) Reprocessing Neonatal Resuscitation Equipment. For full detail on reprocessing use this link https://www.path.org/resources/reprocessing-guidelines-for-basic-neonatal-resuscitation-equipment-in-resource-limited-settings/. Used with permission

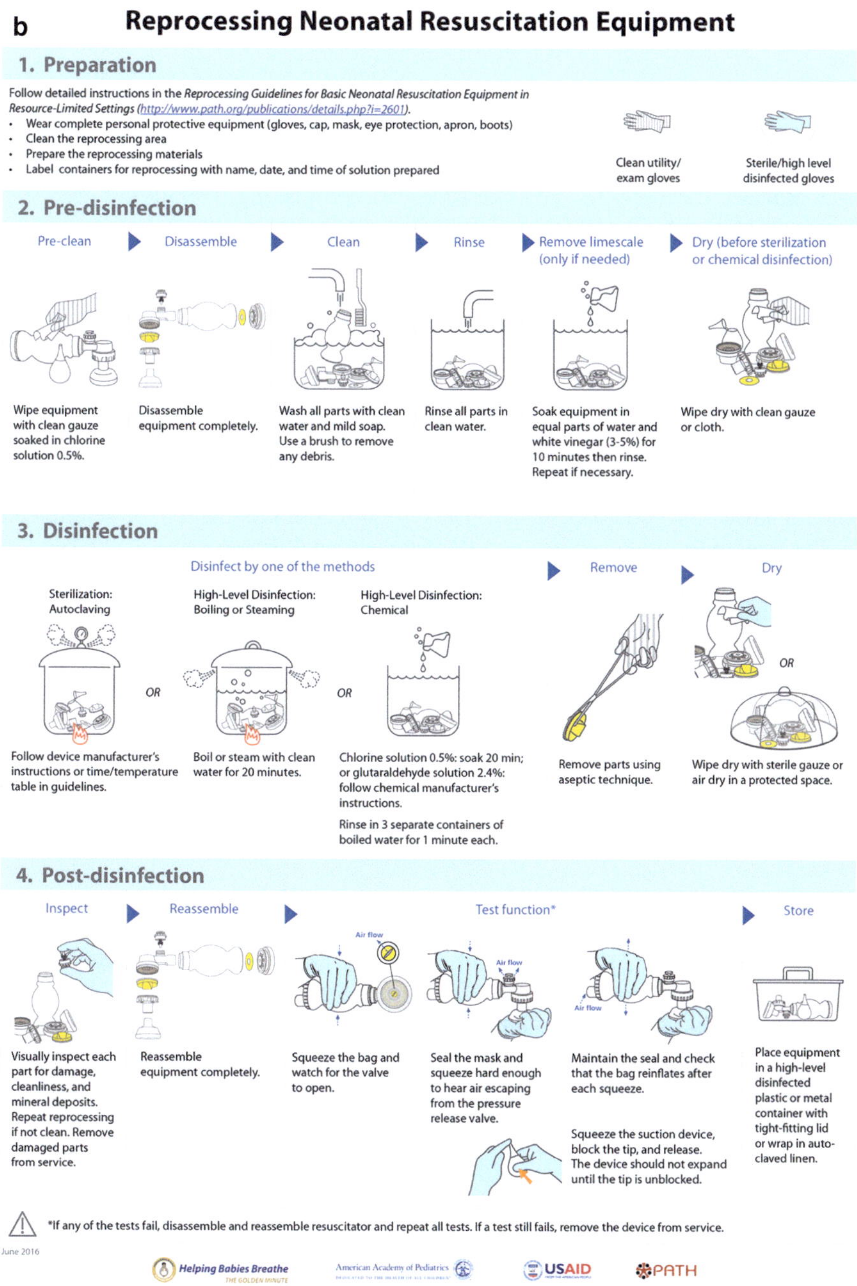

Fig. 1 (continued)

8 Record Keeping

Accurate record keeping is important in all aspects of providing and improving patient care. A shared patient medical record available in the unit for all disciplines, using shared medical terms and chart organization, is essential. The accuracy of the data provides the basis for good bedside decision-making, identifying areas for quality improvement, and is essential for research – all with the goal of improving patient outcomes. Every unit should keep an accurate, daily record of the unit census including the total patient number and important information including diagnoses, demographics, outcomes, and dispositions for all admissions and discharges.

No one type of record keeping is clearly superior. Although electronic medical records (EMR) may improve accuracy and provide some safety alerts, they are expensive, require significant technical infrastructure, and are time intensive, which can decrease physician and nurse time at the bedside. The use of well-organized, complete, printed medical records has proved to be sufficient and universally suitable for advancing good patient care. The type of record keeping will be determined by the availability of resources and trained personnel. Irrespective of the type of record keeping, the data recorded in the individual patient medical record should include daily vital signs, all fluid inputs and outputs, medications and route of administration, important laboratory results, daily notes from all disciplines, event summaries, admission history and physical exams, and discharge summaries. A printed example of a bedside ICU patient record is provided (Fig. 2a, b).

9 Evaluating Clinical Care

Every unit should have a system in place to evaluate clinical outcomes and quality of care. This is best accomplished by regularly scheduled review of individual cases, adverse events, morbidity, and mortality and/or by problem-based discussions. The purpose of review is to monitor outcomes, constructively problem solve, and identify areas where clinical care and outcomes can be improved. Reviews are most effective if they are multidisciplinary including physicians, nursing, and appropriate ancillary staff. Using the formal quality improvement (QI) process is an effective way to examine and change clinical practice and outcomes.

10 Training/Education

Ongoing educational activities for all physician and nursing providers are necessary to maintain up-to-date knowledge about disease physiology, current treatment protocols, and medical advances. This may be accomplished by case-based teaching, topic presentations, journal clubs, daily rounds, grand rounds, and individual

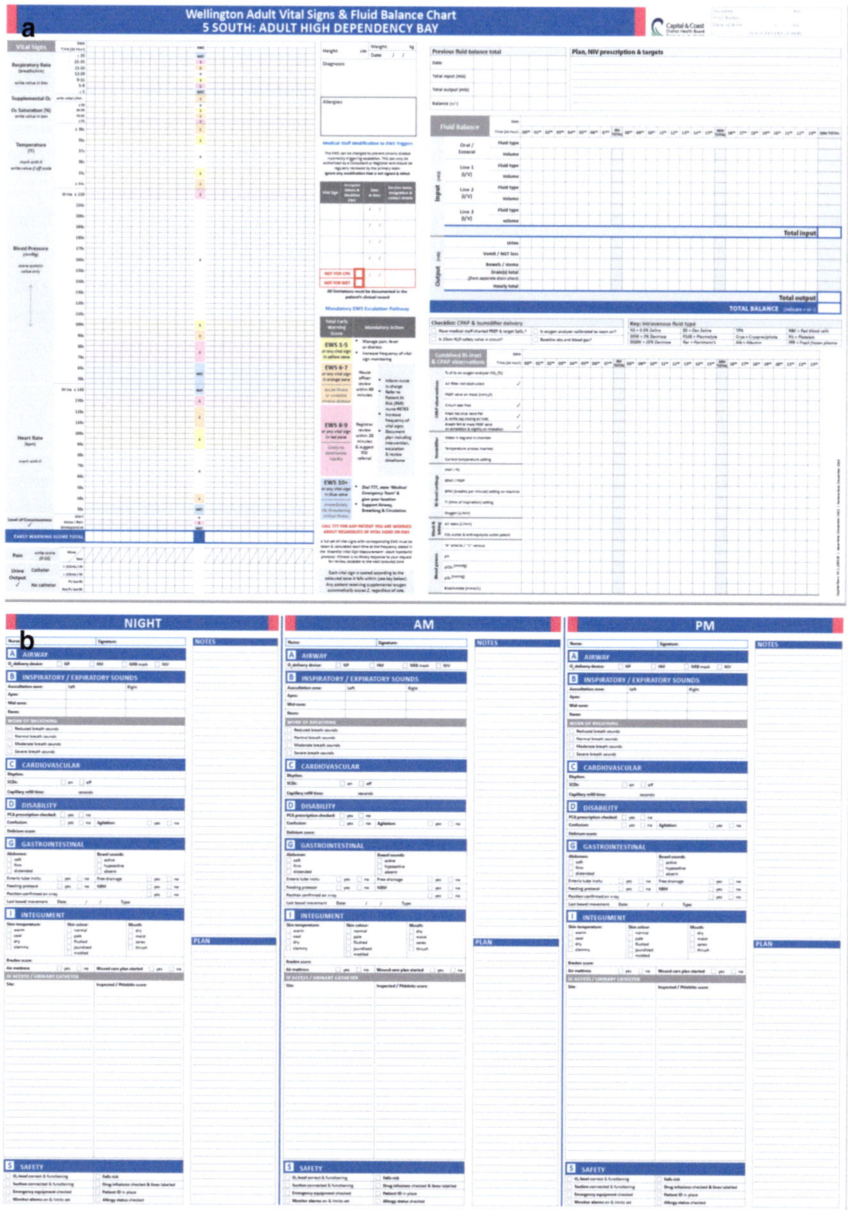

Fig. 2 (**a**) Example of bedside record (ews.wellingtonicu.com). (**b**) Example of bedside record (ews.wellingtonicu.com)

participation in workshops, online webinars, conferences, and subspecialty training. Documentation of attendance helps assure provider participation in educational activities and may be required for licensure or to obtain hospital privileges.

11 Challenges

Critical care units in developing countries face a myriad of challenges. These challenges range from a dissonance in vision and/or mission between the unit, institution administration, and the MOH to a simple lack of resources and/or training. Mitigating these challenges starts with a culturally appropriate plan to develop and maintain units that are fully supported by all levels of the healthcare personnel, from bedside staff to high-ranking government officials. Addressing the considerations discussed above early in the development of an HAA will help establish good clinical outcomes, maintain unit morale, and improve the likelihood of long-term unit success.

References

1. WHO. Emergency triage assessment and treatment (ETAT), manual for participants. Geneva: Child Health and Development, Maternal, Newborn, Child and Adolescent Health, and Ageing, World Health Organization; 2005. p. 78.
2. WHO. Guideline: updates on paediatric emergency triage, assessment and treatment: care of critically-ill children. Geneva: World Health Organization; 2016.
3. American Academy of Pediatrics. Helping babies breathe (HBB) facilitator flip chart. 2nd ed. Laerdal: American Academy of Pediatrics; 2017.

Further Reading

American Academy of Pediatrics. Committee of Fetus and Newborn: levels of neonatal care. Pediatrics. 2012;130:587–97.

American Academy of Pediatrics, International Resources. Helping babies breathe. 2nd ed. American Academy of Pediatrics, International Resources; 2016. https://laerdalglobalhealth.com/products/helping-babies-breathe/.

Challenges in critical care in africa: perspectives and solutions. ICU Manag Pract. 12(4). https://healthmanagement.org/c/icu/issuearticle/challenges-in-critical-care-in-africa-perspectives-and-solutions.

Committee on Trauma, American College of Surgeons. Resources for optimal care of the injured patient. 6th ed. Chicago: Committee on Trauma, American College of Surgeons; 2014.

Kwizera A, Dunser M, Nakibuuka J. National intensive care unit bed capacity and ICU patient characteristics in a low income country. BMC Res Notes. 2012;5:475. https://doi.org/10.1186/1756-0500-5475. PMID: 22937769.

Marshall JC, Bosco L, Adhikari NK, Connolly B, Diaz J, Dorman T, Fowler R, Meyfroidt G, Nakagawa S, Pelosi P, Vincent JL, Vollman K, Zimmerman J. What is an intensive care unit? A report of the task force of the World Federation of Societies of Intensive and Critical Care Medicine. J Crit Care. 2017;37:270–6. https://doi.org/10.1016/j.jcrc.2016.07.015.

Negro-Calduch E, Azzopardi-Muscat N, Krishnamurthy RS, Novillo-Ortiz D. Technological progress in electronic health record system optimization: systematic review of systematic literature reviews. Int J Med Inform. 2021;152:104507. https://doi.org/10.1016/j.ijmedinf.2021.104507.

Quality improvement guide. https://actt.albertadoctors.org/file/quality-improvement-guide.pdf.

WHO decontamination and reprocessing of medical devices for health care facilities. https://apps.who.int/iris/bitstream/handle/10665/250232/9789241549851-eng.pdf.

WHO guidelines on hand hygiene in health care: a summary. https://www.who.int/publications/i/item/9789241597906-summary.

World Health Organization. Department of Child and Adolescent Health and Development. Emergency triage and assessment and treatment (ETAT), manual for participants. World Health Organization; 2005. Retrieved from: https://www.who.int/publications/i/item/9241546875.

Neonatal Resuscitation in Resource-Constrained Settings: Sustaining Helping Babies Breathe and Beyond in a Low-Resource Setting

Anne White and Amy R. L. Rule

Abbreviations

CPAP	Continuous positive airway pressure
HBB	Helping Babies Breathe
HLD	High-level disinfection
IO	Intraosseous
IV	Intravenous
LISA	Less invasive surfactant administration
LMA	Laryngeal mask airway
LMIC	Low- and middle-income country
NRP	Neonatal Resuscitation Program
PPV	Positive-pressure ventilation
RDS	Respiratory distress syndrome

1 Case Example

You are called to the bedside of a 38-week gestation infant who was just born. The infant's mother arrived at the hospital in Kenya this morning and proceeded with precipitous delivery. She had limited prenatal care during this pregnancy with only

A. White
Department of Pediatrics, Division of Neonatology, University of Minnesota, Minneapolis, MN, USA

A. R. L. Rule (✉)
Cincinnati Children's Hospital Medical Center, Neonatal and Pediatric Hospitalist, Perinatal Institute | Hospital Medicine | Global Health Center, Cincinnati, OH, USA
e-mail: Amy.Rule@cchmc.org

T. M. Slusher et al. (eds.), *Pediatric Procedural Adaptations for Low-Resource Settings*, https://doi.org/10.1007/978-3-030-99955-1_4

two prenatal visits. She has four older children, including a 12-month-old, and has been on antiretroviral therapy for human immunodeficiency virus since 2018.

The infant is floppy, cyanotic, and apneic with a heart rate less than 100 beats per minute. You dry and stimulate the baby with no response. You dry and stimulate for a few more seconds, and due to lack of spontaneous respirations, you decide to begin positive-pressure ventilation (PPV) using a bag-mask device. After about 1 minute, the infant begins to breathe. His color and tone improve, and heart rate increases to greater than 100 beats per minute. You discontinue positive-pressure ventilation; however, the infant is nasal flaring and grunting and you plan to place him on bubble continuous positive airway pressure (CPAP) (chapter "Bubble CPAP in a Low-Resource Setting"). Your self-inflating bag cannot provide CPAP, so you administer blow-by oxygen while you transport him to the special care unit for further care.

2 Introduction

Despite the great success in reducing asphyxia as a cause of neonatal death in the United States following implementation of the Neonatal Resuscitation Program in 1986 [1], asphyxia remained a top cause of neonatal mortality worldwide, with the largest burden of mortality in low- and middle-income countries (LMICs) [2, 3]. There was some initial concern that management of perinatal hypoxic-ischemic events (asphyxia) required intensive care and thus was not practicable or feasible in most LMIC settings [4]. However, through early experience with NRP, it was found that the initial, basic steps (i.e., drying, stimulation, and bag-mask ventilation) were effective in many cases and thus of great value [5].

Studies demonstrated that about 90% of babies successfully transition to extrauterine life with no intervention; the remaining 10% are born with absent or poor respiratory effort and require some support [5–7]. Of the 10% requiring intervention, 4–7% respond to drying and stimulation, and 3–6% will go on to require positive-pressure ventilation; <1% require advanced resuscitation including intubation, chest compressions, and medications [7]. This suggested that focus on the initial, basic steps of resuscitation could save millions of newborn lives every year.

Reduction of neonatal deaths due to asphyxia became a global priority. Through the American Academy of Pediatrics and partnership with several additional stakeholders, the first edition of the Helping Babies Breathe (HBB) program was published in 2010 [8].

3 The Helping Babies Breathe Program

Helping Babies Breathe (HBB) is an educational skills-based neonatal resuscitation program developed to save newborn lives in low-resource setting [9, 10]. It seeks to address perinatal events and fresh stillbirths as one of the top three causes of neonatal mortality globally, along with infections and prematurity or low birth weight [11]. The program is an outreach of the evidence and knowledge on which the NRP is based [4, 12].

Using an evidence-based, standardized curriculum with education and technology adaptable to the different provider levels and settings where babies are born all over the world, HBB stresses two main teachings: (1) all infants need to be kept clean, warm, and encouraged to breastfeed and (2) an infant who does not breathe needs extra help within the first minute after birth [12].

The HBB workshop kit includes a facilitator flipchart, learner workbooks, and a large poster-sized Action Plan [10, 13]. The Action Plan is a step-by-step algorithm in neonatal resuscitation and is intended to clearly and simply guide the learner through the *evaluation-decision-action* cycle of newborn care and resuscitation [12]. Laerdal Medical introduced a low-cost, high-fidelity neonatal simulator that became standard with the program, in addition to a reusable suction and bag-mask mask device that can be used for real patient care following training (Fig. 1). Notably, the simulator and kit are reusable and designed for use in harsh environments and are far more reasonable in cost than higher fidelity neonatal simulators. They are also easily repaired.

Rapid dissemination and large-scale implementation of HBB were facilitated through the establishment of the Global Development Alliance [4, 12]. Implementation partners traveled to all parts of the world and trained in-country facilitators, a train-the-trainer model, and worked to incorporate guidelines on neonatal resuscitation and basic newborn care into hospitals and local government agendas [4]. Standalone HBB workshops were found to improve provider skills in the short-term but not influence long-term change [4], identifying the need for frequent practice to maintain infrequently performed skills, such as bag-mask ventilation; the recommendation for high-frequency, low-dose simulation would later become standard.

HBB success stories poured in from the field. At one site in Tanzania, post-HBB implementation there was a persistent 47% decrease in early neonatal mortality and 24% reduction in fresh stillbirth [14]. Several additional studies showed reduction in fresh stillbirth rates following HBB implementation [15, 16]. Studies also continued to show the benefit of high-frequency, low-dose simulation with regard to both

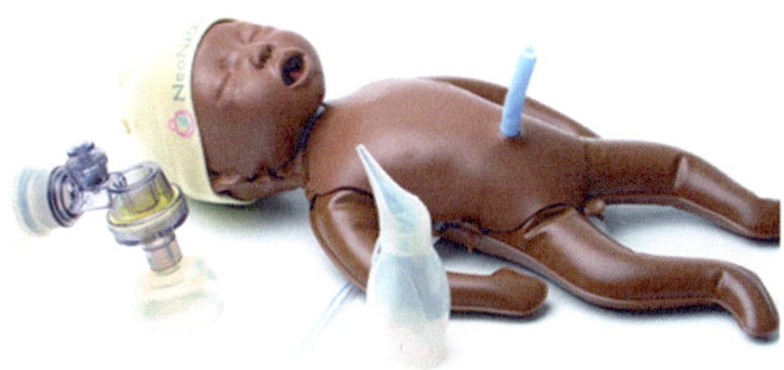

Fig. 1 NeoNatalie™ simulator, bag-mask device, and penguin suction [13]

resuscitation skills and early newborn care, as opposed to longer refresher courses over protracted time intervals [17–20].

HBB underwent revision with several updates to the second edition, which was released in 2018. Scientific updates were included in accordance with the 2015 *International Liaison Committee on Resuscitation Consensus on Science with Treatment Recommendations* and the 2012 WHO *Basic Newborn Resuscitation Guidelines* and the Utstein formula for survival: resuscitation science x educational efficiency x local implementation = survival [21]. Feedback from frontline users was incorporated into the second edition revisions, including a recommendation for routine in-house, high-frequency, low-dose practice [22]. The second edition also differs from the first in the addition of recommendations for the reprocessing (disinfection) of reusable medical equipment [23].

4 The Helping Babies Breathe Action Plan (Second Edition)

The Action Plan contains all of the steps of neonatal resuscitation in the HBB program and is a frequent reference tool throughout the course [9]. The Action Plan is poster-sized and it is helpful to tape to a wall or prop up against an easel during training, for easy visibility and reference by all. The Action Plan is color-blocked into three zones. The Green Zone indicates routine care. The Yellow Zone designates a newborn who needs help to breathe. The Red Zone depicts the need for ongoing respiratory support and consideration of advanced care. The goal is to follow the Action Plan to establish adequate ventilation for every newborn by 60 seconds of life, *The Golden Minute* (Fig. 2).

5 Expanding Care Beyond HBB

As previously described, the widespread dissemination and implementation of the HBB program led to great success in reducing rates of stillbirth and early neonatal mortality in many of the world's most vulnerable locations. HBB has been instituted as the formal neonatal resuscitation guideline from local birth attendants to district hospitals to ministries of health. Some facilities have expressed the capacity for additional care beyond what is described in HBB, and we will discuss a few of those potential interventions here [25]. Of note, expansion of the HBB neonatal resuscitation algorithm is not currently sanctioned by the AAP, and the following interventions could be considered at capable facilities but are not formally endorsed. Facilities with critical care capabilities should consider certification in NRP or the Newborn Life Support course offered by the European Resuscitation Council or national course endorsed by the national pediatric council/organization and the Ministry of Health.

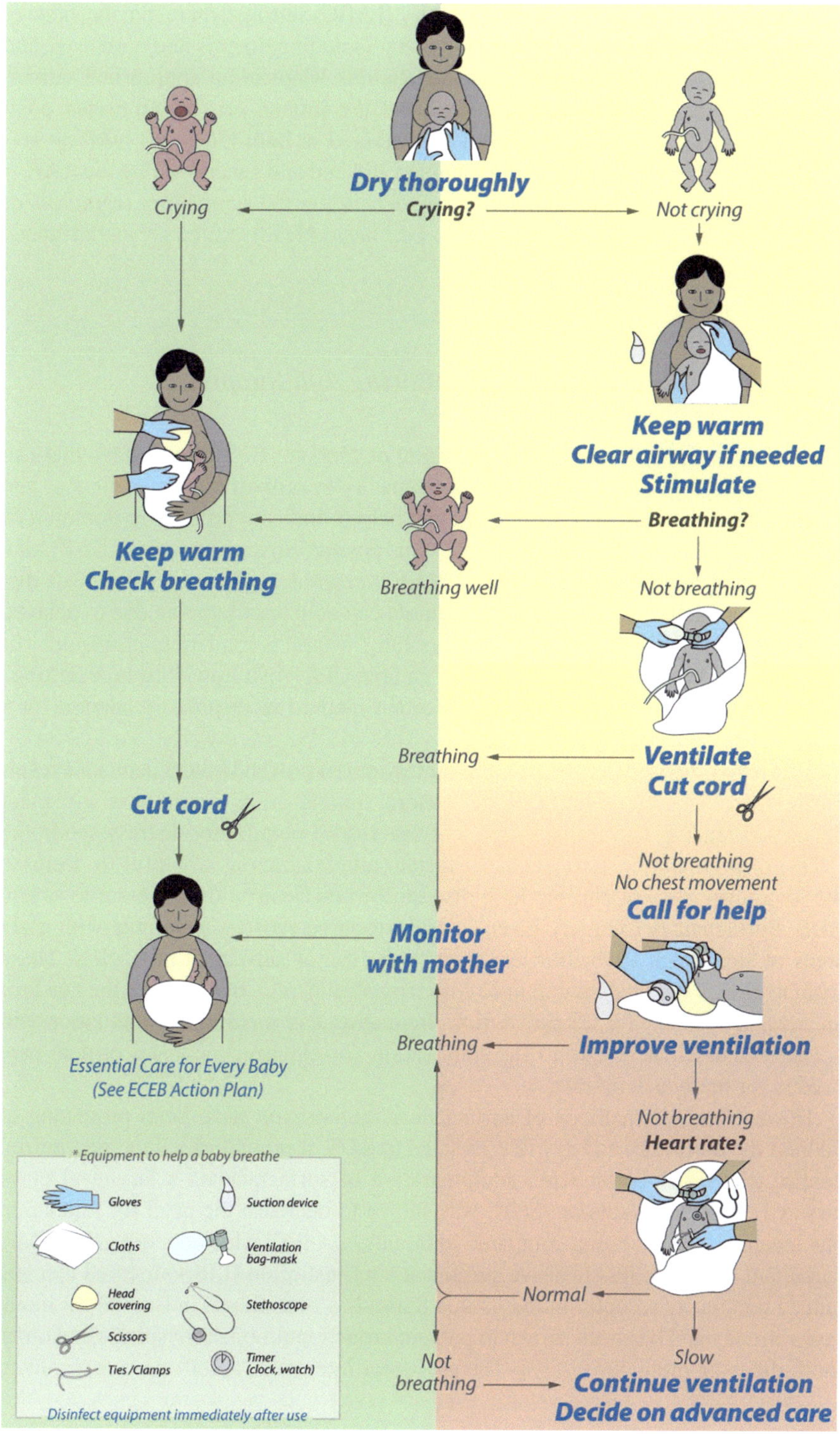

Fig. 2 The Helping Babies Breathe, 2nd Ed. Action plan [24]

In some low- and middle-income country (LMIC) settings, there may be value in starting with HBB for all healthcare providers, including doctors and midwives, and then adding chest compressions and medications when in an appropriate setting, where these interventions are indicated and the infants can be supported post-resuscitation. This is what many providers trained in both HBB and NRP do in a LMIC where there is no such hybrid course validated and sanctioned by the AAP. A benefit of this approach is having all providers doing the same thing regardless of skill set and eventual practice location, i.e., basic health center versus advanced referral center.

5.1 Advanced Respiratory Monitoring and Support

Pulse oximetry and the use of supplemental oxygen are two interventions that can be high yield for facilities that have the capacity to properly apply, maintain, and monitor their use [19]. Pulse oximetry can help to indicate prompting initiation of low-flow supplemental oxygen or continuous positive airway pressure (CPAP), or a pre- and post-ductal difference may signify a newborn with congenital heart disease. Supplemental oxygen via nasal cannula can help treat hypoxia due to delayed transition from intra- to extrauterine life or lung disease secondary to prematurity or infection. CPAP is discussed in chapter "Bubble CPAP in a Low-Resource Setting" in this book and is an effective and important method of respiratory support for a range of neonatal pathology.

Surfactant administration is another intervention proven to aid a neonate's respiratory distress, based on the etiology. Preterm infants are known to have surfactant deficiency leading to varying degrees of severity of respiratory distress syndrome (RDS) of prematurity. Exogenous surfactant administration is helpful to decrease the long-term risks of chronic lung disease for newborns with moderate to severe RDS. Surfactant is routinely given in high-resource settings to infants with early signs of significant RDS. Barriers exist to the use of surfactant in LMICs. These include cost of the medication, need for refrigeration, and, historically, the need for an advanced airway for administration. Intubation and mechanical ventilation will not be discussed here due to the implication for extended neonatal critical care needed for these sick infants.

However, novel methods of surfactant administration have been promising to address the morbidity and mortality related to RDS of prematurity. In a randomized control trial by Roberts et al., administration of surfactant via a laryngeal mask airway (LMA) to infants on CPAP was shown to decrease the need for intubation and mechanical ventilation compared to infants on CPAP who were not given LMA surfactant [26]. The less invasive surfactant administration (LISA) method that has gained popularity recently in the United States has been in use in Europe for many years already and has been shown to prevent bronchopulmonary dysplasia and other morbidities of prematurity [27]. There is great interest in an effective aerosolized mode of surfactant, with studies currently underway. Dosing of surfactant depends on which product is used and should be verified for the product available.

5.2 *Chest Compressions*

Chest compressions are indicated in NRP when the establishment of adequate ventilation does not lead to improvement in a low heart rate. The NRP recommendation is that chest compressions begin after placement of an advanced airway, since the etiology of circulatory collapse in a newborn is often respiratory [28]. If the facility has the capability of placing an advanced airway and providing ongoing critical care, chest compressions may be indicated for a baby with a heart rate less than 60 beats per minute following establishment of the airway. The ratio for chest compressions to breaths is 3–1 with a goal of greater than 100 compressions per minute.

5.3 *Medications and Access*

The use of medications, such as epinephrine, is an additional arm of neonatal resuscitation that may be beneficial in skilled facilities. Epinephrine is indicated in NRP when an infant's heart rate is less than 60 beats per minute after the establishment of a secure airway. Similar to the discussion above regarding chest compressions, epinephrine is maximally beneficial with a secure airway already established. Neonatal medication dosing is weight-based, and an estimated weight must be determined for advanced resuscitation.

Epinephrine is administered either via an endotracheal tube or intravenously, with intravenous the recommended route. For increased simplicity, there are slight changes to the recommended dosing in the newest edition of NRP, published in 2021 [28]. The correct neonatal concentration is 1 mg to 10 mL, or 0.1 mg/mL, followed by a 3 mL normal saline flush. The endotracheal dose of epinephrine is 0.5–1 mL/kg and the preferred intravenous dose is 0.1–0.3 mL/kg (Table 1).

There is a 1 mg/mL epinephrine concentration frequently used in older children and adults that should not be used for neonates if possible due to the high risk of dosing error. If the 1 mg/mL concentration is all that is available, it must be diluted 1:10 with normal saline. For example, if the indicated epinephrine dose is 1 mg which is equal to 1 mL, then 1 mL of medication should be drawn into a syringe and diluted with 9 mL of normal saline.

For a baby with a history of known or suspected blood loss and/or shock and who is not responding to the steps of resuscitation, administration of volume including O negative packed red blood cells may be indicated. Volume should be given in 10 mL/kg aliquots over 5 to 10 minutes.

Table 1 Neonatal resuscitation medications [28]

	Eighth edition	Previous editions
Epinephrine concentration	0.1 mg/mL	1:10,000
Epinephrine dose in mg for IV or IO	0.02 mg/kg[a]	0.01–0.03 mg/kg
Epinephrine dose in volume with the 0.1 mg/mL concentration for IV or IO	0.2 mL/kg	0.1–0.3 mL/kg
Flush after IV or IO	3 mL/kg of normal saline (applies to all weights)	0.5–1 mL of normal saline
Epinephrine dose in volume with the 0.1 mg/mL concentration for endotracheal dose	0.1 mg/kg = 1 mL/kg	0.5–1 mL/kg
If your epinephrine comes as 1 mg/mL (*formerly called 1/1000*), you will need to dilute it to 0.1 mg/mL before administration to neonates. This can be done by using 1 mL of epinephrine 1 mg/mL in 9 mL sterile water for injection, 0.5 mL of epinephrine 1 mg/mL in 4.5 mL sterile water for injection, 0.3 mL of epinephrine 1 mg/mL in 2.7 mL of sterile water for injection, and 0.2 mL of epinephrine 1 mg/mL in 1.8 ml of sterile water for injection if using 3 mL syringe, *but choose only 1 syringe size that is readily available for your hospital and use that all the time*		

[a]Actual dose range not changed but chose one dose to avoid confusion

For epinephrine to be administered via the preferred intravenous route, vascular access must be established. A peripheral venous line placed at delivery is one option. Another option is emergent placement of an intraosseous (IO) or umbilical venous line. IO and umbilical catheters are discussed in separate chapters (Table 1) [28].

Following a resuscitation during which epinephrine is administered, an infant requires intensive ongoing evaluation and management in a special care nursery or neonatal intensive care unit. Ongoing needs include continuous vital sign monitoring, likely invasive mechanical ventilation, and constant provider supervision.

6 Equipment: Purchasing, Maintenance, and Reprocessing

6.1 Purchasing

HBB-specific neonatal resuscitation equipment is manufactured by Laerdal Global Health. Although we have no stock in Laerdal, we appreciate the value and efficacy of the $86 NeoNatalie Complete Kit in comparison to high-technology manikins which cost hundreds and thousands of dollars. The NeoNatalie™ Complete Kit is available for purchase online at laerdalglobalhealth.com.

The educational materials, including the Facilitator Flipchart, Provider Guides, Action Plan Wall Poster, and Reprocessing Poster, are also available for purchase online from Laerdal Global Health. The HBB second edition materials are available from Laerdal Global Health in three languages: English, French, and Spanish. In addition, the materials are available free of charge for download on the American Academy of Pediatrics website in several additional languages including Arabic, Nepali, and Russian. Laerdal Global Health sells materials on a not-for-profit basis to the countries with the highest maternal and neonatal mortalities; other countries may purchase the non-discounted equipment from Laerdal Medical.

6.2 Reprocessing

HBB second edition includes recommendations for the reprocessing (disinfection) of the neonatal resuscitation bag-mask and penguin suction devices. This enables their repeated use for patient care. Proper reprocessing is important not only for infection prevention but also for long-term maintenance of adequately functioning equipment [29]. The recommendations, published by the nongovernmental group of public health innovators at PATH, follow the gold-standard principles of sterilization or high-level disinfection (HLD) described by the Centers for Disease Control and Prevention and World Health Organization and were designed for implementation in low-resource settings [23]. The recommendations are included in the teaching of the HBB second edition, which includes a Reprocessing Poster. Details regarding the materials and steps required for each of the methods of disinfection are available in the PATH guideline, available free of charge for download at https://www.path.org/resources/reprocessing-guidelines-for-basic-neonatal-resuscitation-equipment-in-resource-limited-settings/.

The guideline is not recommended for use with single-use equipment, which does comprise a large amount of the neonatal resuscitation equipment in low-resource settings, largely acquired through donation. No formal recommendations exist for the reprocessing of single-use equipment [30]. Efforts must be made to eliminate reliance on single-use, donated equipment. This can occur through improved delivery of reusable equipment by bolstering local supply chains and advocating for equitable, ethical donation.

7 Conclusion

Incorporating the HBB/HBS program and moving beyond to NRP when resources allow has the potential to help babies survive, thrive, and become contributing members of our world. It requires initial investment, commitment, and dedication including frequent reviewing and practicing. The cost is well worth it as we strive to meet Sustainable Development Goal 3.2 and lower the neonatal mortality to 12 per 1000 live births or below [31].

8 Case Resolution

The infant did well due to the successful resuscitation you provided following the HBB guidelines. She was admitted to your Special Care Baby Unit, placed on bubble CPAP for 24 hours after which time she was weaned to room air. Because of their reprocessing *protocol, your staff cleaned all the equipment including the bag, mask, and suction appropriately and placed them in the correct place in the resuscitation cart. Your team evaluated the baby for HIV and treated according to the guidelines in Kenya. At her first checkup at 1-week discharge, she was doing well.*

References

1. Guyer B, et al. Annual summary of vital statistics-1997. Pediatrics. 1998;102(6):1333–49.
2. Lawn JE, et al. 4 Million neonatal deaths: when? Where? Why? Lancet. 2005;365(9462):891–900.
3. Lawn JE, et al. Two million intrapartum-related stillbirths and neonatal deaths: where, why, and what can be done? Int J Gynaecol Obstet. 2009;107(Suppl 1):S5–18, S19.
4. Niermeyer S, et al. A short history of Helping Babies Breathe: why and how, then and now. Pediatrics. 2020;146(Suppl 2):S101–11.
5. Wall SN, et al. Neonatal resuscitation in low-resource settings: what, who, and how to overcome challenges to scale up? Int J Gynaecol Obstet. 2009;107(Suppl 1):S47–62, S63–4.
6. Barber CA, Wyckoff MH. Use and efficacy of endotracheal versus intravenous epinephrine during neonatal cardiopulmonary resuscitation in the delivery room. Pediatrics. 2006;118(3):1028–34.
7. Perlman JM, Risser R. Cardiopulmonary resuscitation in the delivery room. Associated clinical events. Arch Pediatr Adolesc Med. 1995;149(1):20–5.
8. American Academy of Pediatrics. Clinical reminder: Helping Babies Breathe. American Academy of Pediatrics; 2010.
9. American Academy of Pediatrics. Helping Babies Survive (HBS) – essential care for every baby – facilitator flip chart. Laerdal Global Health; 2014.
10. American Academy of Pediatrics. Helping Babies Breathe (HBB) facilitator flip chart. 2nd ed. Laerdal; 2017.
11. Lawn JE, Wilczynska-Ketende K, Cousens SN. Estimating the causes of 4 million neonatal deaths in the year 2000. Int J Epidemiol. 2006;35(3):706–18.
12. Little G, et al. Neonatal nursing and Helping Babies Breathe: an effective intervention to decrease global neonatal mortality. Newborn Infant Nurs Rev. 2011;11:82–7.
13. Products: Helping Babies Breathe education materials. 2017. Available from: https://shop.laerdalglobalhealth.com/product-category/educational-materials/helping-babies-breathe/.
14. Msemo G, et al. Newborn mortality and fresh stillbirth rates in Tanzania after Helping Babies Breathe training. Pediatrics. 2013;131(2):e353–60.
15. Goldenberg RL, et al. Stillbirths and neonatal mortality as outcomes. Int J Gynaecol Obstet. 2013;123(3):252–3.
16. Kc A, et al. The burden of and factors associated with misclassification of intrapartum stillbirth: evidence from a large scale multicentric observational study. Acta Obstet Gynecol Scand. 2020;99(3):303–11.
17. Evans CL, et al. Peer-assisted learning after onsite, low-dose, high-frequency training and practice on simulators to prevent and treat postpartum hemorrhage and neonatal asphyxia: a pragmatic trial in 12 districts in Uganda. PLoS One. 2018;13(12):e0207909.

18. Rule ARL, et al. Using quality improvement to decrease birth asphyxia rates after 'Helping Babies Breathe' training in Kenya. Acta Paediatr. 2017;106(10):1666–73.
19. Weiner GMZJ. Textbook of neonatal resuscitation (NRP), vol. 326. 7th ed. Elk Grove Village: American Academy of Pediatrics; 2016.
20. Budhathoki SS, et al. Does the Helping Babies Breathe Programme impact on neonatal resuscitation care practices? Results from systematic review and meta-analysis. Acta Paediatr. 2019;108(5):806–13.
21. Global Resuscitation Alliance, Utstein formula of survival. 2017 [cited 20 Sept 2021]. Available from: https://www.globalresuscitationalliance.org/utstein/.
22. Kamath-Rayne BD, et al. Improvements in the delivery of resuscitation and newborn care after Helping Babies Breathe training. J Perinatol. 2017;37(10):1153–60.
23. PATH. Reprocessing guidelines for basic neonatal resuscitation equipment in resource-limited settings. Seattle: PATH; 2016.
24. American Academy of Pediatrics. Action plan: Helping Babies Breathe. 2nd ed. American Academy of Pediatrics; 2016.
25. Umphrey L, et al. When Helping Babies Breathe is not enough: designing a novel, mid-level neonatal resuscitation algorithm for medecins sans frontieres field teams working in low-resource hospital settings. Neonatology. 2018;114(2):112–23.
26. Roberts KD, et al. Laryngeal mask airway for surfactant administration in neonates: a randomized, controlled trial. J Pediatr. 2018;193:40–46 e1.
27. Aldana-Aguirre JC, et al. Less invasive surfactant administration versus intubation for surfactant delivery in preterm infants with respiratory distress syndrome: a systematic review and meta-analysis. Arch Dis Child Fetal Neonatal Ed. 2017;102(1):F17–23.
28. Weiner GM, et al. Textbook of neonatal resuscitation. 8th ed. American Academy of Pediatrics; 2021. p. 377.
29. Eslami P, Bucher S, Mungai R. Improper reprocessing of neonatal resuscitation equipment in rural Kenya compromises function: recommendations for more effective implementation of Helping Babies Breathe. Resuscitation. 2015;91:e5–6.
30. CDC. Reuse of single-use medical devices: guideline for disinfection and sterilization in healthcare facilities. 2008 [18 Sept 2016, 20 Sept 2021]. Available from: https://www.cdc.gov/infectioncontrol/guidelines/disinfection/reuse-of-devices.html.
31. Reference sustainable development goals. Available from: https://sdgs.un.org/goals.

Further Reading

American Academy of Pediatrics. Essential care for every baby: facilitator flip chart. Helping Babies Survive 2015. Available at: http://internationalresources.aap.org/Resource/.

American Academy of Pediatrics. Essential care for small baby: facilitator flip chart. Helping Babies Survive 2015. Available at: http://internationalresources.aap.org/Resource/.

American Academy of Pediatrics. Helping Babies Breathe, 2nd ed. Provider guide. Helping Babies Survive 2015. Available at: http://internationalresources.aap.org/Resource/.

Ersdal HL, Mduma E, Svensen E, Perlman JM. Early initiation of basic resuscitation interventions including face mask ventilation may reduce birth asphyxia related mortality in low-income countries: a prospective descriptive observational study. Resuscitation. 2012;8:869–73.

Laerdal Global Health. Products: Helping Babies Breathe. 2017. Available at: https://laerdalglobalhealth.com/products/helping-babies-breathe/.

Rule ARL, Tabangin M, Cheruiyot D, Mueri P, Kamath-Rayne BD. The call and the challenge of pediatric resuscitation and simulation research in low-resource settings. Simul Healthc. 2017; https://doi.org/10.1097/SIH.0000000000000260.

Phototherapy in a Low-Resource Setting

Isa Abdulkadir, Clark Sleeth, and Udochukwu M. Diala

Abbreviations

AAP	American Academy of Pediatrics
ABE	Acute bilirubin encephalopathy
AC	Alternating current
BBS	Bronze baby syndrome
BSA	Body surface area
DC	Direct current
EBT	Exchange blood transfusion
FSPT	Filtered sunlight phototherapy
KSD	Kernicterus spectrum disorder
LED	Light-emitting diode
LMICs	Low- and middle-income countries
PT	Phototherapy
TSB	Total serum bilirubin

I. Abdulkadir (✉)
Department of Paediatrics, Division of Neonatology, Ahmadu Bello University, Zaria, Nigeria
e-mail: isaabdulkadir@abu.edu.ng

C. Sleeth
Tenwek Mission Hospital, Department of Pediatrics, Tenwek Mission Hospital, Bomet, Kenya

Departments of Internal Medicine and Pediatrics Lexington, University of Kentucky, Lexington, KY, USA

U. M. Diala
Department of Paediatrics, University of Jos, Jos, Nigeria

T. M. Slusher et al. (eds.), *Pediatric Procedural Adaptations for Low-Resource Settings*, https://doi.org/10.1007/978-3-030-99955-1_5

1 Case Example

A 4-day-old premature baby girl with an estimated gestational age of 32 weeks is being transferred to your facility in Kenya, after admission to an outside facility. At the outside facility, she was noted to be dehydrated, irritable, and jaundiced. Her weight was 1670 g. Intravenous access could not be established: heel stick glucose was 3.8 mmol/L and bilirubin level was 14 mg/dL (239 μmol/L). The referral center noted that this was below their recommended exchange blood transfusion (EBT) level of 15–18 mg/dL (257–308 μmol/L). The neonate was started on phototherapy (PT) with a locally made fluorescent unit; a dose of IM benzylpenicillin and IM gentamicin (two common antibiotics used in newborns) were given. She was fed via a nasogastric tube. The following morning, despite PT, the bilirubin had risen to 15 mg/dL (257 μmol/L). She was transferred to your facility for possible EBT.

On arrival at your facility, the baby is noted to be feeding poorly and is somewhat irritable but has normal muscle tone, cry, and facial exam. The baby is immediately placed under intensive PT with a locally made light-emitting diode (LED) unit which had been recently tested to deliver irradiance of 36 μW/cm²/nm. Peripheral IV access is established and labs are drawn. EBT is planned but no exchange blood transfusion kit is available, and the blood bank is out of type O blood as the hospital had just taken care of multiple victims of a motor vehicle accident. One additional PT LED unit is added. Four hours later, while awaiting blood donation, typing, and cross-matching, a second bilirubin is drawn which shows that bilirubin has dropped to 12 mg/dL (205 μmol/L). You wonder if the prior PT had a therapeutic irradiance.

2 Introduction

Worldwide, 24 million infants are at risk for severe hyperbilirubinemia. Of these at least 480,700 globally are at risk of extreme hyperbilirubinemia and possible acute bilirubin encephalopathy. Of those who live, 75,400 are at risk for lifelong sequelae or kernicterus spectrum disorder (KSD) [1], most occurring in low- and middle-income countries (LMICs). Acute bilirubin encephalopathy (ABE) remains an important cause of neonatal morbidity and accounts for 5–14% of neonatal deaths [2, 3]. Effective phototherapy (PT) is the cornerstone of successful management of neonatal unconjugated hyperbilirubinemia.

Countries should be encouraged to develop their own appropriate guidelines for both PT and EBTs based on specific risk categories such as the percent of the population with G6PD deficiency, availability of anti-D for rhesus disease, availability of intensive PT, electricity, and blood for EBTs. If countries do not have specific country guidelines and are choosing to use other countries' guidelines such as the American Academy of Pediatrics (AAP) guidelines to determine the need for PT or

EBTs, modifications may be appropriate. For many LMICs excluding the low-risk category if using the AAP guidelines may be appropriate.

An astounding variety of commercial and locally made PT units are in use in resource-limited settings [4]. Problems with the maintenance and setup of both locally constructed and commercially made units, limited availability and high cost of commercial units, and issues with the design of locally made units all contribute to the high reported rates of suboptimal PT in resource-limited settings.

Light sources for locally made PT units are typically either LEDs or fluorescent tubes. Filtered sunlight may be another option in austere settings without reliable or consistent electricity pending further testing and in accordance with local guidelines and regulations. Here we will review some practical points in the design and construction of locally made PT units using these modalities, as well as principles of maintenance applicable to both locally made units and commercial devices.

3 Science of Phototherapy

PT for neonatal jaundice has been in use since the 1950s. In 1958, Cremmer et al. published a paper fully describing its use [5]. Bilirubin absorbs light which enhances the conversion of the toxic, fat-soluble, unconjugated bilirubin through photoisomerization to photoisomers, which are then conjugated in the liver to nontoxic water-soluble forms that can be excreted in stool and urine [6, 7]. The extent to which PT can efficiently impact bilirubin levels is greatly influenced by the following factors: irradiance of the PT device, pre-therapy serum bilirubin levels, surface exposure, and duration of PT [4, 8, 9]. PT is conventionally delivered with the device at a distance overhead from the infant. Other methods of delivering PT include the bed or blanket method where the baby is laid on the PT device or the device is wrapped on the back of the neonate. Double PT refers to use of an overhead PT device and an additional device including a second unit below or beside the neonate.

The efficacy of PT is foremost a function of the quality and intensity of the light, as represented by the wavelength, which should be within the range of 400–520 nm [9]. This contributes significantly to the irradiance delivered by the device at the surface of intended therapy. The irradiance is the outcome of the interplay between the wavelength of the lamps used (a function of the type of light and its intensity), the distance of the light source from the newborn, and the baby's surface area exposed to the light [4, 9, 10]. The irradiance decreases exponentially as the distance of the PT device from the baby increases. The desire for improved efficacy has led to evolution of different device designs. Since the 1950s, light sources used in devices include halogen lamps, fluorescent lamps, and – in the 1990s – light-emitting diode (LED) lamps [11–13]. The superior performance of LED lamps' intensity/wavelength, half-life, thermal emission, and performance has been clearly demonstrated. Lately, filtered sunlight therapy is currently being evaluated as a source of phototherapy and has shown promising results particularly in settings with abundance of sunlight [14].

Therapy targets when providing PT for infants weighing at least 2000 grams and or GA ≥35 weeks are irradiance of at least 10 μW/cm²/nm for conventional PT and 30 μW/cm²/nm and above for intensive PT. Lower levels for intensive PT are advised for preterm neonates particularly those less than 1000 g [15–18]. The higher the irradiance, the larger the decline in bilirubin levels, particularly at high starting serum bilirubin levels.

Overall, the clinician determines the desired dose of PT by prescribing the irradiance over the period the neonate needs to be treated with a given PT device, while considering other factors such as the pre-treatment serum bilirubin levels, rate of rise, and availability of support facility for monitoring. As we continue to understand PT better including potential toxicities related to its use based on various factors such as the size of the neonate, type of light, irradiance level, and duration of treatment, it is important to view PT as you would any other drug. PT should be dosed according to risk category of the neonate versus risk of the PT. In LMICs, the clinician must also weigh in other factors such as quality of PT available, reliability of electricity, distance to a referral center able to do an EBT if needed, gestational age of the neonate, and their particular risk factors such as setup for rhesus disease or G6PD deficiency. Dosing of PT is done measuring the irradiance of the device at the footprint or intended surface of PT using an irradiance meter. Several commercial meters are available, though can be cost prohibitive in low-resource settings.

Even as PT has been available and effectively used over the last seven decades as a relatively inexpensive, safe, and noninvasive method of treating neonatal hyperbilirubinemia, the inequalities in health and health resource distribution have left resource-constrained countries vulnerable and deprived. This results from lack of availability, affordability, accessibility, timeliness, and sustainability of PT services in low- and middle-income countries where the risk of severe neonatal jaundice and its potential complications remain quite high and widespread [4]. In addition, inconsistency in use and the unintentional use of devices providing inadequate irradiance pose challenges even in high-resource settings [19].

More and more attention, therefore, is currently being focused on addressing availability of efficient PT devices with efforts aimed at in-country production of devices. This, coupled with ensuring that PT services are available at all times, accessible, affordable, and timely alongside optimal use of devices, will bring about the much-desired near elimination of severe neonatal hyperbilirubinemia and its sequelae in low-resource settings.

3.1 Suggested Resources for Facilities Using Phototherapy

1. A working PT device
2. A way to measure bilirubin level quickly and reliably
3. An irradiance meter

4. A reliable electricity supply source (if not possible consider exploring the possibility of filtered sunlight PT)
5. A neonatal thermo-friendly environment
6. A protocol to guide treatment
7. BIND IIR score sheet

4 Indications

Generally, PT is indicated in neonates with:

- Elevated serum bilirubin per in-country guidelines or adapted high-income country guidelines
- Rapidly rising serum bilirubin levels (more than 0.2 mg/dL/hour (3.4 μmol/L/hour) or more than 5 mg/dL/day (86 μmol/L/day) or any jaundice in the first 24 hours
- Hyperbilirubinemia with signs of acute bilirubin encephalopathy (ideally while preparing for an exchange blood transfusion)
- Post exchange transfusion

4.1 Contraindications

PT does not have many contraindications, though there are causes of hyperbilirubinemia that it will not be effective for such as primarily direct hyperbilirubinemia or biliary atresia.

4.2 Technique

Equipment, supplies, and construction of PT units are listed under the two types of phototherapy units below.

5 Light-Emitting Diodes

5.1 Equipment/Supply List for LED

Light-emitting diodes, or LEDs, have several advantages over other light sources. The diodes maintain their brightness well over time, meaning less maintenance and lower costs of operation. This also means that having an irradiance measuring device on hand is not an absolute requirement; if the PT device can be measured once in situ at the time of installation and its intensity found to be adequate, it will generally remain within target for several years of typical use. LEDs also have lower power consumption than halogen or fluorescent devices of similar intensity. This means that battery backup is a possibility. Lower power consumption results in less heat production, which allows the devices to be installed closer to the infant without overheating the baby (although heat production is still considerable and needs to be accounted for).

In design and construction of an LED PT unit, there are three components to consider: the lights, the power supply (also called the driver), and the enclosure as noted below.

1. *Lights* – LEDs come in many form factors and colors. LED bulbs typically have the driver built in (see below), but more frequently for PT, an LED without an integrated driver is used, as the overall cost tends to be lower and you have more flexibility in construction. Any type of LED form factor can be made to work, but the most common and least expensive type of LED is surface-mounted devices (SMD), which are categorized based on their size. A convenient type for construction of PT units is blue SMD 5050 strips (5050 means each LED is 5 mm by 5 mm), which are typically supplied in 5-meter strips containing 60 LEDs per meter. These can be cut to length and then soldered, and usually come with an adhesive backing to facilitate installation. Another consideration in choosing LED form factor is how even of a light they cast; more uniform is better. As for color, dedicated blue LEDs are the best (what is marketed as blue LEDs are indium gallium nitride and have a peak wavelength of 450–475 nm); "color-changing" LEDs actually have three different colored LEDs in them, only one of which is blue. "White" LEDs have a blue diode combined with one or more other color, and can be substituted if that is all is available, the "cooler" the color tone, the better (if indicated, these will typically have a "color temperature" of 5000 K), but it is difficult to make generalizations as there is much variation between manufacturers and models.
2. *Power Supply* – LEDs use direct current (DC), so if your electricity source is mainly alternating current (AC), then a power supply (often called a driver) is needed. These are readily available commercially and come in two types, constant current or constant voltage. Which type you need depends on the LED circuitry. Most LED strips have matched resistors built into the circuit and are intended for a constant voltage power supply; these will specify the voltage for which they were designed, typically 12 V, whereas LEDs with drivers integrated into the circuit are usually constant current drivers. Although there are efficiency advantages to constant current drivers, constant voltage drivers have more flexibility in device design, are less expensive and more readily available, and can be repurposed from other electronic devices, such as 12 V "brick-type" laptop power supplies. When choosing a constant voltage driver, the LEDs must be designed for constant voltage and the driver must match that voltage; the wattage

should be at least the rated power draw of the LEDs. Recall that watts = volts × amperes. For instance, 12 V SMD 5050 strips typically need 72 W for a 5-m, 300-LED strip (supplied by a constant voltage of 12 V, 6A power supply). Additional LEDs can be added up to the current capacity of the driver, after which it reduces the current to all the LEDs, causing them to dim. For more information on constant current drivers, there are a number of good technical discussions available on the Internet.

3. *Enclosure* – an ideal enclosure is sturdy and protects the PT electronics, is able to be set up close to the patient, and provides for reasonable heat dissipation. Some enclosures may have reflectors or cloth curtains built in to maximize light on the patient. Due to availability and cost, most locally made PT units use a combination of plywood and plexiglass. A variation on the enclosure is to create a second "bed" that the baby lies on so that PT shines on both the front and back of the infant; care must be taken to ensure the baby does not overheat.

LED units need very little upkeep beyond keeping them clean. A surge protector is a reasonable investment to protect the driver. If an irradiance meter is not available, replacing the LEDs every 2 years with typical usage (5000 hours of use) is a very conservative maintenance schedule [20].

See the Resource section of this chapter for a link to plans for a locally constructed LED PT unit in use at one of the chapter author's hospitals, with a total cost of $35 USD (2020) per unit, including labor cost. Below are two examples of homemade LED phototherapy devices (Figs. 1 and 2).

Example of a locally constructed LED PT unit in use at one of the author's institutions, tested to provide an irradiance of 34–38 μW/cm²/nm. The photograph to the left is of an infant in an incubator and the one to the right shows a stand for an infant in a cot; both are of the same design of unit. A switch reduces the intensity to 20 μW/cm²/nm for use in premature infants.

Source: Authors (CS)

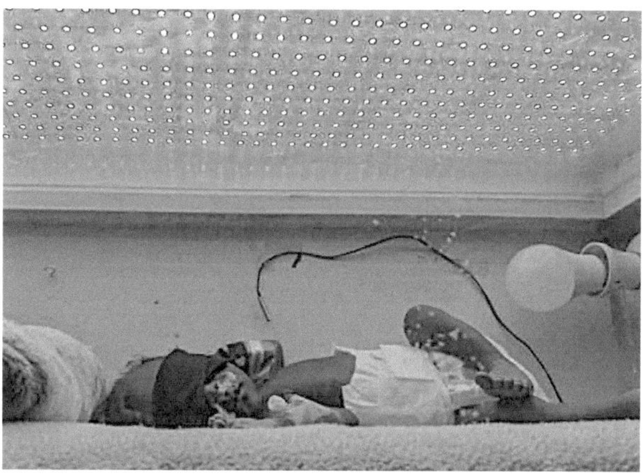

Fig. 1 Example 1 of an adaptation for LED phototherapy device

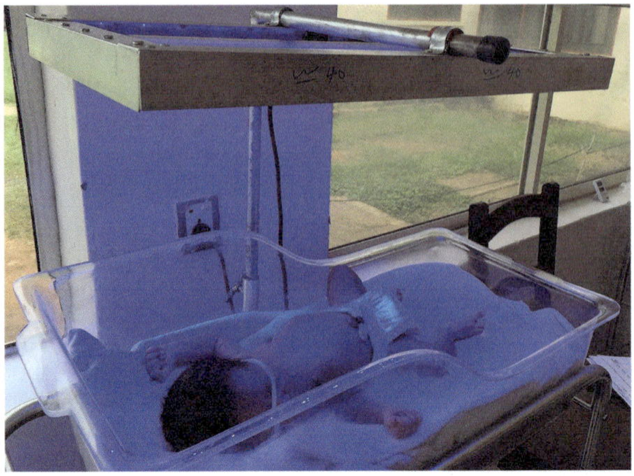

Fig. 2 Example 2 of an adaptation for LED phototherapy device. (Note distance between neonate and phototherapy often greater than with fluorescent tube phototherapy because LED phototherapy often much more intense)

6 Fluorescent Tube Units

6.1 Equipment/Supply List for Fluorescent Units

Fluorescent tubes as a light source have the advantage of relatively good availability, and blue fluorescent tubes (of varying quality) can often be found in the local commercial market. Compared to LEDs, however, they require much more maintenance, resulting in much higher overall operating costs, as well as diligence to maintain intensity either by regular measurement of irradiance and targeted replacement or else scheduled replacement of tubes. This applies to both commercial and locally made models.

1. *Lights* – Compared to LEDs, there is much more variation in the intensity and spectrum of light produced by fluorescent tubes. Special PT blue fluorescent tubes are, as would be expected, the most suited for construction of PT units; they are also typically unavailable in resource-limited settings. Commodity blue fluorescent tubes can often be found on the open market; a typical price is around $30 USD per tube. If using commodity blue fluorescent tubes, approximately 150–200 W of power (e.g., seven to ten 20-watt tubes) will provide between 10 and 20 μW/cm^2/nm of intensity in a typical installation. It is difficult to get to intensive PT levels (>30 μW/cm^2/nm) using nonspecialized tubes due to mounting constraints. If using white fluorescent tubes, a similar setup would be expected to deliver intensities in the 5–10-μW/cm^2/nm range. However, these are very broad generalizations, and individual results may be very different depending on the specific equipment used.
2. *Enclosure* – Constructing the mounting enclosure has similar considerations as for a LED device, except that heat production is more of an issue.
3. *Maintenance* – As for maintenance, there is more variation in the rate of decay of irradiance of fluorescent tubes compared with LEDS. An irradiance meter is very helpful; if not available, a conservative replacement schedule is every 6 weeks of typical use (500 hours assuming it is on 50% of the time) [21]. An

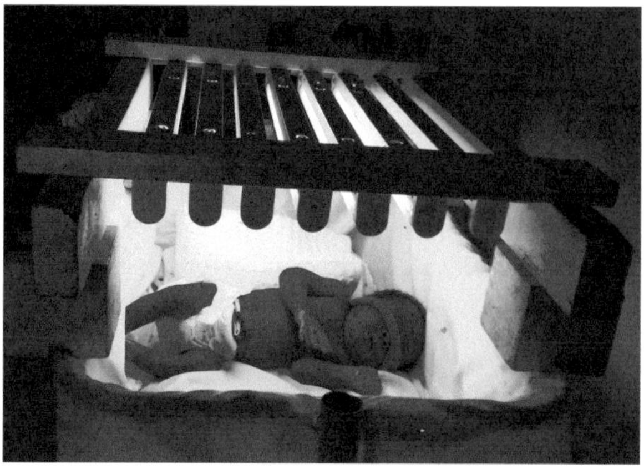

Fig. 3 Homemade fluorescent phototherapy unit

hour meter, often sold as an engine accessory, is a very useful adjunct. As with an LED device, a surge protector is also a reasonable investment. See example of a homemade fluorescent phototherapy unit (Fig. 3).

A locally constructed fluorescent unit that illustrates several issues. Note the large distance between the tubes and the baby and the number of tubes (one had burnt out and was yet to be replaced), the absence of reflectors, and that an eye shield was not on the infant. This unit was measured to have an intensity of 6 μW/cm²/nm. Source: Authors (CS).

7 Filtered Sunlight Phototherapy (FSPT)

7.1 Equipment/Supply List for FSPT

- Appropriate tested window tinting film such as Air Blue 80 (for other choices and information on selecting and testing films, see Vreman et al.) [22]
- Polycarbonate panel-walled room with windows and doors that open and close for ventilation (without exposing the patient to direct sun)
- PCV pipe-constructed canopy frames that support window tinting film stretched over them for either multiple neonate (usually up to n = six) or single neonate canopies (include illustrations)
- Optional but helpful
  - Solar powered fan
  - Device for reading or recording room/canopy ambient temperatures continuously

Sunlight is a low-cost universally available modality that requires little infrastructure. The main limitations are the weather, which on occasion prevents FSPT, and of course it is limited to sunny daylight hours. It is critical to monitor the neonate's temperature and respond appropriately in order to avoid hypo- or hyperthermia. Many days with light rain still have adequate irradiance for FSPT. Sunlight includes a full spectrum of light, including both the blue light helpful for PT and harmful ultraviolet radiation, and consequently must be filtered. To construct an area for sunlight PT, a "greenhouse"-like structure is built out of tested window tinting inside a polycarbonate room or used to form a canopy, tent, or room (Fig. 4). Ways to ensure safe neonatal temperatures in the locations FSPT is most needed, where there are usually a limited number of healthcare providers, are currently under investigation. Additionally, as with all forms of therapy, appropriate governmental regulations must be followed and permission sought as appropriate in each country.

7.2 *Instructions for Use*

7.2.1 Measuring Phototherapy

One of the determinants of the efficiency of PT is the irradiance of the device at a distance from the surface of intended therapy; this is greatly influenced by the intensity and wavelength of the lamp or light source [11, 12, 23]. As in every therapy, the irradiance for therapy should be prescribed, measured, and set. The irradiance of a PT device is determined using an irradiance meter. Different devices come with specific meters for measuring irradiance. It is best, where available, to use the meter specific for a given device [24]. However, where specific meters are not available, the Ohmeda Biliblanket Meter II™ has been used widely and had been a good choice for measuring irradiance across different brands of PT including homemade devices. To measure the irradiance of a device where the usual overhead method of PT is employed:

1. Power on the PT device.
2. Allow time for the device to come fully on with a warm up period of at least 15 minutes.

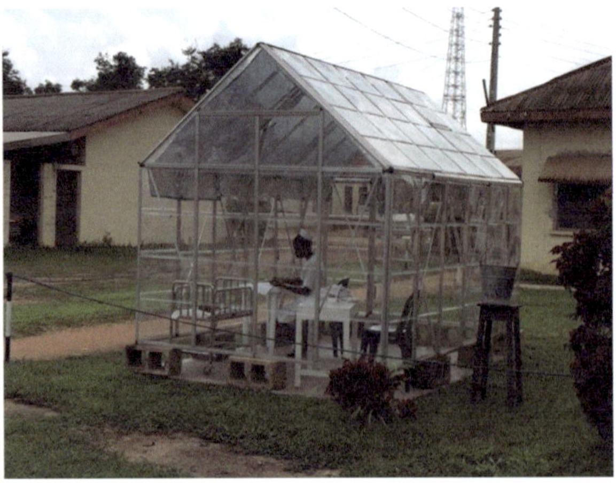

Fig. 4 Example of FSPT room (Courtesy of Drs. Slusher and Gbadero)

3. Place the irradiance measuring meter at a defined distance under the PT device.
4. Determine that the sensor area of the irradiance meter is located midway and centrally situated under the PT device. Use a box to place the irradiance meter at the approximate height of the infant.
5. With some irradiance meters, a mesh can be attached to increase the effective range, in this case from 26 to 67 $\mu W/cm^2/nm$ (Fig. 5).
6. Power on the meter device.
7. Allow measurement until meter reading remains unfluctuating.
8. If needed, convert to the correct units. Some devices report irradiance in $\mu W/cm^2$, in which case the result must be divided by the spectrum bandwidth measured (e.g., if a device measures in the spectrum of 422–499 nm, and reports intensity at 2696 $\mu W/cm^2$, then the irradiance in $\mu W/cm^2/nm$ is 2696/(499–422) = 35.4 $\mu W/cm^2/nm$).
9. Record the irradiance of the PT device at the distance of measurement.

Where the desired irradiance is not obtained, the PT device can be adjusted toward the meter until the desired irradiance for therapy is attained. The distance at which the desired irradiance set is achieved should be such that the therapy is safe and comfortable for the neonate, free of risk of injury or heating, and at the same time permits for close monitoring, optimal nursing care, and observation of the neonate. To measure irradiance accurately, the following should be noted:

1. Avoid taking measurements at points toward the extreme ends in the footprint of the device.
2. Use an appropriate meter.
3. Allow the meter to stabilize before reading the measurement.
4. Ensure all lamps are lit and fully on without flickering.

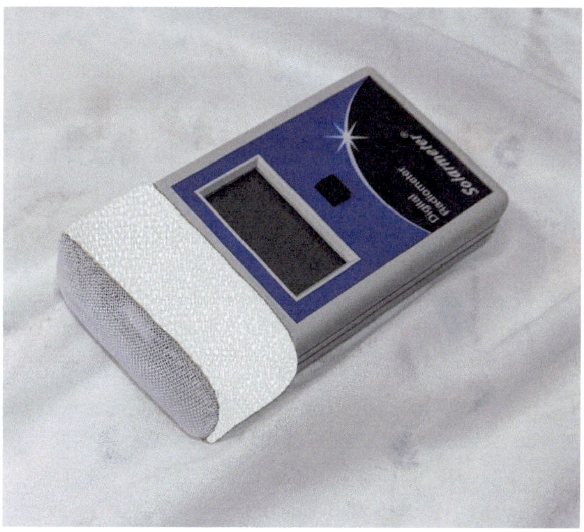

Fig. 5 Example of an irradiance meter with a mesh attached (Courtesy of Dr. Sleeth)

If sharing an irradiance meter with other facilities, irradiance may be measured at scheduled times at set distances allowing the clinicians to simply choose a PT unit, set the height appropriately based on the most recent irradiance measurement, and proceed with PT. It is desired that irradiance of PT devices is measured and determined before infant is placed under device. The use of distance to approximate desired irradiance may, however, be misleading and result in overestimation of irradiance, while the actual irradiance is much lower than approximated. This occurs in the following instances:

1. Waning of light intensity with inadequate voltage. Depending on the lamp source, the intensity of the lamps may be significantly affected. This is pronounced with fluorescent tubes compared to LED lamps where the effect is minimal due to their low energy consumption.
2. Lamp half-life expended. Over time, the irradiance of devices diminishes with the decay of the lamps as their half-life is approached. The half-lives of the different lamps vary with LED lamps having 30–50 times the half-life of fluorescent tubes. As the lamps decay, the irradiance of the same PT device measured at a specific distance diminishes over time. The age of the light source affects the quality of PT because of decay of spectral irradiance that is universally observed with use [21]. The rate of decay depends on the type of light source with LED (40,000–50,000 hours) poised to have much longer lifespans than fluorescent tubes (1000 hours) or halogen lamps. Some devices have timers that cumulate the usage hours. For local devices, charting usage hour may help track lamp half-life.
3. Use of barriers in the path of the footprint of the device. The use of Perspex plastic, plexiglass, or glass sheets between the device and the surface of intended therapy, as with incubators, decreases the irradiance of the device at a comparative distance without the barrier [25].

Determining irradiance of PT devices is an important component of providing efficient PT. Some researchers are beginning to explore developing low-cost irradiance meters to bridge this gap [26]. In resource-constrained settings, though measurement of irradiance remains challenging due to the high cost of irradiance meters, protocols for provision of PT should include regular, periodic measurement of irradiance of PT devices in use.

7.2.2 General Principle of Optimizing Phototherapy

Effectiveness is often assessed by the rate of reduction in serum bilirubin of infants receiving PT resulting in shorter hospital stays and less need for exchange transfusion. Several factors contribute to efficacy of PT, namely:

1. Intrinsic characteristics of the PT device such as the spectral wavelength, spectral irradiance at the level of the skin, the treatable percentage body surface area, and age of light source

2. Extrinsic PT device factors such as distance between device and the patient, use of reflectors, aligning the footprint of the light, and prevention of interception of light by objects used to care for the patient such as caps, diapers, eye shields, electrodes, or dust on surfaces between light sources and the patient [27]
3. Duration of treatment
4. Patient characteristics such as severity of jaundice, presence of hemolysis, body surface area, skin pigmentation, as well as skin thickness

During treatment for neonatal jaundice, PT can be optimized by manipulating some of the intrinsic and extrinsic characteristics of PT devices.

7.2.3 Treatable Percentage of Body Surface Area (BSA)

The concept of treatable percentage of BSA is important because it presents a more practical approach to irradiance footprint and situates the irradiance measurement in the context of the beam from the light source. The BSA of an infant is difficult to accurately measure due to its irregularity, but Vreman et al. described a method of estimating it through drawing a 2D silhouette of an average 30-week infant (preterm BSA) and 37-week infant (term BSA) and using that to estimate the treatable BSA. Studies report that different PT devices produce light beams with different BSAs [28, 29]. Using treatable BSA, the mean irradiance deliverable by a PT device is calculated from all the irradiance values found within a hypothetical silhouette placed on the footprint grid. Factors that determine the treatable BSA include spread of units of the light source and orientation of these units. Another important factor that should be considered when optimizing treatable BSA is distance from the PT device. With most devices producing divergent light beams, treatable BSA increases with increasing distances away from the device.

7.2.4 Minimizing Distance Between Device and the Patient

PT irradiance can be increased by decreasing the distance from the infant's skin. The distance from the skin varies with different manufacturers and commonly ranges from 35 to 45 cm for many patented overhead PT devices that use LED light to provide intensive PT. However, a closer distance of 10–15 cm has been recommended to achieve PT in the near intensive ranges when using light sources with lower irradiance, as commonly experienced in resource-constrained communities [10, 30]. Carrying out PT at such close distances from the skin poses a risk of hyperthermia. When PT is done at close distances, the clinician must monitor the temperature of the infant and adjust the PT lamps upward if the infant is becoming febrile.

7.2.5 Use of Reflectors

Irradiance is universally improved by the use of reflectors around the light source. Reflectors help to direct reflected light to the skin as well as reduce rays that would have otherwise been absorbed by those surfaces. Reflectors have been produced by coating surfaces with materials, painting surfaces white, or even simply using a white curtain around the device [31, 32].

7.2.6 Surface Area of the Skin Exposed to Phototherapy

The area of the skin exposed is another important factor that contributes to optimizing PT. The wider the skin surface exposed, the more rapid the decline in bilirubin levels. PT provided via the traditional overhead devices covers virtually one plane of the total BSA of the treated infant at a time and is often referred to as single-sided PT. With the advent of fiber-optic wraparound devices such as Biliblanket (Ohmeda, Fairfield, CT) and Wallaby II Preterm/Term (Healthdyne Technologies), treatable skin area has been increased by placing the infant on the Biliblanket while also offering overhead PT. Newer devices such as Firefly (MTTS, Asia) also provide double-sided PT. When compared to single-sided PT, double-sided PT (also referred to as whole body PT) provides improved irradiance by increasing treatable BSA. Studies have demonstrated an increased rate of decline in total serum bilirubin (TSB) and reduction in duration of PT and length of hospital stay [33–35]. An example of an infant undergoing LED phototherapy with body exposed is seen in Fig. 6. If an infant is nearing EBT level or has ABE, the diaper may be removed until TSB falls. Figure 6 shows a non-patented LED device using three tubes of nine 2-watt LED lights evenly spaced apart. The device has silver reflectors; the use of a white curtain around the device increases reflection. Also note the close distance of light source to the infant.

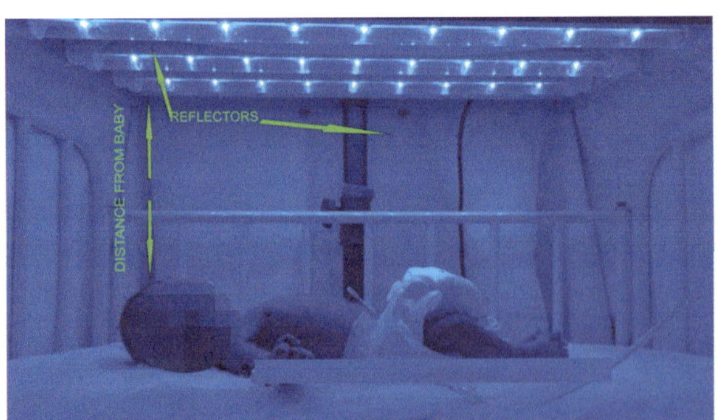

Fig. 6 An infant undergoing intensive PT using LED light source and reflectors

7.2.7 Duration of Treatment

Continuous PT (maintaining the jaundiced neonate under PT, to optimize exposure to radiant energy, virtually all the time with minimal interruptions only during feeding or care) has been shown to be more effective in reducing TSB, resulting in shorter hospital stay when compared to intermittent PT (discontinuation of PT at specific intervals of times and duration to reduce exposure to radiant energy) [36]. However, a study that described a 1-hour, 30-minutes on and 30-minutes off cycle as continuous PT and 1-hour on and 1-hour off cycle as intermittent PT demonstrated non-inferiority in efficacy of intermittent PT. Therefore, intermittent PT with short interval off cycles might be an acceptable treatment option in populations with concerns of adverse outcome such as in extremely preterms [37], or in situations where the number of PT units is limited.

7.3 Complications of Phototherapy

PT is generally considered to be very safe. Temporary side effects include:

1. Temperature instability:
   - Hyperthermia is commonly experienced with the older devices that use fluorescent or halogen light sources and have to be placed close to the baby to deliver acceptable irradiance. When constructing locally fabricated devices, provision of vents reduces the risk of overheating during PT.
   - Hypothermia is a particular risk for premature infants due to need for being unbundled and not doing kangaroo care in most PT units
2. Loose stools from intestinal hypermotility.
3. Dehydration. There are increased insensible losses during PT which could lead to dehydration, especially in neonates who are experiencing feeding difficulties. Therefore, attention should be placed on ensuring adequate breastfeeding. Intravenous fluids or supplementary feeds are not necessary unless the child is severely dehydrated or has other conditions precluding effective breastfeeding.
4. Rashes.
5. Bronze baby syndrome (BBS). This rare phenomenon has been observed in infants with both conjugated and unconjugated hyperbilirubinemia receiving PT. It is characterized by a gray-brown discoloration of the skin and urine during PT. The cause of BBS is still unknown and thought to be as a result of certain photosiomers of bilirubin, copper porphyrins, or even biliverdin [38, 39]. BBS is harmless and usually resolves within a few weeks of discontinuing PT.

6. Retinal damage. This is usually prevented by using a shield to cover the eyes while taking care not to occlude the nares. It is important to ensure that eye shields are properly applied and do not slip leaving the eye uncovered or causing noisy breathing.
7. DNA breakage. There is weak evidence in support of increased risk of damage of genetic materials in the long run. However, this is the rationale for shielding the gonads using trimmed diapers.
8. Hypocalcemia. This is occasionally noticed in premature babies and thought to be mediated by altered melatonin metabolism.
9. Extremely low birth weight (<750 g) outcome differences. Due to unknown cause, there is an increased mortality risk in this weight category that must be weighed against and balanced with improved neurologic outcome data [40].

8 Case Resolution

Two hours later, another bilirubin was drawn; bilirubin had dropped further to 10 mg/dL (172 µmol/L), which was now below EBT levels. The lab notifies you that O blood is finally available, but the EBT is deferred because the TSB has dropped below the EBT level and there is no evidence of moderate to severe ABE. The baby was treated with homemade LED PT with irradiance of 36 µW/cm^2/nm with 2 PT units. Her bilirubin level continued to decline on serial measurements and she was managed for concomitant sepsis and dehydration. PT was discontinued on day 4 of admission. The baby fully recovered and was discharged home on hospital day 15. Her neurological exam was grossly intact at follow-up and a hearing screen was normal.

References

1. Bhutani VK, et al. Neonatal hyperbilirubinemia and Rhesus disease of the newborn: incidence and impairment estimates for 2010 at regional and global levels. Pediatr Res. 2013;74(Suppl 1):86–100.
2. Diala UM, et al. Patterns of acute bilirubin encephalopathy in Nigeria: a multicenter pre-intervention study. J Perinatol. 2018;38(7):873–80.
3. Bhutani VK, et al. The need to implement effective phototherapy in resource-constrained settings. Semin Perinatol. 2011;35(3):192–7.
4. Abdulkadir I, Adebiyi MN, Adeoye G, Ogala WN. An evaluation of phototherapy services in newborn units in Kaduna State Nigeria. Niger J Paediatr. 2018:45(2):76–80.
5. Cremer RJ, Perryman PW, Richards DH. Influence of light on the hyperbilirubinaemia of infants. Lancet. 1958;1(7030):1094–7.
6. Vandborg PK, et al. Dose-response relationship of phototherapy for hyperbilirubinemia. Pediatrics. 2012;130(2):e352–7.
7. Tan KL. The nature of the dose-response relationship of phototherapy for neonatal hyperbilirubinemia. J Pediatr. 1977;90(3):448–52.

8. Abdulkadir I, Adebiyi NM, Hassan L, Abdullahi F, Ogala WN, Slusher TM, Vreman JH. Irradiance levels of phototherapy devices fabricated in Nigeria. Niger J Paediatr. 2019;45(4):180–4.
9. Vreman HJ, Wong RJ, Stevenson DK. Phototherapy: current methods and future directions. Semin Perinatol. 2004;28(5):326–33.
10. Diala UM, et al. Factors influencing irradiance of locally fabricated phototherapy devices in Jos, north-central Nigeria. Trop Doct. 2018;48(2):142–6.
11. WHO. ONTOP-IN 2012: phototherapy units: phototherapy units. Geneva: World Health Organization; 2012.
12. WHO. ONTOP-IN 2012: phototherapy job aids: phototherapy unit. Geneva: World Health Organization; 2012.
13. Wentworth, S. Neonatal phototherapy – today's lights, lamps and devices. 2005.
14. Slusher TM, et al. Filtered sunlight versus intensive electric powered phototherapy in moderate-to-severe neonatal hyperbilirubinaemia: a randomised controlled non-inferiority trial. Lancet Glob Health. 2018;6(10):e1122–31.
15. Maisels MJ, Watchko JF. Treatment of jaundice in low birthweight infants. Arch Dis Child Fetal Neonatal Ed. 2003;88(6):F459–63.
16. Maisels MJ, et al. An approach to the management of hyperbilirubinemia in the preterm infant less than 35 weeks of gestation. J Perinatol. 2012;32(9):660–4.
17. National Collaborating Centre for Women's and Children's Health. National Institute for Health and Clinical Excellence: guidance. In: *Neonatal Jaundice*. London: RCOG Press; 2010. Copyright © 2010, Royal College of Obstetricians and Gynaecologists: London.
18. American Academy of Pediatrics Subcommittee on Hyperbilirubinemia. Management of hyperbilirubinemia in the newborn infant 35 or more weeks of gestation. Pediatrics. 2004;114(1):297.
19. Borden AR, et al. Variation in the phototherapy practices and irradiance of devices in a major metropolitan area. Neonatology. 2018;113(3):269–74.
20. Olusanya B, et al. The burden and management of neonatal jaundice in Nigeria: a scoping review of the literature. Niger J Clin Pract. 2016;19(1):1–17.
21. Olusanya BO, et al. Irradiance decay in fluorescent and light-emitting diode-based phototherapy devices: a pilot study. J Trop Pediatr. 2016;62(5):421–4.
22. Vreman HJ, et al. Evaluation of window-tinting films for sunlight phototherapy. J Trop Pediatr. 2013;59(6):496–501.
23. Abdulkadir I, et al. Making locally fabricated phototherapy devices work better. J Trop Pediatr. 2020;66(1):24–8.
24. Vreman HJ. Phototherapy: the challenge to accurately measure irradiance. Indian Pediatr. 2010;47(2):127–8.
25. Ismail MT, Horn AR. The effect of device position and use of transparent covers on the irradiance distribution of LED phototherapy devices. S Afr J Child Health. 2020;14:87–93.
26. Powell P, Satrom K, Abdulkadir I, Slusher TM, DeWitt G. Smartphone enabled phototherapy irradiance meter for the care of the jaundiced neonates in low-resource regions. In: Proceedings of the 2020 design of medical devices conference. 2020: Minneapolis, MN, USA.
27. Cline BK, et al. Phototherapy device effectiveness in Nigeria: irradiance assessment and potential for improvement. J Trop Pediatr. 2013;59(4):321–5.
28. Vreman HJ, et al. Standardized bench method for evaluating the efficacy of phototherapy devices. Acta Paediatr. 2008;97(3):308–16.
29. Subramanian S, et al. Evaluation of phototherapy devices used for neonatal hyperbilirubinemia. Indian Pediatr. 2011;48(9):689–96.
30. Owa JA, et al. Irradiance readings of phototherapy equipment: Nigeria. Indian J Pediatr. 2011;78(8):996–8.
31. Kurniasih A, Tjipta GD, Ali M, Azlin E, Sianturi P. Effectiveness of phototherapy with reflecting curtains on neonatal jaundice. Paedoatr Indones. 2011;51(5):256–61.

32. Satrom K, Slusher T, Satrom J. Effectiveness of phototherapy units in Cameroon. J Trop Pediatr. 2014;60(3):264–6.
33. Arnolda G, et al. A comparison of the effectiveness of three LED phototherapy machines, single- and double-sided, for treating neonatal jaundice in a low resource setting. PLoS One. 2018;13(10):e0205432.
34. Amadi HO, et al. Comparative outcome of overhead and total body phototherapy for treatment of severe neonatal jaundice in Nigeria. Paediatr Int Child Health. 2020;40(1):16–24.
35. Nizam MA, et al. Efficacy of double versus single phototherapy in treatment of neonatal jaundice: a meta-analysis. Eur J Pediatr. 2020;179(6):865–74.
36. Zhou S, et al. Analysis of therapeutic effect of intermittent and continuous phototherapy on neonatal hemolytic jaundice. Exp Ther Med. 2019;17(5):4007–12.
37. Niknafs P, Mortazavi AA, Torabinejad MH, Bahman-Bijari B, Niknads N. Intermittent versus continuous phototherapy for reducing neonatal hyperbilirubinemia. Iran J Pediatr. 2008;18(3):251–6.
38. Le Pichon JB, et al. The neurological sequelae of neonatal hyperbilirubinemia: definitions, diagnosis and treatment of the kernicterus spectrum disorders (KSDs). Curr Pediatr Rev. 2017;13(3):199–209.
39. McDonagh AF. Bilirubin, copper-porphyrins, and the bronze-baby syndrome. J Pediatr. 2011;158(1):160–4.
40. Tyson JE, et al. Does aggressive phototherapy increase mortality while decreasing profound impairment among the smallest and sickest newborns? J Perinatol. 2012;32(9):677–84.

Additional Resource

https://www.icuworkshop.org/projects/phototherapy-units.

Umbilical Venous Catheter Placement in a Low-Resource Setting

Chinyere Ezeaka, Iretiola Bamikeolu Fajolu, and Beatrice Ezenwa

Abbreviations

BW	Birth weight
EBT	Exchange blood transfusion
IV	Intravenous access
LGA	Large for gestational age
LMICs	Low- and middle-income countries
PICC	Peripherally inserted central catheter
UVC	Umbilical venous catheter

1 Case Example 1

Baby girl Ojo is a 4.5 kg infant born after a prolonged labor not breathing or crying at birth in your emergency room in Togo. She does not respond to bag mask ventilation or to bag mask ventilation with chest compressions. You are planning to give epinephrine 0.1 mg/mL (formerly called 1/10,000) IV emergently but an IV catheter cannot easily be placed. The local provider wants to place an umbilical venous catheter (UVC), which they are proficient in performing, but the store has been out of commercial umbilical catheters for the past 3 months. You wonder what other options you have for umbilical vein access.

C. Ezeaka (✉)
Department of Paediatrics, Division of Neonatology, University of Lagos, Lagos, Nigeria
e-mail: vezeaka@unilag.edu.ng

I. B. Fajolu · B. Ezenwa
Department of Paediatrics, Lagos University Teaching Hospital (LUTH), Lagos, Nigeria

T. M. Slusher et al. (eds.), *Pediatric Procedural Adaptations for Low-Resource Settings*, https://doi.org/10.1007/978-3-030-99955-1_6

2 Case Example 2

Baby girl Chelsie is an extremely preterm infant delivered at 26 weeks' gestation to a 35-year-old with no prenatal care by spontaneous vaginal delivery in Nigeria. At delivery, Chelsie was limp but her tone improved after the initial resuscitation. You noted that she was pale and having respiratory distress. You placed her on your low-cost bubble continuous positive airway pressure device (chapter "Bubble CPAP in a Low-Resource Setting"). You perform a point-of-care random blood sugar which was 20 mg/dl (1.1 mmol/L). Urgent vascular access was needed and two attempts at peripheral intravenous (IV) access were unsuccessful. You decide to place an umbilical venous catheter (UVC) but commercial UVCs are out of stock. You wonder what other options you have for umbilical vein access.

3 Introduction

Umbilical venous catheters (UVCs) are the most common type of access in emergent or urgent situations or for prolonged use in LMICs when ongoing peripheral access is not believed to be possible or in the absence of peripherally inserted central catheters. The umbilical cord has three vessels (two arteries and one vein). The vein is usually situated *above* the two arteries at the 12 o'clock position. It is thin-walled and patulous when compared to the thick-walled, smaller caliber arteries. The process of inserting a catheter into the umbilical vein must be carried out by a trained and competent healthcare provider who observes strict aseptic procedure. As with all other procedures in this book, only healthcare practitioners trained to place UVCs should be performing this procedure. The tip of a correctly inserted UVC should be in the inferior vena cava. Studies have shown UVC insertion to be a useful and safe alternative to peripherally inserted central catheters (PICCs) in trained hands [1]. The UVC as an intravenous access route can be utilized in the newborn until the 14th day of life, but becomes more difficult after 5–7 days of life.

4 Challenges to Umbilical Catheterization in LMICs

Many LMICs utilize a fee-for-service healthcare model, where families pay out of pocket for medical services. This may impact on the access to the correct umbilical catheter type as may the actual availability of commercial UVCs. The ideal catheter type is a multi-lumen polyvinyl catheter which enables administration of different drugs and fluids. This is important in avoiding unfavorable drug-drug interactions [2]. These ideal catheters are often unavailable or too costly. A nasogastric tube can be substituted; however, risk of substituting feeding tubes for commercial umbilical venous catheters is not well studied but has been done for decades in many low-resource settings. The risk profile may not be comparable between the commercial UVC and feeding tube but this is not well documented.

5 UVC Indications/Uses/Benefits

- UVCs are the preferred initial venous access in infants <1000 g in many settings.
- Vascular access during resuscitation.
- Technical difficulties in establishing a peripheral access when IV access is essential.
- For emergencies up to the seventh–tenth day of life (occasionally older in the hands of experienced provider).
- Exchange blood transfusion (EBT).
- Central venous pressure monitoring.
- Administration of hypertonic solutions and other medications that need central venous administration (e.g., glucose >12.5%, parenteral nutrition, or inotropes).

6 UVC Contraindications

Contraindications for inserting a UVC include:

- Infants with necrotizing enterocolitis
- Umbilical sepsis or omphalitis
- Major anterior abdominal wall defects such as gastroschisis or omphalocele

6.1 UVC Equipment/Supplies (*Fig. 1*)

1. Source of heat such as radiant warmer.
2. Sterile gloves and gown.
3. Sterile drapes – in an emergency, you can use the sterile inside of sterile glove packaging.
4. Instrument pack – EBT tray or dressing packs ideally include a vein dilator.

   Umbilical catheter – commercial multiple lumen is preferred in infants <1000 g or extremely sick; commercial single lumen catheter (3.5F if birth weight <1500 g; 5.0F if birth weight ≥1500 g) is preferred for short-term usage if available; *sterile size 5 or 6 feeding tube can be used if umbilical vein catheter is unavailable or in an emergency. If planning to use a sterile feeding tube as a UVC, test to make sure that a syringe will attach to the feeding tube before*

Gloves (sterile)	Must
Umbilical tie, Clamp, or Clean String	Must
Drape(s) or inside of glove paper	Must
Cleaning solution (chlorohexidine, alcohol, spirits, other	Must (except dire emergency in delivery room)
5F, 6F NG tube (any size neonate); 8F term	Must
10 mL syringe (5-20 mL will work)	Must
2 three-way stopcocks	Very helpful but can make do with 1 stopcock or even none but increases infectious risk as have to disconnect multiple times
IV tubing to make waste tubing	Must if using 2 stopcocks
Blood giving set with filter	Must
Vein dilator	Very helpful but can often get in fresh cords without this
Small Forceps	Helpful but usually not essential for UVC; Must have if also placing a Umbilical Artery Catheter
Tape or suture if placing high and leaving in place	Must have if leaving line in place
X-ray or Ultrasound if leaving UVC in place	Need to confirm placement

Fig. 1 Equipment/supplies needed for UVC/EBT

inserting. Newer feeding tubes may attach only to oral syringes. If a newer feeding tubes that will not attach to regular syringes are the only potential UVC catheter available and the need for access is emergent, the healthcare provider may cut the oral syringe adapter off the sterile feeding tube and carefully insert a sterile 18 g needle into the lumen of the feeding tube. Be careful not to puncture the tube. Before using the tube, flush the tube to ensure there is not a leak in the tube. Do not leave this tube modification in the long term as it could potential separate in an unmonitored situation (Fig. 2a, b).

5. Three-way tap if available.
6. Syringes (5–10 cc).
7. 0.9% NaCl flushing fluid.
8. Cleaning agents: 2% aqueous chlorhexidine solution as skin preparation or povidone-iodine; dilute 1:1 with sterile water if infant is <750 g and 70% alcohol (methylated spirit).
9. Intravenous infusion giving sets (Solusets) or infusion pumps.
10. Size 22 sterile scalpel blade.
11. Umbilical tape or clean ties/string if tape is unavailable.
12. Atraumatic suture (3/0 silk on a cutting-edge needle) if placing a high UVC that will not be removed immediately after the resuscitation or exchange blood transfusion.
13. Skin plasters or tape.

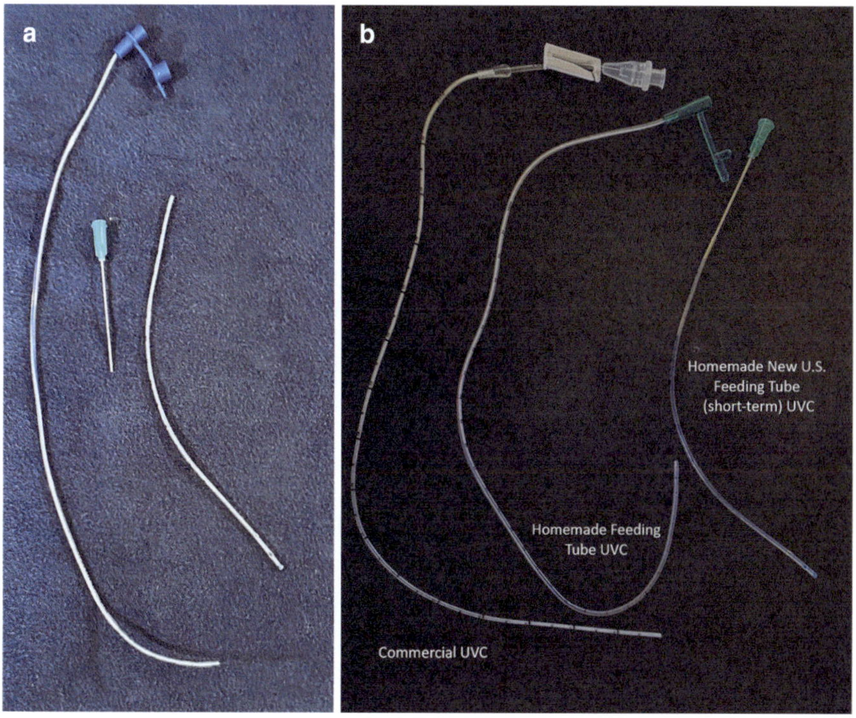

Fig. 2 (**a**) Supplies for modifying feeding tubes for temporary UVC. (**b**) Examples of Commercial and Homemade UVCs

7 UVC Procedural Technique

This procedure should be done only by providers trained in doing the procedure and with proper informed consent, except when needed urgently. Some steps are omitted as they are understood by practitioners experienced in placing a UVC.

7.1 Initial Preparation

- Position the infant, keep warm under the radiant warmer if available, and restrain all limbs. If no radiant warmer is available, complete procedure in the warmest location available and monitor the infant's temperature frequently.
- Monitor all vital signs before and during the procedure. If available, place the infant on a continuous pulse oximeter.
- Select appropriate catheter or sterile feeding tube if commercial catheters are unavailable.

- Determine the type of UVC you want to insert: either a low-lying or high-lying catheter.
  - A properly placed *low*-lying UVC is suitable for one-time EBT or in delivery room resuscitation. Hyperosmolar fluids should *not* be infused through a low-lying UVC.
  - *A high*-lying UVC is suitable for LGA babies with hypoglycemia, ongoing access in extreme prematurity, or when prolonged access for some days is required and peripheral venous access is not possible.
- *Low*-lying catheters are inserted about 3–5 cm into the umbilical vein or just until blood return is seen in the catheter. Stop inserting the catheter as soon as you get good blood return. If the catheter is advanced beyond level of first blood return, the catheter may be in the liver. A catheter in the liver is unsafe and should never be used.
- The *high*-lying UVC is inserted using the formula below to estimate the length of catheter to be inserted. Four alternative methods for determining the length of insertion are included below. Remember to add the length of the stump to the measured distance.
  - Plot on a graph found in a neonatal handbook which used the distance from infant's shoulder to the level of umbilicus.
  - 0.66 × distance from infant's shoulder to the level of umbilicus
  - [2/3 the distance from infant's shoulder to the level of umbilicus]
  - [BW(kg) × 2] + 5]
- Offer pain relief (drops of oral sucrose drops up to 1–2 mL).

7.2 Sterile Preparation

- Follow all standard sterile procedures.
- Loosely tie a single knot using clean (sterile if available) cotton tape around the base of the umbilicus. Secure enough to maintain hemostasis but not to prevent passage of catheter. Use the wrap-wrap or double wrap tie method to keep the tie or string from slipping. You may also insert a purse-string suture at the base of the umbilical cord through the Wharton's jelly for hemostasis. The tape or string may be applied before cleaning, but if this is done, the tape or string should also be included in the cleaning process.
- Drape the umbilical stump with sterile towels if available.
- Place sterile sheet with a hole in the center over the cord. Pull the cord through the hole – *in emergency the drape can be the inside of the sterile glove pack with hole cut or torn in the middle* (Fig. 3).

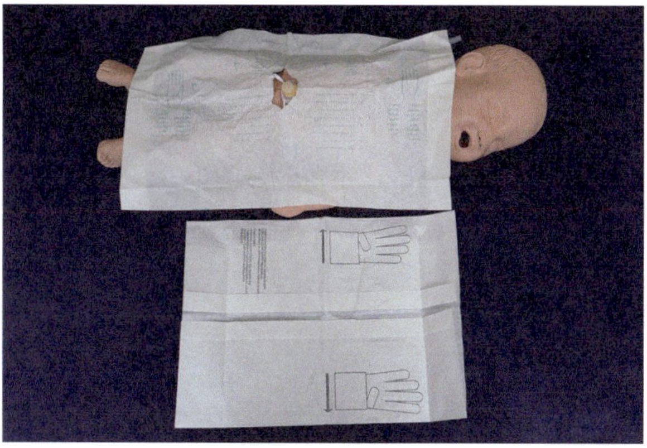

Fig. 3 Example of how to use inside of sterile glove package as sterile drape

7.3 *Catheter Placement*

1. Trim the umbilical cord to about 1–2 cm from the abdomen in a single cut using a straight blade.
2. Immobilize the cord by grasping the cut edges with two artery forceps (if available) at 3 and 9 o'clock, taking care not to include the vessels.
3. Identify the umbilical vein, insert the tip of an iris forceps or a dilator into the lumen, and gently and repeatedly dilate the vein by allowing the forceps to spring open (although ideal to dilate as describe above, it is often possible in an emergency to insert a sterile feeding tube without a dilator as feeding tubes are generally a little stiffer than a commercial UVC and may go in without dilating the vein first).
4. Gently introduce the primed catheter into the vein, advancing cautiously in a cephalad direction. Be careful not to create a false passage.
5. For a low-lying UVC, the tip must lie completely below the liver (i.e., 3–5 cm + stump length). This is called either a low-lying or short UVC. Catheters at this position can be used for short-term purposes such as for emergency resuscitation or exchange blood transfusion only. *Avoid placement of catheters in the portal circulation!*
6. For a high-lying UVC, advance the catheter to the desired length as earlier calculated. The desired final position of the tip of the high-lying UVC catheter should be in the inferior vena cava at the level of the diaphragm (between T8 and T9). This can be confirmed with an imaging study (X-ray or beside ultrasound) after insertion.

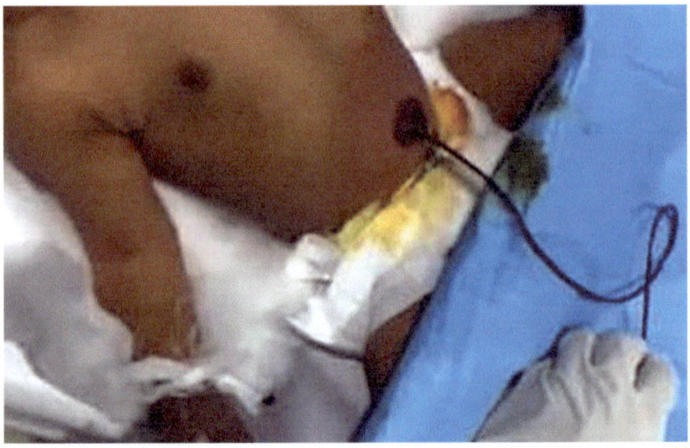

Fig. 4 Example of inserted UVC and free flow of blood

A correctly inserted catheter will yield free flow of blood in the withdrawing syringe and will pass freely without resistance (Fig. 4).

7. *Pitfalls:* If catheter will not advance beyond 4–5 cm and blood cannot be withdrawn, it is likely that a false passage has been created. Remove catheter and seek advice from a more experienced senior person. If possible, consult a surgeon or senior person able to place a central line or do an umbilical venous cut-down.

7.4 Securing Catheter

- Low-lying lines for emergent use in the delivery room or for single exchange blood transfusions may be held in place by the operator/provider and do not need to be sutured or secured.
- High-lying lines should be secured with 3.0 silk suture and/or bridge taping (Fig. 5a, b).
- Place two sutures into the cord, one on either side of the catheter, and then tie a purse string around the catheter to secure it in place and achieve hemostasis.

Catheter Placement Confirmation An abdominal X-ray or ultrasound to check the position of the catheter prior to use is mandatory except in low-lying UVC or in an emergency. The UVC goes straight up on the X-ray, unlike a UAC which forms a loop. If the catheter tip position of a "long" UVC is too high (inside the right atrium), it can be pulled back appropriately. X-ray or ultrasound should be repeated after repositioning [3]. Ultrasound-guided catheter placement is associated with

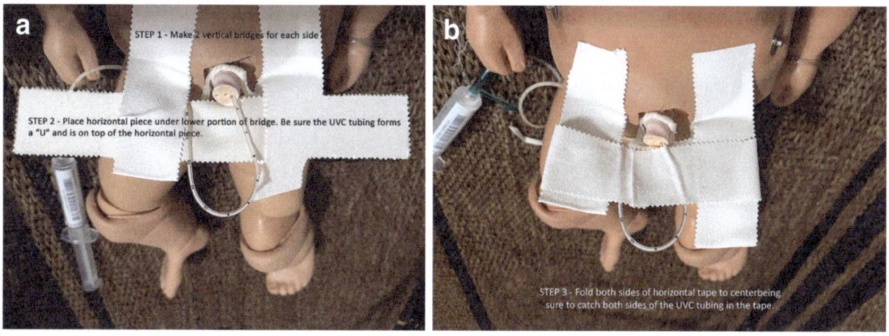

Fig. 5 Steps to tape a UVC in place (**a**) First half of bridge tape. (**b**) Final bridge tape

more success and less complications and overall, is more cost-effective than conventional catheter placement. Post-catheterization monitoring of the catheter placement requires X-ray to assess the position and correct placement of the UVC or ultrasound. Ultrasound has been shown to be superior to thoraco-abdominal X-ray in determining UVC tip position [4]. Ultrasound is also feasible as a guide especially with post-insertion migration which may occur after initial assessment with X-ray [5, 6]. If the tip is below the diaphragm once sterility is broken, a fresh catheter should be reinserted to avoid contamination. Start infusion as soon as the position is confirmed.

7.5 *Instructions for Use*

7.5.1 Care of the UVC

- Catheter may remain in place for up to 7 days. After 7 days, the risk of infection increases.
- Aseptic techniques must be observed while using the UVC for infusions and drugs.
- Daily observe the cord stump and UVC site for evidence of infection or erythema.
- Continuous infusion of intravenous fluids is necessary to maintain patency of the UVC.
- Review need for catheter daily and when possible replace with PICC line or a peripheral line if available.

7.5.2 Indications for UVC Removal

- UVC access no longer required.
- Concern about sepsis.
- Catheter has exceeded 7 days.
- After resuscitation or EBT is completed (low-lying UVC).

7.5.3 Procedure for Catheter Removal

- This is also an aseptic procedure. Scrub and put on gown and gloves.
- Clean the cord with cleaning solutions – povidone-iodine or 2% chlorhexidine solution.
- Turn the infusion off.
- Withdraw the catheter gradually in a single action.
- Send the tip for culture if infection is suspected.
- If bleeding occurs while the umbilical tie or string is in place, pull the tie just tight enough to stop the bleeding. If the tie has fallen off, press firmly just above the umbilicus until 1–2 minutes after the bleeding has stopped.
- Nurse infant in the supine position for at least 4 hours after removal of the catheter with the abdomen visible for inspection, not covering the umbilicus with a nappy/diaper or dressing, so that any inadvertent bleeding from the umbilicus will not go unnoticed.

7.6 Complications

- Sepsis [7].
- Bleeding due to disconnection of tubing; always use a Luer lock or screw on connection when attaching the catheter to the infusion lines.
- Perforation; never cut off the rounded end of any indwelling catheter.
- Clot formation, embolism, and spasm.
- Effects of catheter mispositioning – cardiac arrhythmias, hepatic necrosis, or portal hypertension.
- Cardiac tamponade.

8 Case Resolution 1

A UVC was quickly inserted using a 5 Fr sterile nasogastric tube using sterile gloves and glove paper for the drape after quickly prepping and cutting the cord. One dose of epinephrine was given. CPR was continued for 1 minute. The heart rate rose to 120 BPM. The infant started to cry and breathe well. The resuscitation was stopped. The catheter was removed after the resuscitation without securement. Ten days later, the infant went home with the mother with plans for close follow-up as an outpatient.

9 Case Resolution 2

A radio-opaque nasogastric tube is inserted using the calculation for high UVC and an X-ray is done to confirm placement. Catheter was secured using the bridging tape. When it became apparent that the UVC would not be able to be removed in 1–2 days, it was sutured and bridge tape removed. The UVC was removed after 7 days when a peripheral line is inserted. She did well and was discharged on day of life 30 in KMC (chapter "Kangaroo Mother Care in a Low-Resource Setting") rotating between family members after the grandmother made her KMC holder and family was comfortable with her care. She returned 3 days later doing well.

References

1. Konstantinidi A, et al. Umbilical venous catheters and peripherally inserted central catheters: are they equally safe in VLBW infants? A non-randomized single center study. Medicina (Kaunas). 2019;55(8):442.
2. Bradley JS, et al. Intravenous ceftriaxone and calcium in the neonate: assessing the risk for cardiopulmonary adverse events. Pediatrics. 2009;123(4):e609–13.
3. El-Maadawy S, El-Atawi K, Elhalik M. Role of bedside ultrasound in determining the position of umbilical venous catheters. J Clin Neonatol. 2015;4(3):173–7.
4. Michel F, et al. Comparison of ultrasound and X-ray in determining the position of umbilical venous catheters. Resuscitation. 2012;83(6):705–9.

5. Dubbink-Verheij GH, et al. Inadvertent migration of umbilical venous catheters often leads to malposition. Neonatology. 2019;115(3):205–10.
6. Guzman-de la Garza FJ, et al. [Ultrasound-guided umbilical venous catheterisation: a cost-effectiveness analysis]. An Pediatr (Engl Ed), 2020. 92(4): 215–21.
7. Gordon A, Greenhalgh M, McGuire W. Early planned removal of umbilical venous catheters to prevent infection in newborn infants. Cochrane Database Syst Rev. 2017;10:CD012142.

Exchange Blood Transfusions for Severe Hyperbilirubinemia in Resource-Limited Settings

Katherine Satrom, David Shwe, and Fatima Usman

Abbreviations

AAP	American Academy of Pediatrics
ACD	Acid citrate dextrose
BIND	Bilirubin-induced neurologic dysfunction
CPD	Citrate phosphate dextrose
EBT	Exchange blood transfusion
EDTA	Ethylenediaminetetraacetic acid
IVIG	Intravenous immunoglobulin
KSD	Kernicterus spectrum disorder
NPO	Nil per os
RhD	Rhesus disease
TSB	Total serum bilirubin
UVC	Umbilical venous catheter

K. Satrom (✉)
Department of Pediatrics, Division of Neonatology, University of Minnesota, Minneapolis, MN, USA
e-mail: ksatrom@umn.edu

D. Shwe
Department of Paediatrics, University of Jos, Jos, Nigeria

F. Usman
Department of Paediatrics, Bayero University, Kano, Nigeria

T. M. Slusher et al. (eds.), *Pediatric Procedural Adaptations for Low-Resource Settings*, https://doi.org/10.1007/978-3-030-99955-1_7

1 Case

A 5-day-old now 2.5 kg infant born at 36 weeks' gestation presents to your hospital in Jos, Nigeria, with yellow eyes, fever, poor feeding, and high-pitched cry for 1 day. Her history is significant for late preterm delivery due to preterm rupture of membranes with prolonged labor, limited prenatal care, and reportedly delayed first cry for 1 hour after birth despite stimulation. She was wrapped in a cloth that smelled strongly of camphor balls, also known as "moth balls" or naphthalene balls. Blood group of both parents is O positive. On exam you note an ill-appearing infant with fever, scleral icterus, and jaundice noted up to the palms and soles using the Kramer's dermal scale for jaundice. Bilirubin-induced neurologic dysfunction (BIND II) score is 8/12. Neurologic exam reveals lethargy with refusal to suck on gloved finger; paralysis of upward gaze; opisthotonos; scissoring of arms, and legs; intermittent seizure-like activity; and apnea. Her exam is otherwise within normal limits. Her laboratory work-up is positive for a total serum bilirubin, 35 mg/dL (599 μmol/L, direct bilirubin 2.0 mg/dL (34.2 μmol/L), and a complete blood count with leukocytes of 2500 with 80% neutrophils, platelet count of 75 K, and a hematocrit of 28%. You are doing a study on the relationship of neonatal sepsis and glucose-6-phosphate dehydrogenase deficiency (G6PDD) and are able to get a screening test done which reveals that she is G6PD deficient and a bedside CRP which is 90 mg/L (normal for your lab is <10 mg/L), cultures are pending, and early CSF studies are within normal limits.

Your diagnosis is severe acute bilirubin encephalopathy with anemia secondary to probable sepsis and G6PD deficiency in a late preterm infant. You conclude you need an emergent exchange blood transfusion and ask the father to find a blood donor while you place the neonate under your best phototherapy and treat her for sepsis with appropriate antibiotics. You note that you have used up all the donated exchange blood transfusion kits you had in your nursery.

2 Introduction

Exchange blood transfusion (EBT) is an emergency procedure for the treatment of severe unconjugated hyperbilirubinemia unresponsive to intensive phototherapy or when the total serum bilirubin (TSB) is above the cutoff for exchange on the EBT nomogram for your hospital/country/region or in any neonate with moderate-severe acute bilirubin encephalopathy (ABE) regardless of the TSB [1, 2]. It is used in conjunction with phototherapy for maximum effect in order to prevent, reverse, or limit the progression of severe unconjugated hyperbilirubinemia to encephalopathy or even death [3]. It was first described in 1921 by Dr. Bruce Robertson, a Canadian surgeon, and was first used in 1924 by Dr. J.L. MacDonald to treat erythroblastosis fetalis [4]. The procedure is aseptic, involving an incremental removal of the neonate's blood through an umbilical or peripheral vessel [5] while simultaneously replacing it with donor-compatible blood in a single or double volume exchange [6].

The frequency of EBTs has markedly reduced in high-income countries because of lower incidence of severe hyperbilirubinemia [7–9], and an increased vigilant approach. It however is still widely practiced in low-resource settings particularly in Sub-Saharan Africa and East Asia [10–12] due to the high burden of disease, delayed recognition of its onset, late presentation, lack of hospital facilities for effective TSB monitoring and phototherapy, inadequate clinical expertise in some settings, and poor logistic support [13].

A review of annual data trend for EBT in Eastern Europe showed an evident decline from 54 to 8 EBTs per year [14]. Similarly, a report on the serial prevalence of extreme hyperbilirubinemia and rescue EBTs in California over a 5-year period showed a significant decrease in the incidence and rate of severe hyperbilirubinemia and EBT, respectively [15]. This is in contrast to what obtains in low- and middle-income countries (LMICs) where a high EBT prevalence ranging between 5.3% and 46.9% are being reported [16–20].

3 Indications for Exchange Blood Transfusion

Therapeutic:

- Severe hyperbilirubinemia (TSB >20–30 mg/dl or 342–513 µmol/L) as an adjunct to phototherapy. The exact level of TSB to perform an EBT should be determined by local in-country guidelines when available factoring in the quality of phototherapy available, the stability of electricity, and condition of the neonate.
- Moderate hyperbilirubinemia (TSB 15–18 mg/dl or 257–308 µmol/L) with significant anemia (hematocrit <30%) or prematurity. Again, use in-country guidelines whenever possible and again consider same factors as above.
- Any infant with hyperbilirubinemia with evidence of moderate-severe ABE (BIND II score ≥3) irrespective of the level of serum bilirubin.
- Rate of rise of TSB >0.5 mg/dL/hr. (8.6 µmol/L) or 5 mg/dL/day (86 µmol/L/day) continuing after beginning intensive phototherapy.

Prophylactic for polycythemia (partial volume exchange transfusion, i.e., replace with normal saline):

(a) Central hematocrit of >65 with symptoms related to hyperviscosity and resultant poor perfusion and include lethargy, poor feeding, hypotonia, seizures, cyanosis, respiratory distress, necrotizing enterocolitis, hypoglycemia, and thrombocytopenia, among others
(b) Central hematocrit of >70 even without symptoms

For very low birth weight neonates (<1500 g) or extremely low birth weight (<1000 g) neonates, consider performing an EBT using the following rules: neonates >2000 g with TSB 10 mg/dl (171 µmol/L) by 24 hrs of age, 15 mg/dl

(257 μmol/L) by 48 hrs, or 20 mg/dl (342 μmol/L) at any age. Another simple rule for determining the EBT level in preterm neonates is to use a cutoff of a TSB which is greater than or equal to the body weight in grams divided by 100, e.g., for a weight of 1500 g, EBT is suggested at 15 mg/dl (257 μmol/L). Again, for any preterm infant, use local in-country guidelines when available and consider other factors as noted in the quality of phototherapy, availability of electricity, and condition of the neonate. All values for EBT should be directed by facility, region, or country guidelines whenever possible and clinician input based on their knowledge of the quality of the phototherapy, reliability of electricity, availability of blood, and other relevant local factors as determined per the clinicians carrying for the neonates. All levels mentioned in this chapter are rough guidelines. Care should always be directed by the clinicians caring for each neonate.

The American Academy of Pediatrics (AAP) guidelines recommend appropriate risk prediction for severe hyperbilirubinemia using hour specific nomogram [21], and exchange blood transfusion guideline charts [1] based on gestational age (GA), postnatal age (in hours), and antecedent risk factors, namely, isoimmune hemolysis, G6PD deficiency, asphyxia, sepsis, and acidosis designating into low-, medium-, and high-risk categories to determine the need for EBT. However, note that these are the American guidelines are often not the appropriate guidelines for LMICs. If AAP guidelines are used in LMICs because of the lack of local or in-country guidelines, consider deleting the low-risk category and consider all neonates to be at least moderate risk. Each country/region should be encouraged to develop their own guidelines appropriate to their setting.

4 Contraindications

- Primary conjugated/direct hyperbilirubinemia without a concerning unconjugated/indirect TSB (with most nomograms including the AAP nomograms, do not subtract the conjugated/direct fraction from the total to determine the exchange levels).
- Porphyria

5 Benefits

EBT remains one of the most reliable and effective treatment options especially in resource-limited settings for preventing bilirubin encephalopathy. Although it is not without its complications, it plays an important role in management of severe unconjugated hyperbilirubinemia. These include the following:

- EBT often speeds up recovery and reduces the duration of hospital stay by lowering unconjugated bilirubin to nontoxic levels faster than other bilirubin lowering strategies [3].

– It may prevent acute bilirubin encephalopathy (ABE) and lifelong neurodevelopmental disability (kernicterus spectrum disorder) associated with bilirubin encephalopathy.
– In severe hyperbilirubinemia due to hemolytic disease of the newborn, EBT lowers the concentration of immune antibodies and sensitized red cells in circulation, thus reducing the rate of hemolysis.
– Remotely, EBT has the potential to have a high impact on community, social, and economic progress by reducing the cost of continuing care for a disabled child which may ultimately decrease the burden on an already overstretched health system and the economy.

6 Steps to Set up

Preparation for EBT

(i) Consent
(ii) Counseling
(iii) EBT checklist
(iv) Setting up the environment

6.1 Procedure Supplies

1. Fresh whole blood: Generally, O, rhesus (Rh)-specific blood less than 72 hours old cross-matched against maternal and infant serum is most often used in LMICs. Use Rh negative for Rh-mediated hemolysis (mother Rh-negative, infant Rh-positive) or if the infant is Rh-negative. Heparinized blood fresh blood (<24 hours old) is ideal but often not an option is the most ideal. Blood preserved with acid citrate dextrose (ACD) or citrate phosphate dextrose (CPD) can also be used. If blood banking resources allow, reconstituted PRBCs can also be used as is usually done in high-income countries. All blood must be screened for HIV, hepatitis B, hepatitis C, and syphilis. Blood from donors with sickle cell trait should not be used whenever possible as blood from donors with sickle cell trait can sickle when it becomes acidotic. Blood giving set with a filter is also essential.
2. Umbilical vein catheterization kit (or sterile feeding tube 5–8 fr), cleaning solution, sterile gloves, umbilical tie or equivalent, three to five syringes (5 ml,10 ml, or 20 mL depending on infant weight and availability of syringes), stopcocks (two three-way), adhesive plaster/tape, gauze, blood bag, and discard basin. Small artery forceps and vein dilator are also helpful.
3. Procedure table, blood warmer, stop clock, input and output charts, towels, radiant warmer, gauze, tape, stethoscope, thermometer, pulse oximeter if available, and blood giving set

4. Baseline labs: type and cross match, hemoglobin, platelet count, basic metabolic panel, calcium level, and TSB at the time the EBT is begun. Calcium gluconate 10% if using blood anticoagulated with ethylenediaminetetraacetic acid (EDTA).
5. Sterile water for injection or normal saline for injection for diluting and flushing calcium.

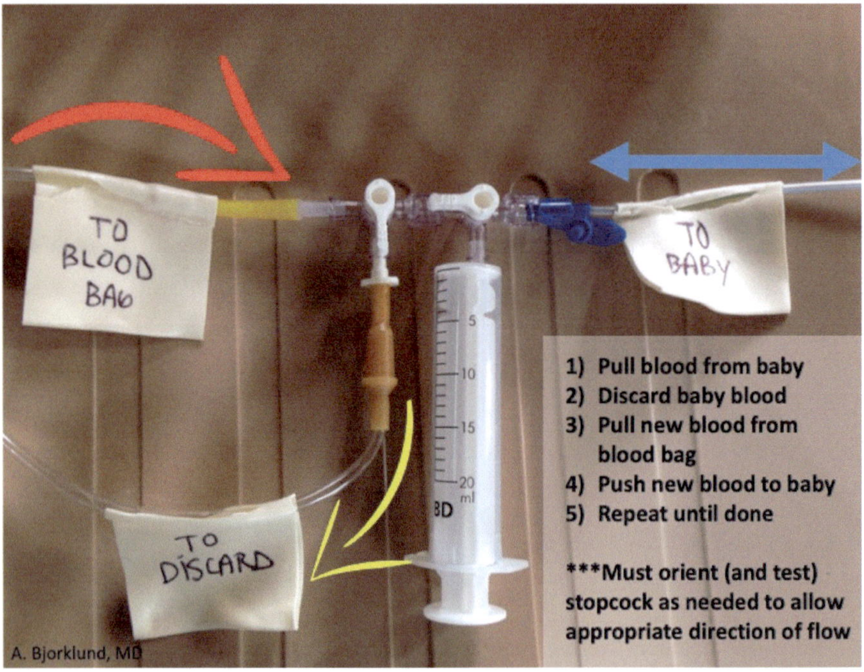

Modified Exchange Blood Transfusion Kit

6.2 Pre-procedure Preparations

1. Determine total volume of blood for exchange transfusion. For double volume exchange, twice the neonates' blood volume is calculated at 160 mL/kg of blood, assuming a total neonate blood volume of 80mls/kg up to 1 unit of whole blood. Do not exceed 1 unit of whole blood per EBT. For bigger neonates, you may only use a 1.0–1.5 volume exchange instead of a double volume EBT.
2. Calculate the volume per aliquot to be used depending on patient weight (not to exceed >10% of total blood volume). Generally, for neonates >3 kg, use 20 mL aliquots; for 2–3 kg, use 15 mL aliquots; for 1–2 kg, use 10 mL; and for <1 kg, use 5 mL. This can be alerted as needed by the clinician based on the stability of the neonate and the size of syringes available.
3. Set up procedure supplies, ensuring correct orientation/positioning and labeling of equipment for easy access and identification.

4. Notify unit staff and identify two supporting personnel for the procedure, making a total of at least three persons conducting the procedure.
5. Ensure patient's pre-procedure vitals are done and within normal limits.
6. Ensure a warm and conducive ambient temperature (25°C to 30°C) by shutting windows, switching off fans, or using radiant warmer.
7. Ideally, enteral feeding should be discontinued at least 4 hours before and after the procedure to avoid procedure-induced vomiting and aspiration of gastric content. However, do not delay EBT in a neonate exhibiting signs of ABE or with an extremely elevated TSB. As soon as blood is available, begin the EBT. If needed, place a gastric tube and aspirate the gastric contents. Place the neonate on glucose-containing fluids. At least two people should cross-check, confirm, and document details on blood to be used match the patient's, verifying compatibility.

6.3 Patient Preparation

1. Place neonate in restraints (swaddling the upper body using a towel while keeping the abdomen exposed) on a firm surface/table in supine position and keep warm using caps, socks, and mittens.
2. Measure the baseline vitals, namely, temperature, pulse rate and volume, respiratory rate, and oxygen saturation including blood glucose level
3. Place UVC (see chapter "Umbilical Venous Catheter Placement in a Low-Resource Setting" for details). Generally, a low-lying UVC is used, but if repeated EBTs are likely, then a high UVC may be placed verifying the position with either an X-ray or ultrasound. See chapter "Umbilical Venous Catheter Placement in a Low-Resource Setting" for details on placement of a UVC.
4. Take pre-procedure samples for serum bilirubin and hematocrit.

6.4 Procedural Steps

Again, as with all procedures described in this book, only healthcare workers trained on how to do an EBT should be doing them unsupervised. Healthcare workers not previously trained on how to do an EBT must be trained either in their country or by local experts before attempting to do it by themselves.

Strict aseptic precautions must be observed during the procedure. The push and pull technique via an umbilical vein is the commonest method used in low-resource settings. Umbilical artery catheterization (UAC) for withdrawing blood with a peripheral vein for infusing blood can also be used if umbilical vein cannulation is not feasible. Extreme caution should be exercised when using umbilical artery access to avoid introducing any air into the line as this is high risk for air embolus. If supplies and expertise allow, both a UVC and UAC may be placed with two operators performing the EBT simultaneously. One operator draws from the UAC, while another operator gives blood through the UVC. Using both a UAC and UVC at the same time is rarely an option in a LMIC due to both resources and staffing.

6.5 *Procedure*

1. The exchange transfusion tubing should be set up so that blood is drawn from the neonate and discarded, while blood is drawn from the blood bag via the given set and infused into the neonate.
2. Use the predetermined sized syringe noting that this may be limited by the availability of syringe sizes in your hospital. For our 2.5 kg neonate, we would have ideally used a 20 mL syringe and drawn and given back 15 mL per cycle; however, the largest syringe available was 10 mL syringes. The neonate's blood is removed in aliquots through the tube in the umbilical vein and replaced by an equal volume of blood in a cyclical manner without breaking the circuit until the whole calculated EBT volume has been exchanged.
3. An assistant must record the amount removed and amount given with each cycle. The operator must state how much they have withdrawn or infused each time they withdraw or infuse blood. This should be recorded and periodically tallied on a piece of paper. The assistant should inform the operator when they are at 100 mL of blood exchanged.
4. Because stat ionized calcium levels are rarely available and continuous ECG/EKG recording is also rarely available, most practitioners give 1 mL of 10% calcium gluconate after each 100 mL of blood exchanged. This should be given through the UVC via slow push over at least 10 minutes while monitoring the heart rate to prevent bradycardia. If continuous pulse oximetry is not available, have the assistant listen to the heart rate during the calcium infusion and inform the practitioners immediately if the heart rate begins to fall. If the heart rate starts to fall, stop the calcium infusion and wait for the heart rate to recover before resuming the calcium infusion. Flush UVC before and after calcium is given. It may be helpful to dilute 1 ml of calcium with 9 mL of sterile water to make it easier to give the infusion slowly. Remember to flush slowly after the calcium infusion as there is often enough calcium in the UVC to cause bradycardia if flushed rapidly.
5. Blood that is being transfused must be periodically agitated to prevent settling of red cells which can cause plasma to remain in the blood bag toward the end of the procedure, resulting in anemia. If the neonate is anemic at the beginning of the procedure, it may be appropriate to give an extra 10 mL/kg of blood in over the last two to three pushes of the EBT (i.e., for our 2.5 kg neonate, we chose to give 25 mL more blood out than in, so for the last three push-pulls, we took out 10 cc each time and gave in 20 mL, 20 mL, and 15 mL).
6. Monitoring of vital signs every 15–30 mins during the procedure is advocated with continuous pulse oximetry if available otherwise a stethoscope can be taped to the chest.

7. Take samples for post-EBT serum bilirubin, calcium (if available in your lab), and hematocrit at the end of the procedure.
8. The duration of the procedure should be between 60 and 90 minutes (occasionally 120 minutes). Each cycle should take about 3 minutes.

6.5.1 Determinants of EBT Effectiveness

1. Volume of blood for exchange: The larger the volume of blood exchanged, the greater the fraction of toxic bilirubin removed from the neonate's circulation. Double volume EBT is better and is recommended for severe hyperbilirubinemia. Generally, however, limit the amount exchanged to 1 unit per exchange.
2. Rate of exchange: Rapid EBT can compromise the hemodynamic stability of the neonate leading to bradycardia and reduced renal and cerebral blood flows. In addition, citrated blood may not get sufficient time for hepatic metabolism, thus causing decreases in blood PH and potentially causing elevated cerebral edema.
3. Duration of the EBT procedure:

6.5.2 Post-EBT Care

1. Monitoring:

   (a) Observe for color change particularly cyanosis, apnea, or seizures.
   (b) Vital signs (temperature, heart rate, respiratory rate, oxygen saturation, blood pressure) should be closely monitored every 30 minutes for 2 hours, then hourly for the next 2 hours, 4 hourly for the next 8 hours, and then 6 hourly for the next 24 hours.
   (c) Abdominal girth. This measurement is taken at baseline and then compared with two-hourly measurements. Measurements are taken at fixed, reproducible anatomic landmarks. Measurement 2–3 cm distal to xiphoid process may be used.
   (d) Bowel sounds.
   (e) Strict input and output check assuring adequate output of 1–2 mL/kg/hour.
   (f) Random blood glucose check to detect hypoglycemia.
   (g) Continue to monitor serial bilirubin levels at 2, 4, and 6 hours after the EBT until bilirubin level begins to fall at which time bilirubin levels maybe spaced to 6–12 hours depending on actual bilirubin level, condition of the infant and rate of decline.
2. Neonate should remain nil per os (NPO) for the next 4 hours.
3. If neonate is on parenteral medications (antibiotics, anticonvulsants), they should be continued. Check with pharmacy or look up to determine which medications need to be re-dosed or given after EBT.
4. Commence topical application of 4% chlorhexidine gel if available per guidelines in country/region for newborn cord care.
5. Continue phototherapy until TSB falls below 40% of critical value.

6. Continued parent/caregiver communication and counseling.

6.6 *Follow-Up*

- Hearing screen prior to discharge if possible otherwise refer to a center that can do a hearing test as soon as feasible after discharge.
- Developmental follow-up if available

7 Risks and Potential Complications

Although EBT is a relatively safe procedure, it may be associated with adverse events which can be asymptomatic, transient, or long term [22], varying in severity from mild to life threatening [23]. As noted above, it must only be done by a provider experienced and trained to do EBTs. Learners must therefore be taught by an experienced provider and supervised throughout the entire procedure. The risk of mortality associated with EBT is low, i.e., 0.1–0.5% [24], while that for morbidity ranges between 12% and 74% depending on the severity of the underlying disease condition, route used for exchange blood transfusion, and the volume of blood exchanged [16, 25–29]. These potential complications include:

1. Umbilical and other central line-associated complications
    - Bleeding from umbilical stump due to improperly ligated cord, coagulation abnormalities caused by EBT, sepsis, lack of Vitamin K1, and/or underlying pathology
    - Infection from lack of aseptic techniques
    - Thromboembolic complications from coagulopathies
    - Vessel spasm and/or perforation
    - Necrotizing enterocolitis
    - Cardiac arrhythmias related to electrolyte disturbances, volume shifts, and/or catheter position
    - Hepatic necrosis and/or cirrhosis from pressure effect of the EBT tube in the hepatic vessel
    - Lower extremity gangrene due to disruption of blood supply from vessel spasm
2. Blood product-associated complications
    - Thrombocytopenia from using old blood
    - Anemia from low blood donor hematocrit
    - Infection (i.e., HIV, CMV, malaria, syphilis, hepatitis, bacteria)
    - Electrolyte and acid/base disturbances
        - Hyperkalemia from using old or hemolyzed blood for EBT

  - Hypocalcemia and hypomagnesemia due to the calcium and magnesium chelating effect of citrate in the anticoagulants acid citrate dextrose (ACD) and citrate phosphate dextrose (CPD) in blood bag
  - Acidosis due to the high acid content of blood anticoagulants

- Increase in non-esterified fatty acid level which may affect coagulation and albumin binding if heparinized donor blood is used
- Immediate transfusion reactions (anaphylactic, hemolytic, febrile, etc.) and delayed transfusion reactions (graft-versus-host disease if not using irradiated blood)
- Hypothermia from using cold blood
- Rebound hypoglycemia after EBT from the high glucose content of the anticoagulants in blood bag

3. Procedure-related complications

- Anemia from lysed blood during the push and pull technique
- Hypothermia from cold environmental temperature
- Hypovolemia or overload resulting in heart failure and/or pulmonary edema due to hemodynamic changes caused by the push and pull technique, over- or under-transfusion
- Increased cerebral blood flow and intracranial pressure resulting from too rapid procedure

4. Human-related risks

- Errors in charting the number of cycles done
- Incorrect blood volume replacement during the push and pull technique

7.1 Additional Pearls

- Always start phototherapy before blood is available for EBT and continue phototherapy after the procedure. Use the best phototherapy available preferably with an irradiance of at least 30 microwatts per cm squared per nanometer.
- Albumin, if available, given 1–2 hours prior to EBT may increase the efficiency but is controversial.
- Intravenous immunoglobulin (IVIG) should be considered for neonates with rhesus disease and hyperbilirubinemia if available.
- Use a room heater and blood warmer (if available) during the procedure to prevent hypothermia in the neonate. If no blood warmer available, then allow the mother to hold the wrapped blood under her arm to warm while preparing for the EBT or very carefully warm in warm (not hot) water to room temperature.
- Each person should verbalize when they are starting and stopping their task.
- Have a recorder to document and tally the aliquots, timing, vital signs, and labs.
- The longer the duration of the procedure, the better the efficacy of the EBT. Too rapid an exchange increases the risk of complications.

Table 1 BIND II (bilirubin-induced neurologic dysfunction) score – modification of the BIND M score

BIND II (bilirubin-induced neurologic dysfunction) score		
Clinical sign (score most severe sign)	Score	Severity
Mental status		
Normal	0	None
Sleepy but arousable Decreased feeding	1	Mild
Lethargy Poor suck Irritable/jittery with short-term strong suck	2	Moderate
Semi-coma Apnea Seizures Coma	3	Severe
Muscle tone		
Normal	0	None
Persistent mild hypotonia	1	Mild
Moderate hypotonia Moderate hypertonia Increasing arching of neck and trunk on stimulation without spasms of arms and legs and without trismus (consistent with tetanus not ABE)	2	Moderate
Persistent retrocollis Opisthotonos Crossing or scissoring of arms or legs but without spasms of arms and legs and without trismus	3	Severe
Cry pattern		
Normal	0	None
High-pitched	1	Mild
Shrill	2	Moderate
Oculomotor/eye movements/facies		
Normal	0	None, mild
Sun-setting Paralysis of upward gaze Disconjugate eye movements Blank stare Aimless eye movements	3	Severe
Total BIND II (ABE score)		

Mild ABE 1–3, reversible; moderate ABE 4–6, maybe reversible with RX; severe > 6, largely irreversible even with treatment (Modified from the BIND M [30])

- EBT can be repeated depending on clinical signs and post-procedure bilirubin levels.
- Always use a BIND II score (Table 1) on each neonate before and after an EBT and document the score in the chart. This allows for better follow-up and better communication about ABE/KSD among healthcare providers caring for these children over time.

8 Case Summary

This neonate received an exchange transfusion that was initiated within 4 hours of admission. Except for mild hypocalcemia and mild hypoglycemia, which were monitored and corrected appropriately, she tolerated the procedure well. She was treated for sepsis. Her bilirubin continued to trend down with phototherapy. At follow-up her hearing test was significant for mild hearing loss, and her development demonstrated mild motor delay for which follow-up was recommended. Her family was counseled regarding the need for next pregnancy to be closely monitored and to have the next neonate born at a referral hospital capable of providing immediate intensive phototherapy and rapid EBT if needed. Additionally the family was counseled re appropriate care and products to avoid due to the risk for hemolysis in neonates/children/adults with G6PD deficiency.

9 For Further Reading

- SUGARPREP video demonstration of Exchange Transfusion [31].
- Global Child Health; Newborn Care Chapter – Slusher T, et al.

References

1. American Academy of Pediatrics Subcommittee on, H., Management of hyperbilirubinemia in the newborn infant 35 or more weeks of gestation. Pediatrics. 2004;114(1):297–316.
2. Stevenson DK, Maisels MJ, Watchko J. Care of the jaundiced neonate. New York: McGraw-Hill Medical; 2012.
3. Watchko JF, Tiribelli C. Bilirubin-induced neurologic damage–mechanisms and management approaches. N Engl J Med. 2013;369(21):2021–30.
4. Pochedly C. History of the exchange transfusion; its use in treatment of erythroblastosis fetalis. Bull Hist Med. 1970;44(5):450–60.
5. Chen HN, Lee ML, Tsao LY. Exchange transfusion using peripheral vessels is safe and effective in newborn infants. Pediatrics. 2008;122(4):e905–10.
6. Thayyil S, Milligan DW. Single versus double volume exchange transfusion in jaundiced newborn infants. Cochrane Database Syst Rev. 2006;4:CD004592.
7. Manning D, et al. Prospective surveillance study of severe hyperbilirubinaemia in the newborn in the UK and Ireland. Arch Dis Child Fetal Neonatal Ed. 2007;92(5):F342–6.
8. McGillivray A, Evans N. Severe neonatal jaundice: is it a rare event in Australia? J Paediatr Child Health. 2012;48(9):801–7.
9. Ebbesen F, et al. Extreme hyperbilirubinaemia in term and near-term infants in Denmark. Acta Paediatr. 2005;94(1):59–64.
10. Slusher TM, et al. Burden of severe neonatal jaundice: a systematic review and meta-analysis. BMJ Paediatr Open. 2017;1(1):e000105.
11. Greco C, et al. Neonatal jaundice in low- and middle-income countries: lessons and future directions from the 2015 Don Ostrow Trieste yellow retreat. Neonatology. 2016;110(3):172–80.

12. Usman F, Diala U, Shapiro SM, Le Pichon JB, Slusher TM. Acute bilirubin encephalopathy and its progression to kernicterus: current perspective. Res Rep Neonatol. 2017;8:33–44.
13. Mabogunje CA, Olaifa SM, Olusanya BO. Facility-based constraints to exchange transfusions for neonatal hyperbilirubinemia in resource-limited settings. World J Clin Pediatr. 2016;5(2):182–90.
14. Bujandric N, Grujic J. Exchange transfusion for severe neonatal hyperbilirubinemia: 17 Years' experience from Vojvodina, Serbia. Indian J Hematol Blood Transfus. 2016;32(2):208–14.
15. Bhutani VK, et al. Extreme hyperbilirubinemia and rescue exchange transfusion in California from 2007 to 2012. J Perinatol. 2016;36(10):853–7.
16. Behjati S, et al. Adverse events associated with neonatal exchange transfusion for hyperbilirubinemia. Indian J Pediatr. 2009;76(1):83–5.
17. Pius S, Bello M, Mava Y, Djossi S, Ambe JP. Prevalence of exchange blood transfusion in severe hyperbilirubinaemia and outcome at the University of Maiduguri Teaching Hospital Maiduguri, Northeastern Nigeria. Nigerian J Paediatrics. 2017;44(2):50–5.
18. Owa JA, Ogunlesi TA. Why we are still doing so many exchange blood transfusion for neonatal jaundice in Nigeria. World J Pediatr. 2009;5(1):51–5.
19. Onyearugha CN, Onyire NB, Ugboma HAA. Neonatal jaundice: prevalence and associated factors as seen in federal medical Centre Abakaliki, Southeast Nigeria. J Clin Med Res. 2011;3(3):40–5.
20. Ibekwe RC, Ibekwe MU, Muoneke VU. Outcome of exchange blood transfusions done for neonatal jaundice in Abakaliki, South eastern Nigeria. J Clin Neonatol. 2012;1(1):34–7.
21. Bhutani VK, Johnson L, Sivieri EM. Predictive ability of a predischarge hour-specific serum bilirubin for subsequent significant hyperbilirubinemia in healthy term and near-term newborns. Pediatrics. 1999;103(1):6–14.
22. Sabzehei MK, Basiri B, Shokouhi M. Complications of exchange transfusion in hospitalized neonates in two neonatal centers in Hamadan, a five-year experience. J Compr Pediatrics. 2015;6(2):4–8.
23. Smits-Wintjens VE, et al. Neonatal morbidity after exchange transfusion for red cell alloimmune hemolytic disease. Neonatology. 2013;103(2):141–7.
24. Kaplan M, Wong R, Eric S, Stevenson DK. Neonatal jaundice and liver disease. In: Fanaroff A, Martin RJ, Walsh MC, editors. Neonatal-perinatal medicine: diseases of the fetus and infant. Mosby (Philadelphia, PA); 2010. p. 1478–81.
25. Jackson JC. Adverse events associated with exchange transfusion in healthy and ill newborns. Pediatrics. 1997;99(5):E7.
26. Badiee Z. Exchange transfusion in neonatal hyperbilirubinaemia: experience in Isfahan, Iran. Singapore Med J. 2007;48(5):421–3.
27. Davutoglu M, et al. The etiology of severe neonatal hyperbilirubinemia and complications of exchange transfusion. Turk J Pediatr. 2010;52(2):163–6.
28. Ip S, et al. An evidence-based review of important issues concerning neonatal hyperbilirubinemia. Pediatrics. 2004;114(1):e130–53.
29. Patra K, et al. Adverse events associated with neonatal exchange transfusion in the 1990s. J Pediatr. 2004;144(5):626–31.
30. Radmacher PG, et al. A modified bilirubin-induced neurologic dysfunction (BIND-M) algorithm is useful in evaluating severity of jaundice in a resource-limited setting. BMC Pediatr. 2015;15:28.
31. Lees TPM, Slusher M. SUGARPREP: curricular resources for global health educators. [cited 2021 9/12/2021]; Available from: https://sugarprep.org/videos/#Exchange_Blood_Transfusion.

Breastfeeding Support Devices in Low-Resource Settings

Beverly Ann Curtis and Margaret Nakakeeto-Kijjambu

Abbreviations

CRCT	Creamatocrit
NG	Nasogastric
UNICEF	United Nations International Children's Emergency Fund
WHO	World Health Organization

1 Case I Example

Baby boy Adroa was born at 36 weeks' gestation after spontaneous labor. His birth weight is 5 lb. 2 oz (2268 gm). You observe him with his mother on the lying-in ward in Uganda at the first feeding. You notice that Adroa is having difficulty latching. He roots for the breast but cannot seem to achieve a deep latch and suck and it is painful for the mother. His mother states concern that he does "not want to breastfeed." She wonders aloud if "he likes it and how come it hurts?" How can you help Adroa's mother to understand the baby's behavior and to initiate successful breastfeeding?

B. A. Curtis (✉)
Keystone Pediatrics, Chambersburg, PA, USA

M. Nakakeeto-Kijjambu
Ministry of Health and Government Consultant on Neonatal Health Care, Kampala, Uganda

T. M. Slusher et al. (eds.), *Pediatric Procedural Adaptations for Low-Resource Settings*, https://doi.org/10.1007/978-3-030-99955-1_8

2 Introduction

Exclusive breastfeeding (breast milk) is recommended for the first 6 months of life and has significant benefits for infants and mothers. Breastfeeding reduces morbidity and mortality. Breast milk is the best nutrition to improve growth and provide protection against disease. Infants that do not breastfeed, or only partially breastfeed, have a higher risk of mortality due to gastrointestinal infections and other infections. Breastfeeding can be lifesaving, especially in low-resource settings, where sanitation and safe water are often not available [1–3].

Early breastfeeding can also be lifesaving for mothers. It helps prevent maternal bleeding by causing the uterus to contract. It also assists in mother-infant bonding and promotes successful and exclusive breastfeeding by establishing a breast milk supply that meets the infant's needs for nutrition and growth [1, 4, 5].

The World Health Organization (WHO) and UNICEF recommend early initiation of breastfeeding within 1 hour of birth. Exclusively breastfeeding infants for the first 6 months of life allow them to achieve optimal growth, development, and health. After 6 months, infants should receive safe and nutritious foods to meet their evolving nutritional requirements while continuing to breastfeed for up to 2 years or longer [1, 2, 5].

This chapter focuses on some adaptations useful in low-resource areas but is not meant to be a comprehensive review of feeding or breastfeeding. For details on how and when to feed premature and sick neonates, consult additional references such as these [6–8].

3 Breastfeeding Basics

In this chapter, first we will discuss breastfeeding the full-term well infant including positioning for feeding, latching the infant, assessment of milk transfer, and methods to build and maintain milk production.

3.1 Procedure for Feeding the Well Newborn

For full-term or well infants, encourage the first feeding within the first hour of life with skin-to-skin care. If after the first hour the infant is sleepy, wake the infant to feed.

- Teach the mother to stimulate the rooting reflex by having the baby face her and resting the nipple on the infant's top lip under the nose. The infant should open wide and can be moved onto the breast.
- Tap the infant's heels, softly touch their feet, rub their back, or have the mother talk softly to help wake them up.

- Remove the infant's clothing to increase skin-to-skin contact, keeping the diaper in place: this helps wake the baby. Cover the infant's back with a blanket.

Rationale
- *Colostrum (the first milk) is low in fat and high in sugars (carbohydrates). This helps prevent hypoglycemia of the infant because it is easy and quick to digest.*
- *Colostrum is high in antibodies and helps protect the infant from infection.*
- *Early and frequent breast stimulation helps to establish a substantial milk supply that supports continued breastfeeding success.*
- *Skin-to-skin contact improves parent-infant bonding and infant feeding by decreasing newborn stress and increasing milk production. This is important in both the first hour of life and the first few weeks of life.*
- *Skin-to-skin contact stimulates the infant's hunger response. Skin-to-skin contact helps control the infant's temperature and vital sign stability.*

3.1.1 Positioning

Help the mother hold the infant's body close to her body with the infant's nose in the sniffing position with the head slightly tilted up and chin touching mother's breast. The ear, shoulder, and hip should be in line. The infant's feet should be tucked in close to the mother. This technique (Fig. 1) is used no matter how the mother holds the baby for feeding.

Common positions that work well for small infants:

1. Cross-cradle hold: The mother supports infant's body on its side so that the front of the infant's body is touching the front of the mother's body. Her arm or hand guides the infant's mouth toward the nipple, while the opposite hand holds her breast.
2. Under-the-arm hold: The infant is placed on its side, tucked under the arm on the side of the mother's body, with the infant's neck and shoulders supported by the mother's hand (same side). The mother's opposite hand is holding her breast.

Rationale
- This body position for the infant leads to successful breastfeeding, breathing, and attachment (latch).
- Head tilt in a sniffing position places the chin close to the breast tissue for good attachment. This position also prevents aspiration (milk from going into the lungs) by proper positioning of the head and neck [9].
- Small infants have weak neck muscles and large heads compared to their body size. If their head and shoulders are not supported, they will have difficulty staying attached.

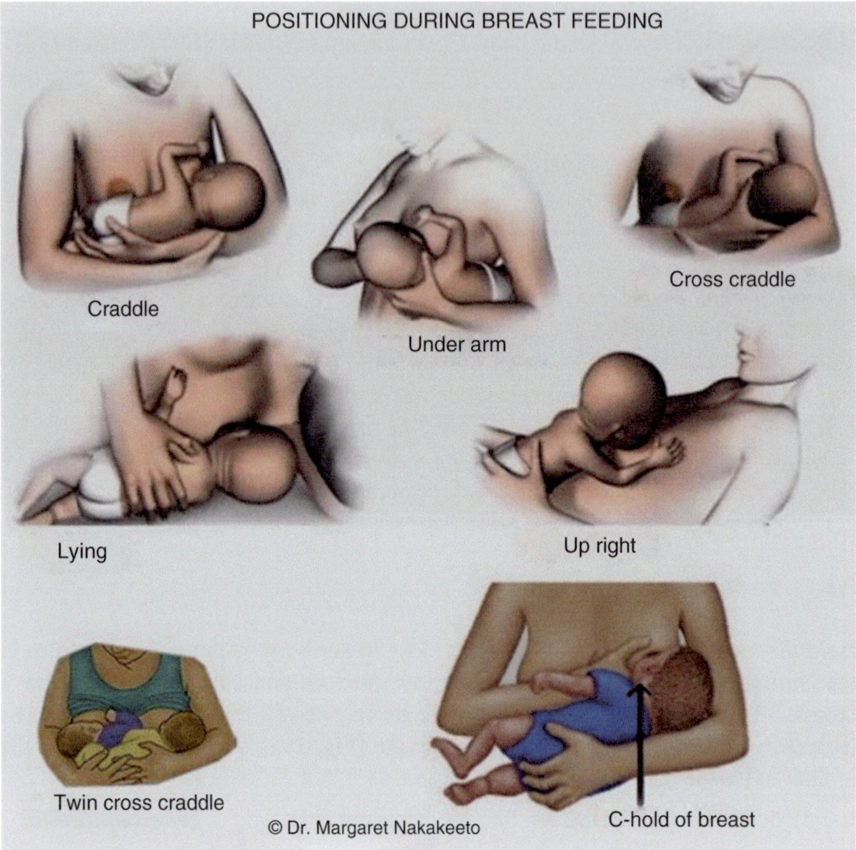

Fig. 1 Positioning during breastfeeding

3.1.2 Methods for Latching

Proper positioning and strong attachment of the infant to the breast is called a "latch" (Fig. 2). The following video from Global Health Media may also be helpful "Attaching your baby at the breast": https://globalhealthmedia.org/portfolio-items/attaching-your-baby-at-the-breast/ [10]:

1. Shape the breast: Teach the mother to shape her breast with her hand, by lightly compressing the breast. The mother's hand should be in the shape of a letter C (Fig. 1).
   - Depending upon the position of the infant's mouth, the mother's hand may need to be rotated so her thumb is in line with the infant's upper lip. Her fingers and thumb should be about 5 cm away from the nipple.
   - When compressed, the oval shape of the breast should match the oval shape of the infant's mouth.
   - Once attached, the mother should *not* release this hold, but continue to compress the breast into this shape during the feeding.

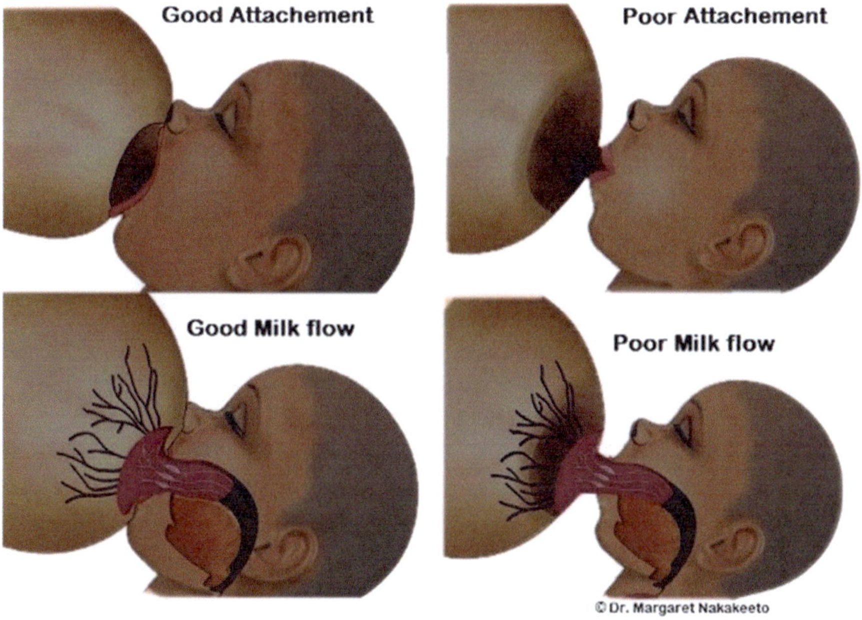

Fig. 2 Breastfeeding latch and attachment

Rationale

- Shaping the breast helps the infant to attach onto the areola rather than just the nipple (Fig. 2). Continuing to hold the breast with compression helps the milk to be expressed and helps the infant stay properly attached.

2. Encourage milk flow: Ask the mother to express a drop of milk, if possible, and rest her nipple gently on the infant's upper lip.

Rationale

- The smell of milk triggers the infant's hunger. This encourages the flow of milk.

3. Establish the latch: When the infant begins to root, and their mouth is wide open, pull the infant onto the breast, with their chin and lower jaw coming into the breast first.
   - The chin and lower jaw should be touching the mother's breast with the entire nipple in the mouth.
   - When the infant is properly positioned at the breast, more of the mother's areola (dark part around the nipple) should be visible above the infant's mouth than below.

- The infant's head should be tilted slightly back, so there is a small space between the infant's chin and chest (Fig. 1). This facilitates good jaw movement for milk transfer.
- The entire nipple should be in the infant's mouth along with as much of the areola as possible.

Rationale
- Proper positioning is necessary for a successful latch and the ability of the infant to remove milk from the breast when sucking.
- Attaching only to the nipple (and not the areola) can cause blistering, breakdown of the skin, and discomfort.
- Maintaining a space between the infant's chin and chest helps to align internal oral anatomy to best protect the infant from milk going into their lungs.
- This position aligns the tongue under the breast tissue.

4. Evaluate comfort: Talk with the mother about any concerns she may have with breastfeeding pain:

    - If attachment is causing pain, break infant's seal by placing a clean finger in between the corner of the infant's mouth and breast tissue. Attempt to reattach (Fig. 2).

Rationale
- Initiation of breastfeeding can be painful if positioning and latching are not appropriately done. It is important to address these problems early to prevent the mother from wanting to stop breastfeeding.
- Ensuring a proper latch will decrease pain.
- Pain may indicate a shallow attachment and need for repositioning.
- Shallow attachment can lead to mother's skin breaking and/or sores on the nipple.

3.1.3 Assessing and Teaching Milk Transfer

Look at the infant's neck to visualize suckling and swallowing; swallow sounds may be heard as well. Watch for movement of the lower jaw. The infant will often start out with fast sucks at the beginning of the feeding. Once the milk is flowing, the infant will change to slow, rhythmic sucking with swallowing and brief pauses to breathe.

- Preterm or small infants may have problems coordinating sucking, swallowing, and breathing. Care must be taken to monitor for choking or apnea with feeding. The breastfeeding should be discontinued if this happens.

- Preterm infants may look like they are sucking but are not able to remove much milk from the breast. The muscles of their mouth and cheeks are not as strong and they are not able to draw out as much milk as term babies.

Rationale
- The lower jaw compresses the underlying milk ducts of the breast, while the lips create a seal around the areola.
- Fast suckling helps the mother's hormones to signal the milk to start flowing.
- Slower, dynamic, rhythmic suckling sustained with a suck, swallow, pause pattern along with breathing is "nutritive" suckling, meaning the infant is taking in more milk.
- For preterm or small infants, sucking is often a reflex. This means they will continue to suck but they are not swallowing the milk (milk will spill from the sides of the mouth or the infant will cough or choke) and do not breathe (observed by not seeing the chest rise, followed by a gasping breath). Both put the infant at risk for aspiration of milk into the lungs.
- Preterm or small infants have weaker muscles and get tired easier than term infants.
- Small infants have smaller mouths and can have difficulty attaching to the areola. Fat pads on the inside of an infant's mouth help to create an airtight attachment, helping to draw out milk.

3.1.4 Feeding Frequency and Cues

- Neonates should be fed about every 2–3 hours or 8–12 times a day [11, 12].
- Breastfeed until the infant is satisfied, usually 10–15 minutes on each breast.
- In the first weeks, if the infant is sleepy, wake them to feed every 3 hours if they are not waking on their own.
- Breastfeed the infant when there are signs of hunger: active and awake, mouthing, or rooting. Crying is a late sign of hunger.

3.2 Common Breastfeeding Problems

While breastfeeding in general goes well, there are some common problems associated with breastfeeding. Table 1 provides an overview of some issues with some specific adaptations for low-resource settings. Inverted nipples can also be an impediment to the implementation of feeding at the breast. Table 2 provides options for treatment.

Table 1 Interventions for common breastfeeding problems

	Procedure	Rationale
Decreased milk supply	Ask the mother how frequently she is breastfeeding or hand expressing her milk At least eight times in a day and night cycle? Encourage the mother to not let the infant sleep longer than a 3-hour period, particularly in the first 2 weeks to 1 month after delivery	The body makes more milk only after the milk in the breast is removed The first month is the most important time to establish a full milk supply for breastfeeding
Pain with breastfeeding – latch	Ask permission to observe the mother breastfeeding and help determine if the infant is attached correctly Is she experiencing pain? Do her breasts feel "full" after the infant has nursed? *Nipple pain video provides more helpful information: Nipple Pain* https://globalhealthmedia.org/portfolio-items/nipple-pain/?portfolioCats=191%2C94%2C13%2C23%2C65 [13]	Improper attachment can lead to decreased milk supply because the infant is not able to empty the breast. This signals the mother's body to make less milk Shallow attachment can cause skin breakdown and blisters. These can lead to infection and make it difficult to remove milk completely from the breast
General maternal breast pain	Ask the mother if her breasts stay full after the infant nurses. Can she feel lumps? Is she experiencing pain in her breast tissue? Teach her to gently massage lumps in breast tissue prior to and during breastfeeding Applying pressure on the lump while the infant is breastfeeding or while she is hand expressing can help the milk to start flowing Apply warm compresses prior to expression and cold compresses to help decrease the swelling following expression of the milk If the mother has a fever, red streaking on her breast tissue, and/or extreme tenderness and pain in her breast tissue, she may have an infection Help her try to express the milk that is clogged, provide comfort measures of cold and hot compresses, and if possible, direct her to be seen by her doctor, as these are signs of infection and she may need treatment	If the mother has full breasts and/or lumps in the breast tissue that are causing her pain, the milk is most likely stuck due to clogged ducts If the milk is not able to be excreted, this signals to the body to make less milk Milk that remains stuck in the breast can lead to an infection of the breast tissue called mastitis Early symptoms are red streaking of the breast tissue, fever, and pain. Antibiotics may be required. It is safe and encouraged to continue to breastfeed

Sources: [5, 9, 11, 14, 15]

3.2.1 Breastfeeding Tips and Pearls

- Begin establishing a milk supply within an hour after birth, with frequent stimulation of the breast by breastfeeding the infant and/or hand expression. Emptying the breasts of milk is important, as this tells the mother's body to make more milk [11, 12].
- Breastfed infants usually nurse every 2–3 hours or 8–12 times a day [11, 12]. Proper positioning and appropriate latch are required for the infant to transfer milk, gain weight, and the mother to build and maintain a milk supply.

Table 2 Inverted nipples

	Procedure	Rationale
1.	Teach the mother to massage her breast, then pinch, and roll fingers directly on nipple When attempting to get the infant to attach, it is especially important for the mother to compress her breast, hold her hand in a "C" shape, and keep her fingers and thumb 5 cm from the nipple	To encourage the nipple to extend out Shaping the breast will help the infant achieve a deeper attachment and hopefully pull the nipple out
2.	Teach the mother to hand express for 5 minutes prior to breastfeeding to start milk flow and help her nipple to come out	Starting the flow of breast milk by hand expression will encourage the milk to flow and draw the nipple out
3.	If other methods do not work, then use a syringe to help pull the nipple out (Fig. 3) Remove the plunger Cut the end off with the tip Place the plunger in the end where the tip was cut off Place the opposite end of the syringe over the nipple Gently pull back on the syringe, using suction to revert the nipple	Back pressure of the syringe will create a suction that may pull the nipple out. Be aware that this may be painful and can cause skin breakdown

Sources: [9, 14]

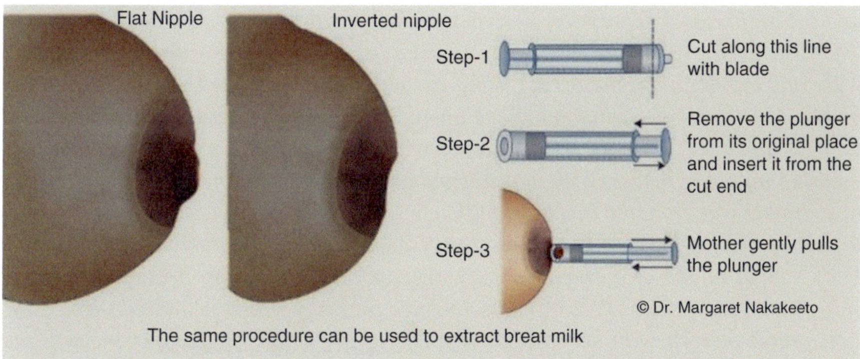

Fig. 3 Inverted nipples

- Assist mothers in hand expression if the infant does not breastfeed well in the first 6 hours of life, to help signal her body to produce milk [2, 3, 14].
- Teach mothers that expected volumes of milk start at drops to milliliters on the first 3 days after birth. Milk comes "in," meaning around 20 ml expressed, on days 3–5. On days 5–14, supply should continue to increase to around 750 ml by day 14. Between 4 and 6 weeks, milk supply is established [2, 11, 12].
- Wake infants, especially those born early, every 3 hours for feeding. They should not sleep longer than 4 hours between feedings [11, 14, 15].
- Making breast milk requires extra energy from the mother. Counsel the mother to eat healthy foods, drink enough water, and rest as much as possible between feedings [5, 12].

- Counsel the mother to drink enough fluids to satisfy her thirst. The amount of hydration depends on the environment and the person. Ten cups a day is a healthy volume [2, 14, 15].
- Have fluids available to the mother while she is breastfeeding. It is common for mothers to experience thirst at onset of let-down, and extra fluids will help the milk flow [12].
- Encourage the mother to leave her breasts open to air and light when possible. This helps to keep the nipples dry, helping to prevent irritation and potential infection [2, 5, 15].
- Nursing pads or cloths can be worn to catch leaking breast milk. These should be changed often. Nipple infections may occur from contact with dried milk on clothes and pads [5, 7, 14].
- A comfortable bra without underwire can be helpful for support if available to the mother [5, 8, 14].

3.3 Case I Resolution

The mother was instructed on how to wake the baby for feedings. She was instructed on the use of the cross-cradle hold ensuring she could move the baby onto the breast and utilize breast compression to assist the baby with transfer of milk. The mother was instructed on how to assess appropriate latch by observing the baby opening wide and moving onto the breast using an asymmetric latch with the chin into the breast and nose with a minimal space away from the breast. She was instructed not to press down on the breast to make an airway as this will cause stress on the nipple creating nipple soreness. With appropriate positioning, with the baby's chin in and nose tilted away from the breast, a sufficient airway was obtained allowing the chin to move freely for better milk expression. The mother was instructed to observe the baby's mouth open at an angle of 160 degrees or more during breastfeeding sessions, ensuring a deep latch. Mother observed the baby with a sustained suck, swallow, pause pattern with six to eight suckles in a row and a pause repeating the pattern for 20 minutes. The mother did not experience nipple pain during latch or with sustained suckle.

3.4 Case Example 2

Malechi born at 37 weeks to a G1P1 O+ mother. Antenatal course was uncomplicated until mother went in to labor 3 weeks prior to her due date. Infant at delivery required brief stimulation and then was stable for the neonatal hospital course. Mother breastfed on demand in the hospital after initial skin-to-skin care. Now mother and baby have been home for 2 weeks, and mother presents to your nearby neighborhood clinic for baby's first exam after a community peer support person thought the baby was not having enough wet diapers and stools. The mother is concerned because he is still very sleepy with feeding and having difficulty waking up. He also cries with gas pains. BW was 2600 grams (5# 12 ounces) and today's weight at 14 days of life is 2500 grams (5 # 8 ounces), 4.3% below BW on day 14 of life. In observing the baby's feeding, you see a baby who is poorly positioned at the breast, latched to the tip of the nipple, very sleepy, and a maternal breast that is soft prior to feedings.

3.5 Building and Maintaining Milk Supply

Some infants may not be able to breastfeed 8 to 12 times in a 24-hour period due to (1) immaturity (lack of coordination, strength, and alertness, (2) respiratory distress, or (3) other medical issues. In such situations, one of the options for the mother is hand expression. Table 3 walks through the process of how to hand express. And delivery of the milk can be via alternative methods including NG tube (Fig. 6), or if

Table 3 Steps and recommendations for hand expression

	Procedure	Rationale
1.	Have the mother wash her hands and breasts with warm water	Hand expression should be performed as a clean procedure to prevent infection
2.	Instruct her to massage her breast tissue in an inward motion toward the nipple (see Fig. 3), like the spokes of a bike	Massaging prior to and during hand expression helps the milk to flow out of the groups of alveoli (also called lobules) down and the ducts (Fig. 4) Helps soften the breast tissue when engorged or full
3.	Teach the mother to hold her breast with a "C"-shaped hand. Her fingers and thumb are placed toward the edge of her areola, about two finger widths from the nipple. Instruct her to: Press her fingers and hand into her breast (toward her chest wall) Then move her fingers toward her thumb. Hold for a few seconds Every minute, massage entire breast (Fig. 4) and repeat "C" hold and continue massage in a downward motion Repeat this motion several times. Milk will not always appear with first to start milk flow	Milk is produced by lactocytes and stored in the alveolus. These are located deep in the breast tissue (Fig. 5). By pressing into her breast tissue, the alveoli empty down into the ducts to be expressed It will take at least two cycles before milk starts to flow down through the ducts from the alveoli Mothers may need encouragement to continue in order to see milk flow Changing hand position on the breast will help to empty ducts in different areas of the breast tissue
4.	Instruct the mother to express for 15 minutes on each breast – even if no breast milk is seen. Teach the mother to perform hand expression every 3 hours if infant is not breastfeeding, even if the infant is also being fed by NG tube after breastfeeding attempts	Frequency of breast stimulation is needed to signal the body to make more milk Fifteen minutes is the average time it takes to empty the breast

(continued)

Table 3 (continued)

	Procedure	Rationale
5.	Place a clean cup under the breast with the nipple in the cup to catch the flow of milk. Expressed breast milk not needed immediately for a feeding can be stored in a clean, covered container	Expressed milk can be given to the infant by alternative feeding methods (e.g., NG tube, cup, bottle) or used for oral care of the infant. (Fig. 6) Infants who are not yet feeding by breast or cup will progress to oral feedings faster if held while being fed by NG tube [12] (see chapter "Kangaroo Mother Care in a Low-Resource Setting" on KMC) See chart below for milk storage times

Sources: [2, 11, 12, 14]

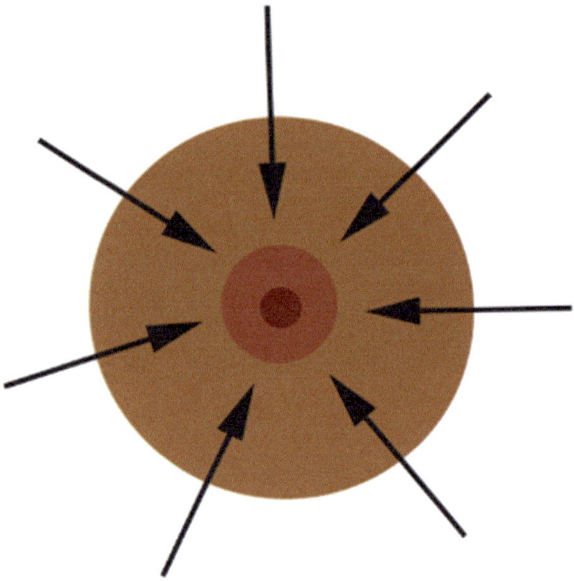

Fig. 4 Hand expression massage motion

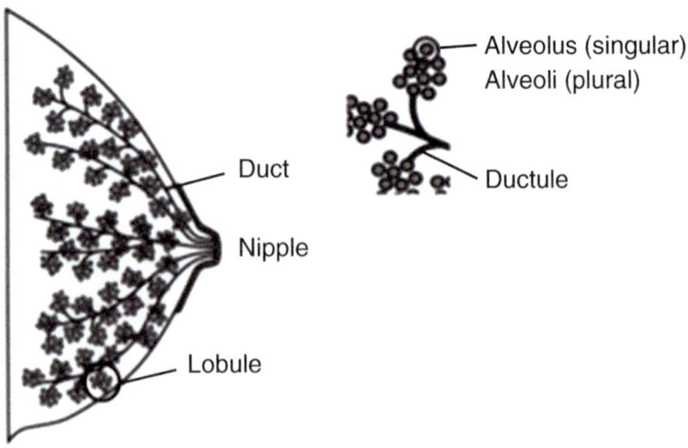

Fig. 5 Breast anatomy. (*Image credit: Mariko Langan*)

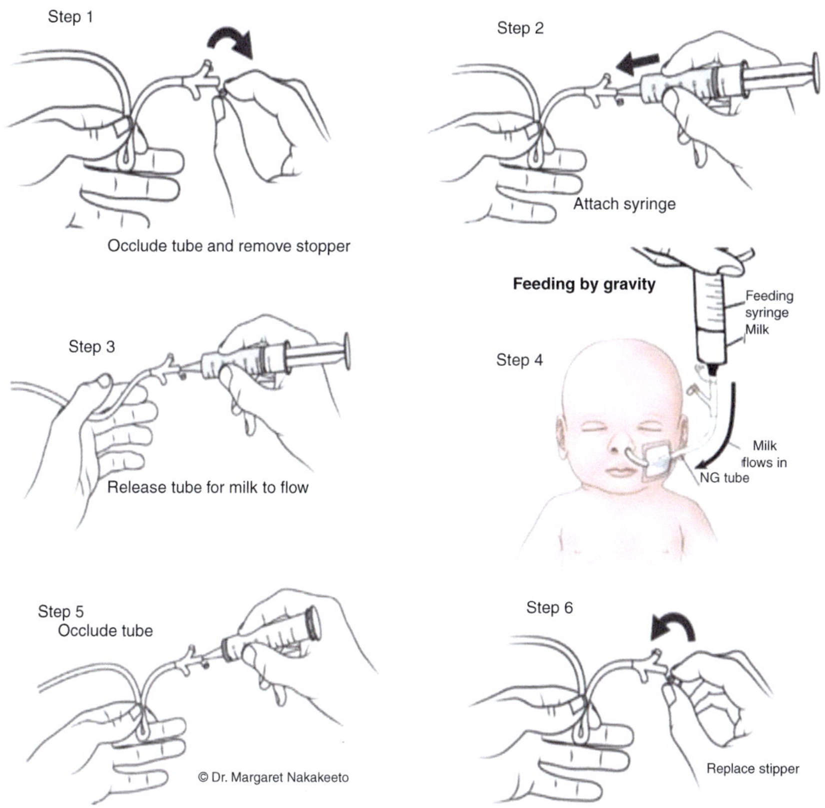

Fig. 6 How to feed an infant using a nasogastric tube. The following Global Health Media video maybe helpful for additional guidance to observe these guidelines in practice [1]: "Breastfeeding the small baby" https://globalhealthmedia.org/portfolio-items/breastfeeding-the-small-baby/. *Sources*: [1, 5, 9, 11, 12, 14, 19]

they are showing feeding cues but lack the strength to transfer milk from the breast, the infant can be offered a cup feeding after breastfeeding attempts. Hold infant in kangaroo mother care (KMC) during NG feeding or following cup feeding. See chapter "Kangaroo Mother Care in a Low-Resource Setting" for more details on KMC as well as this website in addition to the video references below [16]. As the neonate matures, it will be appropriate to transition them to the breast.

Additional resource is the video: hand expression and hand expression for the preterm infant. Again for details beyond the scope of this chapter, see additional resources [6–8, 17, 18].

Rationale

- An infant who is not feeding well from the breast or not ready to breastfeed can still receive the benefits of expressed breast milk.
- Removing the milk from the breast tells the body to make more milk. If the breast is not emptied, the body will gradually make less milk.

3.5.1 Use of Galactogogues

Some mothers experience low milk production. This makes them frustrated and anxious. Anxiety further makes the problem worse. Many mothers have found that some vegetables increased milk production. A vegetable commonly eaten in Eastern and Northern Uganda named "Marakwang" (*Hibiscus sabdariffa*) is used to initiate and/or increase milk production. Normally, milk flow is improved within 2–3 days. We have no scientific evidence but it has worked for many mothers. A study was published in November 2020 from Ghana identifying local foods that are used as galactagogues. Studies have been done elsewhere, but in Uganda these foods are used through community beliefs and observed outcomes [20].

4 Case 2 Resolution

You begin by observing the feeding and instruct the mother on proper positioning and latch in the cross-cradle hold. You explain about observing activity at the breast and how her infant is very sleepy during feedings. You have mother change breasts frequently during feeding to keep baby awake and actively suckling. She feeds for 20 minutes and then hand expresses milk for the infant which she feeds to the infant from a cup. Mother begins to snack on a local vegetable thought to help with milk production and begins to increase her fluid intake. Within 4 days, baby has begun to gain 30 grams per day and mother feels her breasts are fuller before breastfeeding and softer afterward. Within 7 days, baby is actively feeding at the breast with a sustained suck, swallow, pause pattern. Mother is instructed to continue hand expressing after breastfeeds and offering cup feeding after breastfeeds until the baby is fully taking his entire feeding from the breast. Baby's weight and feeding continue to be monitored twice weekly until baby returns to birth weight and has demonstrated appropriate growth. The community health worker notices that the baby is having an appropriate amount of yellow seedy stools and wet diapers. Mother is happy because baby seems to cry less and the gas pains are gone.

5 Case 3

Baby girl Abbo is born at 28 weeks' gestation weighing 1250 grams. She requires bubble CPAP for 3 days but did well and was able to transition to room air on day 5 of life. She is cared for in kangaroo mother care (KMC) (see chapter "Kangaroo Mother Care in a Low-Resource Setting") in the room beside your Special Care Baby Unit in Swaziland by her mother and grandmother using nasogastric tube feeds. Your nurse plots her on the growth chart (Fig. 7) *and notes on day 10 of life and notes she has fallen off the growth chart and now weighs only 1150 grams. Her*

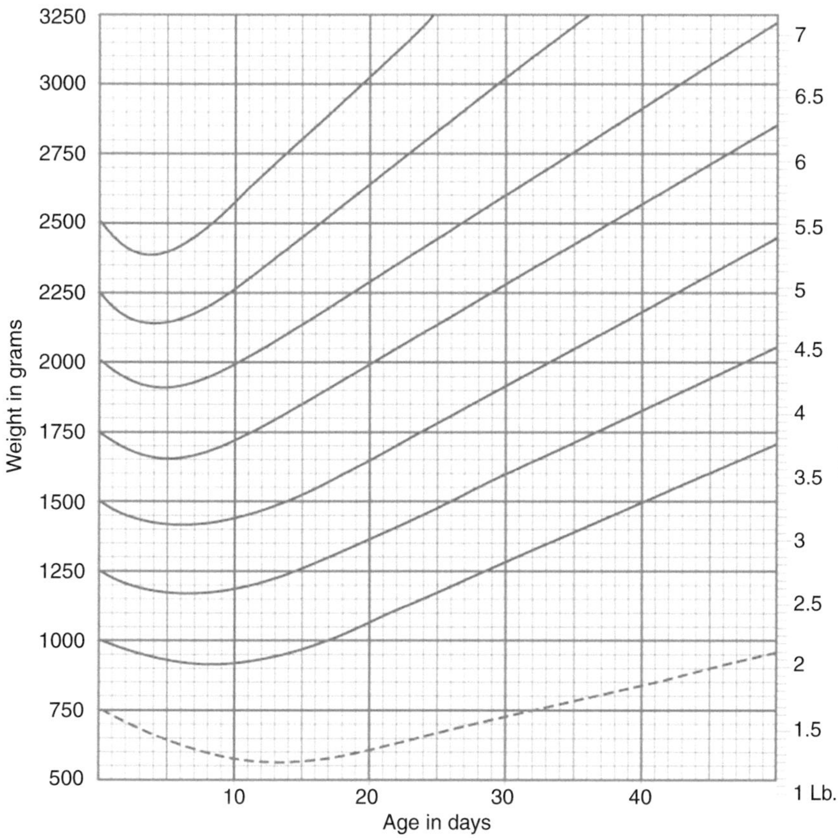

Fig. 7 Example of a growth chart still used in some low-resource setting without access to total parental nutrition and/or breast milk fortifiers [21]

mother states they need to go home soon as they are using their older children's school fees on baby Abbo. She is producing more milk than needed to feed Abbo using a combination of hand expression and the hospital-grade electric breast pump in your nursery with her own pump tubing that she cleans appropriately. Your hospital is baby friendly. How can you attempt to improve Abbo's weight without using formula or other supplement except vitamins?

5.1 Creamatocrit

Breast milk fat content or lipid and caloric concentrations account for the largest part of an infants' energy source. However, individual breast milk specimens may vary in lipid concentration and caloric density, depending upon the time of day when collection occurs, the type of breast milk collection technique utilized and the efficiency of breast milk collection. The creamatocrit (CRCT) is a measurement for estimating the fat content and caloric content of a milk sample. Performing a creamatocrit is a useful evidence-based method to identify the lipid and calories in individual breast milk specimens provided by parents of neonates in special care nurseries. The creamatocrit procedure provides an accurate, rapid, simple, and inexpensive measure of lipid and calorie analysis of individual breast milk samples useful for volume restricted infants, or infants with slow weight gain or growth restriction [4, 11, 15].

5.2 *Measuring a Creamatocrit*

Creamatocrit is done by utilizing a microcentrifuge. A breast milk sample is placed in a microhematocrit tube and spun in a microcentrifuge for 15 minutes. When finished spinning, the layer of fat in the tube is measured as a percentage similar to the measurement of a blood hematocrit. Table 4 provides a detailed step-by-step instruction on how to measure a creamatocrit.

Table 4 Detailed creamatocrit procedure

1. Mother pumps fresh milk into container and shakes well for 5 seconds 2. From this sample, pour about 1/2 cc into a sample cup 3. Mix sample by shaking again for 5 seconds 4. Fill two non-heparinized microhematocrit capillary tubes with milk	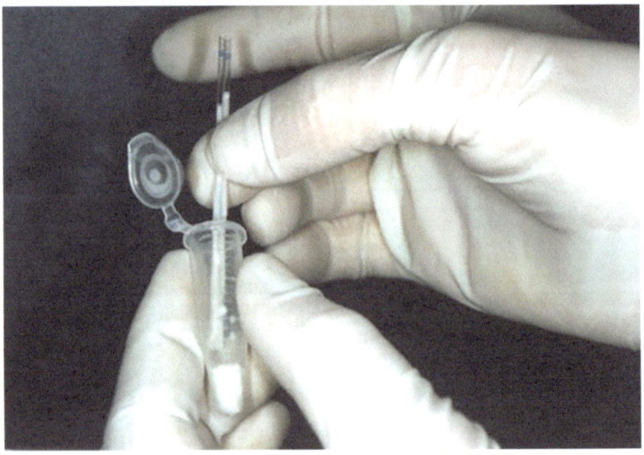

Table 4 (continued)

5. Seal capillary tubes at one end with the Critoseal	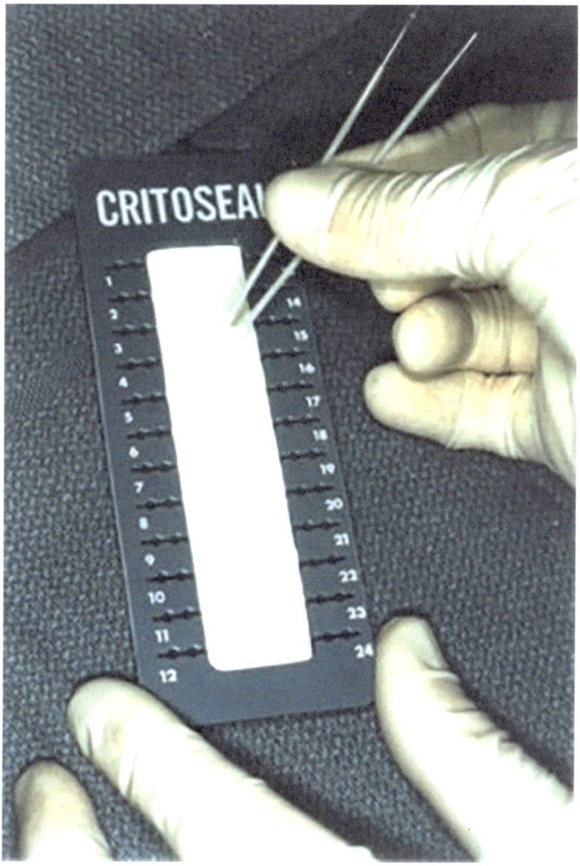
6. Place tubes with sealed end to the outside of the centrifuge, in a counterbalanced position	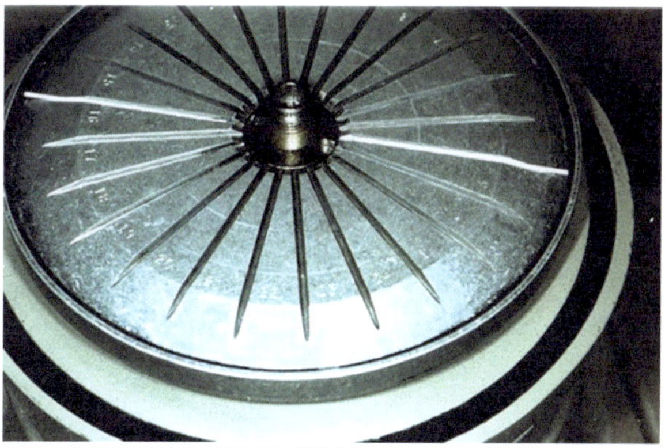

(continued)

Table 4 (continued)

7. Screw lid in place 8. Close top of centrifuge 9. Set timer for 5 minutes 10. When spinning stops, remove tubes from centrifuge	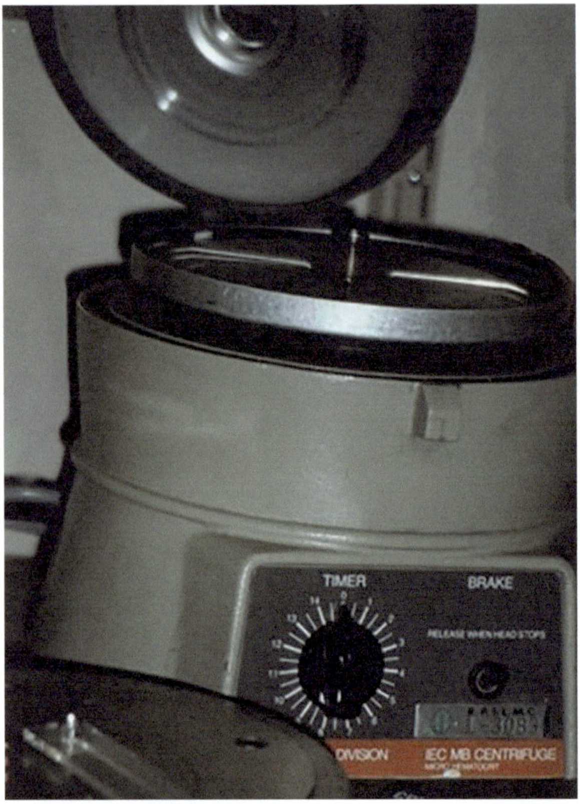
11. Place tubes on hematocrit reader with Critoseal end at the top 12. Place the intersection of sealant and milk at the cross-point of the curved line	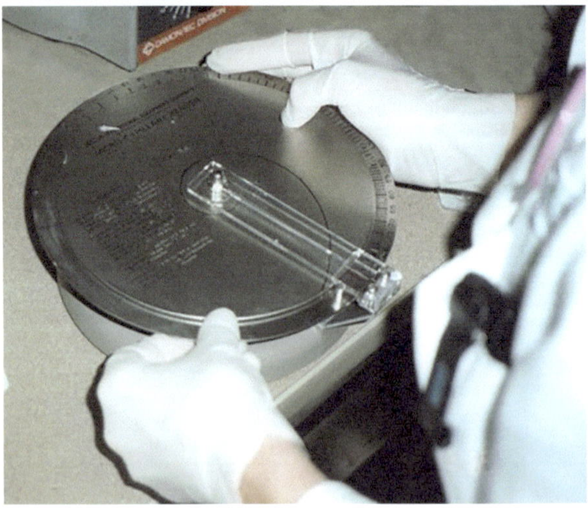

Table 4 (continued)

13. Rotate upper disc so that bottom of curved line intersects *bottom* point of milk in the capillary tube	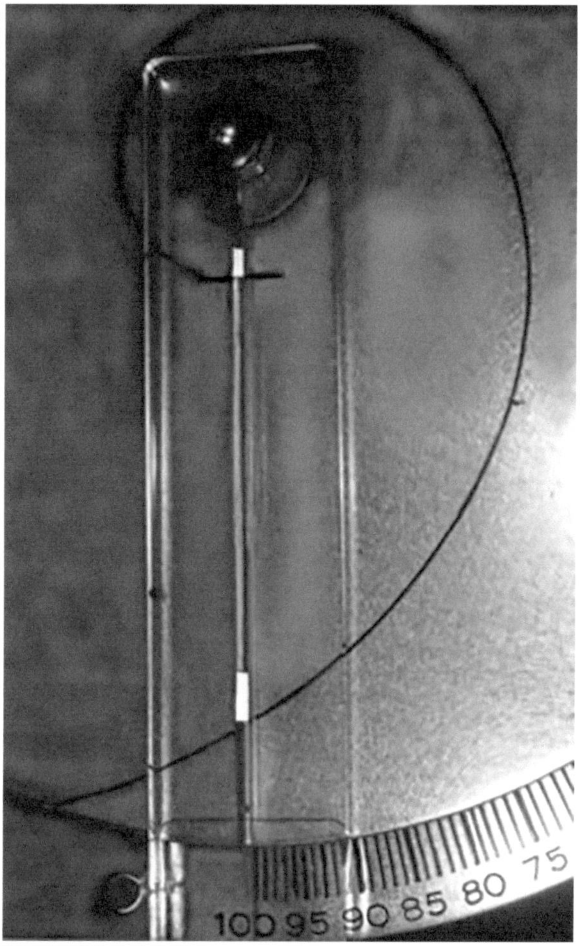
14. Set lower percentage disc at 100%	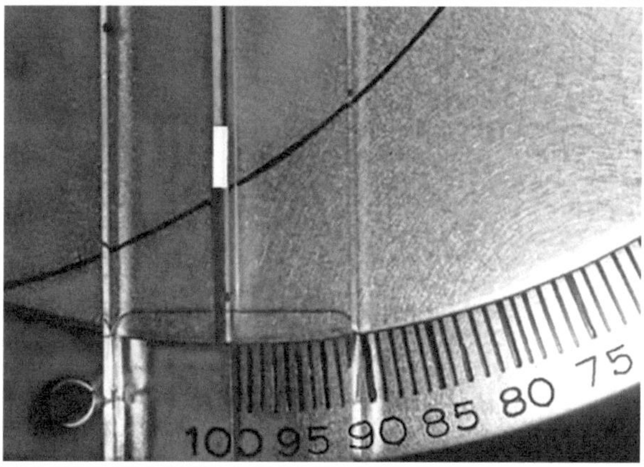

(continued)

Table 4 (continued)

15. Rotate percentage disc until curve line intersects the cream layer of the milk 16. Subtract this percentage (usually 85–95%) from 100%. The result is the creamatocrit (usually 5–15%)	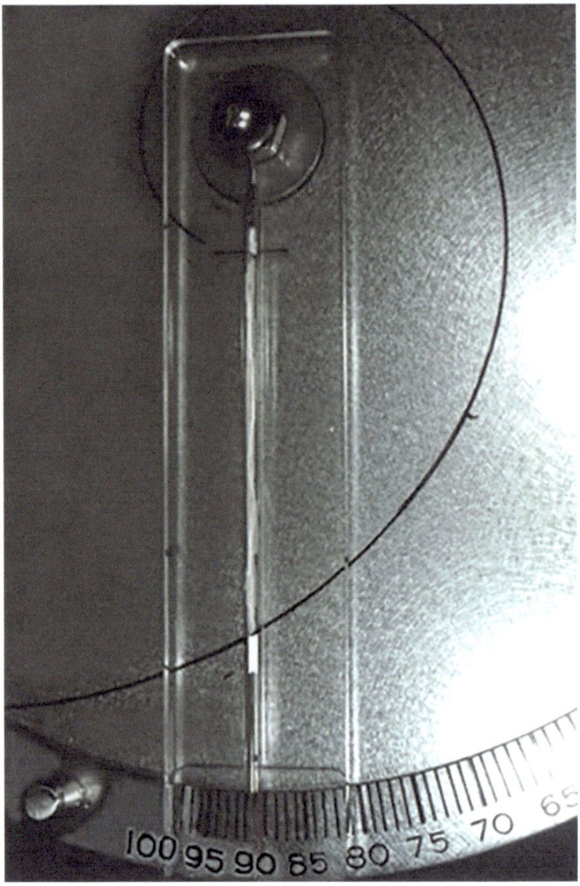

Adapted from Lucas et al. [22]. Procedure and pictures are adapted by and used with permission from Dr. Paula Meier PhD, RN, FAAN Rush University, Chicago, IL, USA

5.3 *Estimating Calories Based on Creamatocrit*

Once the steps to figure out the creamatocrit percentage have been completed, the calories in the breast milk can be estimated based on the measured creamatocrit. See Table 5 for estimations.

Ideally, each center should construct the regression graph based on their own samples as was done by the researchers who developed the Creamatocrit plus™ [11]. The Creamatocrit plus™ is an instrument that does the calculations automatically and eliminates the need for multiple steps and “cumbersome” equipment [11].

Table 5 Creamatocrit and calories

Creamatocrit %	3	4	5	6	7	8	9	10	11	12
Gr of fat/ml	0.017	0.023	0.03	0.037	0.044	0.051	0.058	0.064	0.071	0.078
Cal/ml	0.49	0.56	0.62	0.69	0.76	0.82	0.89	0.96	1.02	1.09
Cal/oz	15.7	17.8	20	22.1	24.3	26.4	28.5	30.7	32.8	34.9
% of Cal – fat	22	37	44	48.2	52.1	56	58.2	60.4	62.6	64

Notes: Based on regression equations in Lucas et al. [22]
For additional details regarding the use of creamatocrit in low-resource settings, consult resources including these [7, 8, 23, 24]

Table 6 Milk storage guidelines

Location	Temperature	Maximum recommended duration
Room temperature	16–29C (60–85F)	4 hours optimal → up to 6–8 hours acceptable under very clean conditions
Refrigerator	4C (39.2F)	4 days optimal → up to 5–8 days under very clean conditions
Freezer	<–4C (24.8F)	6 months optimal → up to 12 months acceptable

Source: ABM Clinical Protocol #8: Human Milk Storage Information for Home Use for Full-Term Infants, Revised 2017 [3]

5.4 *Breast Milk Storage*

Breast milk storage is problematic in many low-resource areas due to the lack of dependable electricity. One of the challenges of using expressed breast milk and promoting the use of hindmilk is that breast milk that is not keep at the proper temperature must be discarded (Table 6) [1]. However, mothers must be encouraged to completely empty their breasts whether using hand expression or electric breast pumps or a combination of both in order to maintain their milk supply over time.

Exercise caution in settings with unreliable freezer temperatures. For details on this and other specifics of breastfeeding and using breast milk in premature and sick infants, consult additional resources such as these [6–8].

6 Case 3 Resolution

Mother is taught now to tell when her breast milk changes from low-fat foremilk to hindmilk. Your nurses run a creamatocrit on her hindmilk collected after 5 minutes of milk expression and note that the hindmilk has a creamatocrit of 9 which translates to a caloric count of approximately 28.5 calories/mL. She begins to feed Abbo this hindmilk with the volume you prescribe topping up with foremilk if she does not have an adequate volume of hindmilk. Abbo grows well and at 16 days is up to 1300 and back on the growth chart. She is discharged on day 20 using nasogastric feeds in KMC care. She will be followed up every 3–5 days in KMC clinic but is expected to do well and to transition without difficulty to cup and spoon and then full breast-feeding at the breast.

6.1 Complications

Complications of breast feeding and the use of breast milk are rare beyond those listed in common problems above. Additional complications are primarily limited to infections such as maternal to child transmission of human immunodeficiency virus (HIV), herpes, or tuberculosis. Some such as MTCT of HIV have been addressed and no longer pose extreme risk to infants. Details of this and other infections are beyond the scope of this book but will worth working to solve as we attempt to use breast milk for the majority of infants globally.

6.2 Conclusion

Breast feeding and use of breast milk is recommended and important worldwide. It is critical to the survival of infants in LMICs. Tackling problems associated with breast feeding and the use of breast milk should be a top priority in our efforts to decrease neonatal morbidty and mortality globally.

References

1. Eglash A, Simon L. ABM clinical protocol #8: human milk storage information for home use for full-term infants, revised 2017. Breastfeed Med. 2017;12(7):390–5.
2. Videos-English, G.H.M.P. Global Health Media Project. c2014–2019; Available from: https://globalhealthmedia.org/videos/.
3. Jones F. In H.M.B.A.o.N. America, editor. Best practices for expressing, storing, and handling human milk in hospitals, homes, and child care settings. HMBANA; 2019.
4. Knake LA, et al. Optimizing the use of human milk cream supplement in very preterm infants: growth and cost outcomes. Nutr Clin Pract. 2020;35(4):689–96.
5. Team, S.C.s.L.S. Providing breastmilk your gift to your baby. Seattle: Seattle Children's Hospital; 2019.
6. Keating EM, Curtis B, Slusher TM. Maternal milk volume and breastmilk expression: implications for diet and nutrition in infants. In: Handbook of dietary and nutritional aspects of human breast milk. Wageningen: Wageningen Academic Publishers; 2013.
7. Slusher T, Vaucher Y, Greenwood C, Powell C, Nakakeeto-Kijjambu M. Newborn care. In: Kamat DMAF, Philip R, editors. Textbook of global child health. 2nd ed. American Academy of Pediatrics; 2015. p. 1050.

8. Slusher T, Vaucher Y, Zamora T, Curtis B. Feeding and fluids in the premature and sick newborn in the low-middle income countries. In: DÖÖ, editor. Contemporary pediatrics. InTech; 2012. p. 27–57.
9. Gardner S, Carter B, Enzman-Hines M, Hernandez J. Breastfeeding the neonate with special needs. In: Merenstein & Gardner's handbook of neonatal intensive care 8th edition an interprofessional approach. Mosby; 2015. p. 419–63.
10. Attaching your baby at the breast. Available from: Globalhealthmedia.org.
11. Meier PP, et al. Accuracy of a user-friendly centrifuge for measuring creamatocrits on mothers' milk in the clinical setting. Breastfeed Med. 2006;1(2):79–87.
12. Team, U.o.W.L.S. Breastfeeding: in the hospital and at home. Seattle: University of Washington Medical Centre; 2017.
13. Nipple Pain. [10/29/2021]. Available from: Globalhealthmedia.org.
14. Genna CW. Supporting sucking skills in breastfeeding infants. Sudberry: Jones and Bartlett Publishers; 2008.
15. Spatz DL, Edwards TM. The use of human Milk and breastfeeding in the neonatal intensive care unit: position statement 3065. Adv Neonatal Care. 2016;16(4):254.
16. Foundacion Canguro. [cited 2021 09/01/2021]; Available from: http://fundacioncanguro.co/PFMMC/en/docs/KMCMM/2.%20THE%20KANGAROO%20POSITION.pdfn.
17. How to Express Breastmilk. Available from: Globalhealthmedia.org.
18. Hand Expression for Preterm Birth. [10/18/2021]; Available from: https://globalhealthmedia.org/videos/expressing-the-first-milk/?portfolioCats=191%2C94%2C13%2C23%2C65.
19. Breastfeeding the small baby. [10/18/2021]; Available from: https://globalhealthmedia.org/videos/breastfeeding-the-small-baby/.
20. U.S. Department of Health and Human Services (DHHS), O.o.W.s.H., Your guide to breastfeeding [Internet], W.D. DHHS, editor. 2011.
21. Dancis J, O'Connell JR, Holt LE Jr. A grid for recording the weight of premature infants. J Pediatr. 1948;33(11):570–2.
22. Lucas A, et al. Creamatocrit: simple clinical technique for estimating fat concentration and energy value of human milk. Br Med J. 1978;1(6119):1018–20.
23. Slusher TM, et al. Comparison of maternal milk (breastmilk) expression methods in an African nursery. Breastfeed Med. 2012;7(2):107–11.
24. Slusher T, et al. Electric breast pump use increases maternal milk volume in African nurseries. J Trop Pediatr. 2007;53(2):125–30.

Kangaroo Mother Care in a Low-Resource Setting

Nathalie Charpak, Louise Tina Day, and Margaret Nakakeeto-Kijjambu

Abbreviations

°C	Degrees centigrade
HIV	Human immunodeficiency virus
KMC	Kangaroo mother care
LBW	Low birth weight
LMICs	Low- and middle-income countries
SDGs	Sustainable Development Goals
STS	Skin-to-skin
WHO	World Health Organization

1 Case

A pregnant woman presents to a rural health center hospital in Uganda in preterm labor. You are visiting for the weekend. The woman is Gravida 1, Para 0, in active labor and estimated to be 30 weeks pregnant. She is treated with tocolytics and

N. Charpak (✉)
Kangaroo Mother Care Program of the San Ignacio University Hospital Senior researcher and Director of the "Fundacion Canguro" in Bogotá, Bogotá, Colombia

L. T. Day
London School Hygiene & Tropical Medicine Maternal and Newborn Group, London, UK
e-mail: louise-tina.day@lshtm.ac.uk

M. Nakakeeto-Kijjambu
Ministry of Health and Government Consultant on Neonatal Health Care, Kampala, Uganda

T. M. Slusher et al. (eds.), *Pediatric Procedural Adaptations for Low-Resource Settings*, https://doi.org/10.1007/978-3-030-99955-1_9

given dexamethasone and labor pains subside for 24 hours after which time labor progresses. She gives birth to a daughter who weighs 1400 grams. She does not have respiratory distress but is unable to suck and therefore to breastfeed. She is placed in an open cot wrapped in blankets. Her temperature at 2 hours of age is 35.0 °C. It is now night and transfer to the capital city Kampala is impossible until the next day. How can you manage this newborn's temperature in this rural health center? How will you transfer the baby and what options for temperature management would you suggest at the referral hospital in Kampala?

2 Introduction

Around 90 percent of preterm and low birth weight babies are born in LMICs. In contrast, 90 percent of the financial investment in health care for preterm babies are in high-income countries. Hypothermia is a leading contributor to neonatal morbidity and mortality worldwide. Prevention and treatment of hypothermia is key to decreasing neonatal death, the single leading contributor to our challenge of reaching the Sustainable Development Goals (SDGs) by the target date of 2030. The World Health Organization (WHO) along with experts like Dr. Charpak continues to emphasize the importance of KMC. The recently released "Tools for the successful scale-up of Kangaroo Mother Care (KMC) in health care facilities and communities" is available online [1].

Care of these "vulnerable" preterm neonates requires a delicate risk-benefit balance of use of sophisticated technology in order to assure these neonates grow into healthy adults both physically and mentally [2].

In 1978, Professor Edgar Rey Sanabria first developed kangaroo mother care (KMC) in Bogota, Columbia. Since then, KMC has been adopted in many countries around the world and at all income levels. It has been shown to have numerous advantages for preterm and low birth weight neonates when modified to meet local requirements. Skin-to-skin (STS) care is now recommended for neonates of all weights immediately after birth to keep the neonate warm, promote bonding, improve cardiorespiratory stability, and humanize care. Continuous STS care is especially advantageous for mortality impact in LMIC with limited or no availability of other standards of care, e.g., incubators where high ratios of neonates per nurse making it essential that mothers and family members provide vital care for their small or preterm patients. KMC has been shown to reduce mortality and severe morbidity particularly morbidity from infection in a systematic review by Lawn et al. [3] and in a cochrane review updated in 2016 (Cochrane Review: Kangaroo mother care to reduce morbidity and mortality in low birthweight infants). In a meta-analysis by Boundy et al., in addition to decreased risk of mortality and infection, it was also shown to decrease the risk of hypothermia, hypoglycemia, apnea, and hospital readmissions as well as to increase exclusive breastfeeding [4]. Physiological improvements were noted by these same authors in respiratory rate, oxygen saturation, and pain measures in premature infants receiving KMC [4]. Additionally, KMC has been shown to promote breastfeeding and exclusive breastfeeding [5]. Not only does it have immediate benefits to these neonates, but amazingly, it has also been shown to have significant benefits 20 years after their course of KMC both on neuroimaging and social and behavioral outcomes [6].

KMC is not limited to LMICs. It is also widely used in high-income countries to improve physiologic stability and facilitate maternal/newborn bonding. STS is now the recommended place to put all stable term and near-term neonates not needing resuscitation immediately after birth [7]. However, even neonates requiring special care can be nursed in KMC. Babies on nasogastric (NGT) feeds (Fig. 1), nasal cannula oxygen (Fig. 2), continuous positive airway pressure (CPAP), and intravenous (IV) cannulas can be placed in KMC as can babies whose mothers have human immunodeficiency virus (HIV) and COVID-19. There are no minimum weight limits or gestational ages. Critically ill neonates on ventilators and with central lines can be placed in KMC intermittently if staff are competent and confident to do so and able to monitor the neonate continuously. Babies may also be place in KMC with conventional phototherapy lights on their backs (Fig. 3) and under filtered sunlight phototherapy.

Some protocols promote the use of KMC twenty-four hours a day, once the infant is stabilized, by rotating care between the mother, father, grandmother and other relatives and family members. An excellent 24/7 protocol, " *Protocol for the care of low birth weight (LBW) and premature infants with the kangaroo Mother care* (KMC) method in a low-income setting (no intensive care unit and no parental

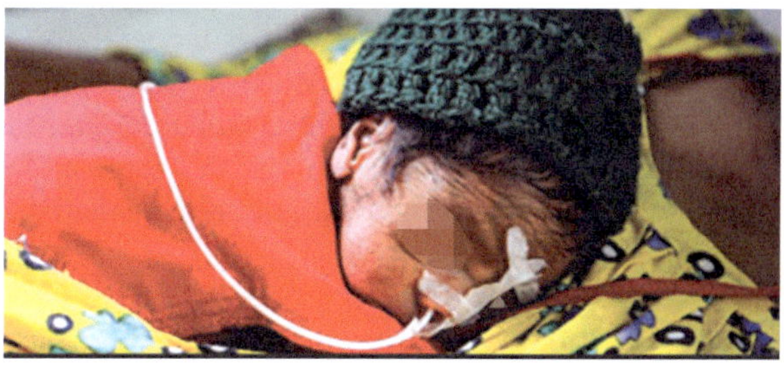

Fig. 1 Baby with NGT in KMC. (Figure used with permission from Dr. Charpak)

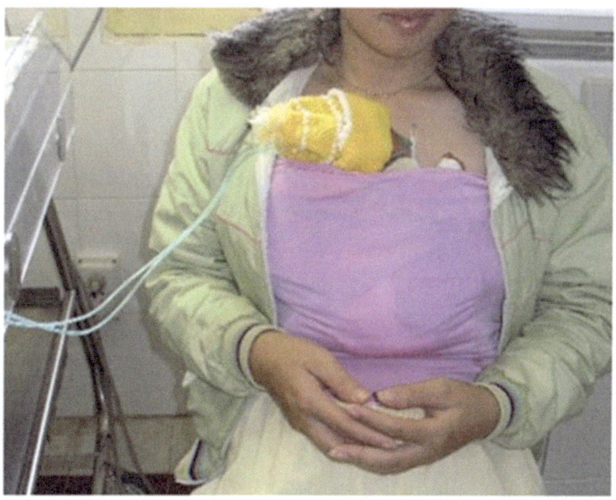

Fig. 2 KMC with baby in oxygen. (Figure used with permission from Dr. Charpak)

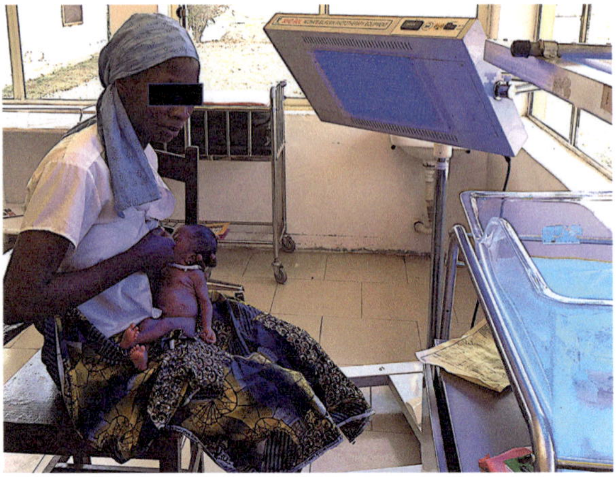

Fig. 3 Baby under phototherapy in KMC. (Figure used with permission from Dr. Slusher)

nutrition)" can be requested by Contacting Dr. Nathalie Charpak or Fundacion Canguro directly [2]. This protocol includes other elements of the KMC package, other protocols alternate between KMC and care in an incubator/isolette or radiant warmer. KMC also provides a viable mode of thermoregulation for transfer of a neonate from a lower level of care to a higher level of care. KMC is a much more effective and dependable way of preventing hypothermia than clothing or blankets.

For KMC to be successful, it is crucial to have both maternal motivation and nursing/medical staff buy-in as well as the willingness/ability to give appropriate maternal education, supervision while in house, and support for ongoing KMC at home. Mothers/other KMC providers will need some means of securing the neonate to their chests. Efforts to ensure that the neonate is comfortable when in KMC should be made, and the family should be confident to continue to provide KMC at home prior to discharge.

3 Indications

- Any neonate less than 37 weeks' gestational age or weighing less than 2500 grams at birth
- Any neonate of any weight or gestation with hypothermia
- Any older infant with hypothermia such as infants who are severely malnourished and unable to maintain normothermia again as long as not requiring care not possible in STS

Table 1 Contraindications/relative contraindication [8]

Relative or absolute contraindications (depending on available options for thermal care)[a]
Neonatal
1. Ongoing need for resuscitation including bag-mask ventilation
2. Cardiorespiratory instability
3. Cyanosis during KMC
4. Neonatal fever (may be worsened by KMC)
5. Umbilical venous or arterial catheters unless adequate healthcare providers for careful continuous monitoring
6. Presence of omphalocele or gastroschisis that is not yet closed or covered
7. Compromised neurological status if tone decreased and/or neonate unable to protect airway
Maternal
1. Maternal fever (may lead to fever in the neonate)
2. Contagious rash or skin lesions
3. Untreated pulmonary tuberculosis
4. Uncontrolled seizures
5. Sedation including not yet recovered from anesthesia
6. Morbid obesity if positioning without obstructing babies airway is not possible

[a] Most contraindications relative if no other means of treating hypothermia or maintaining euthermia/table adapted from Dr. Charpak, Day, and the *Fundacion Canguro* [8]

3.1 Contraindications and Relative Contradictions

Most contraindications are indeed relative and depend on the degree of monitoring and nursing staff available to help with KMC. Listed below (Table 1) are some of the major contraindications and relative contraindications to KMC.

4 Equipment/Supplies

- Hat (knitted hats of varying sizes are a great contribution from charities)
- Wrapper or supporting device to keep the baby secure while allowing the mother or other KMC provider to safely sleep and perform other duties while awake.
- Material (cotton is preferred and Cotton+lycra (10%) is the best to allow the premature infant to have small movements with contention as in the womb of his mother)
- Thread and sewing machine
- Pattern

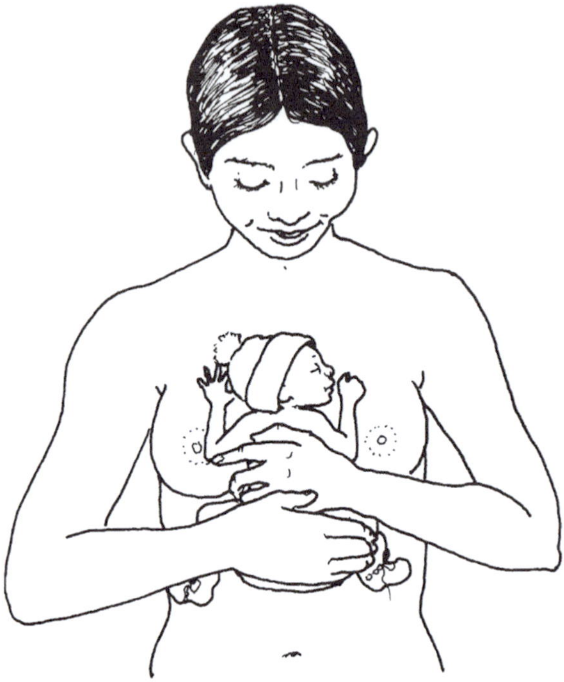

Fig. 4 Position for KMC. (Figure used from the WHO KMC practical guide (2003) https://www.who.int/publications-detail-redirect/9241590351)

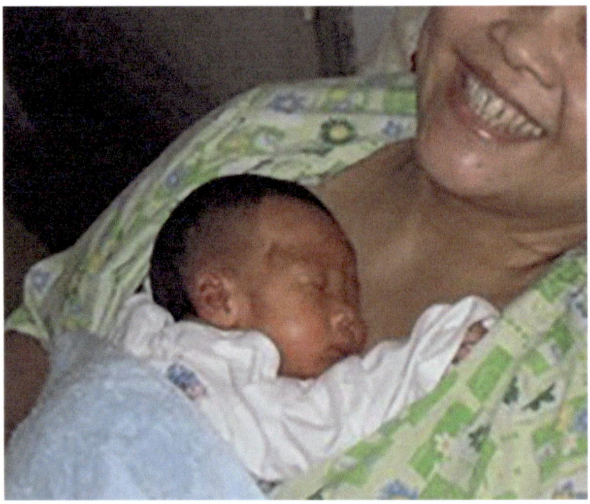

Fig. 5 Baby in KMC. (Figure used with permission from Dr. Charpak)

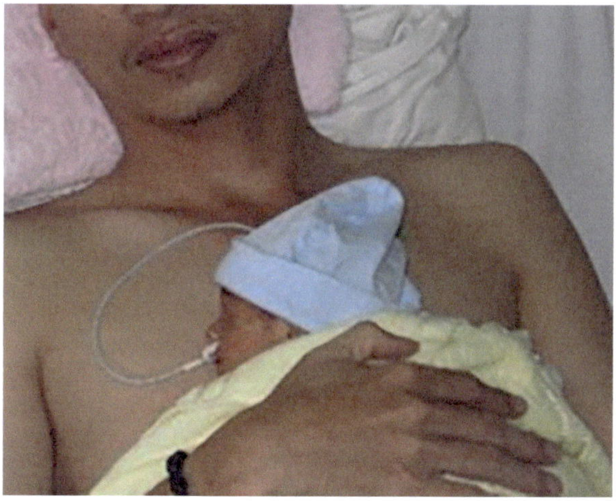

Fig. 6 Family member doing KMC. (Figure used with permission from Dr. Charpak)

5 Technique

- For details on all aspects of KMC, all healthcare providers should receive appropriate training and consult appropriate resources such as Kangaroo Mother Care Training Manual Science and Tenderness [8].
- Briefly, the neonate is placed in a frog-legged position with his/her chest and abdomen STS with the mother's bare chest (Figs. 4 and 5) with the head turned to one side or the other. Generally, it is appropriate for the neonate to have a hat, and diaper on, but to be otherwise unclothed chest and abdomen. Fathers and other family members may also do KMC (Fig. 6).

- During breastfeeding at the breast (when appropriate), the mother can continue to do KMC using a side lying position or "football" hold for the neonate.
- During conventional phototherapy, the neonate may have the phototherapy angled so the light will be on his/her back.
- Older infants placed in STS such as malnourished infants should only do so while the mother is reclining and should be monitored continuously to assure not to fall or obstruct their airway. It is not generally possible or advisable to have them carry their infants/children in STS.

5.1 *Instructions for Support Device/Carrier* [8]

- Must be firm enough to hold the neonate to the chest with minimal to no support from the mother's arms allowing the neonate to stay STS while mother sleeps, feeds herself, walks, and performs small duties.

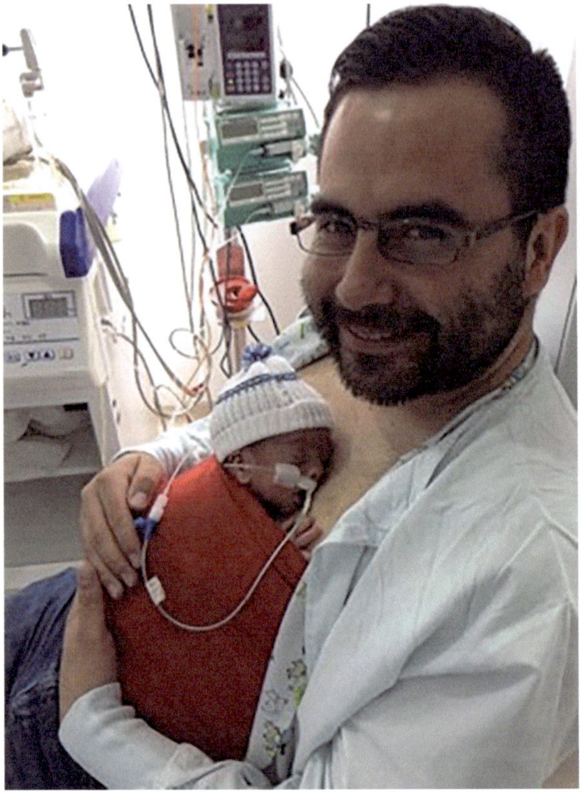

Fig. 7 Father with Lycra Band KMC holder. (Figure used with permission from Dr. Charpak. Dr. L Sarmiento, pediatrician and her husband carried their little Jeronimo born with 30 weeks of gestational age and 1100 g since the first day of life)

- Flexible enough to allow the neonate to move and breathe easily and to be moved into position for breastfeeding (rol of the 10% of lycra).
- Washable.
- Made of locally available material unless commercially sourced.
- Every neonate should have a minimum of two carriers to allow for one to be washed while the other one is used.

Options include:

- Commercial KMC holders such as the CarePlus Preterm Wrap are available from Laerdal (not pictured).
- Lycra Bands are another option for homemade carriers (Figs. 7 and 8).

- Homemade KMC holder which can be sewn out of locally available material such as the one described below. The pattern and design are products of the Kangaroo Mother Care "bag" from LAMB Hospital, Bangladesh (Fig. 9) (www.lambproject.org). A baby in this KMC "bag" is seen below (Fig. 10).

- Blankets or wraps.

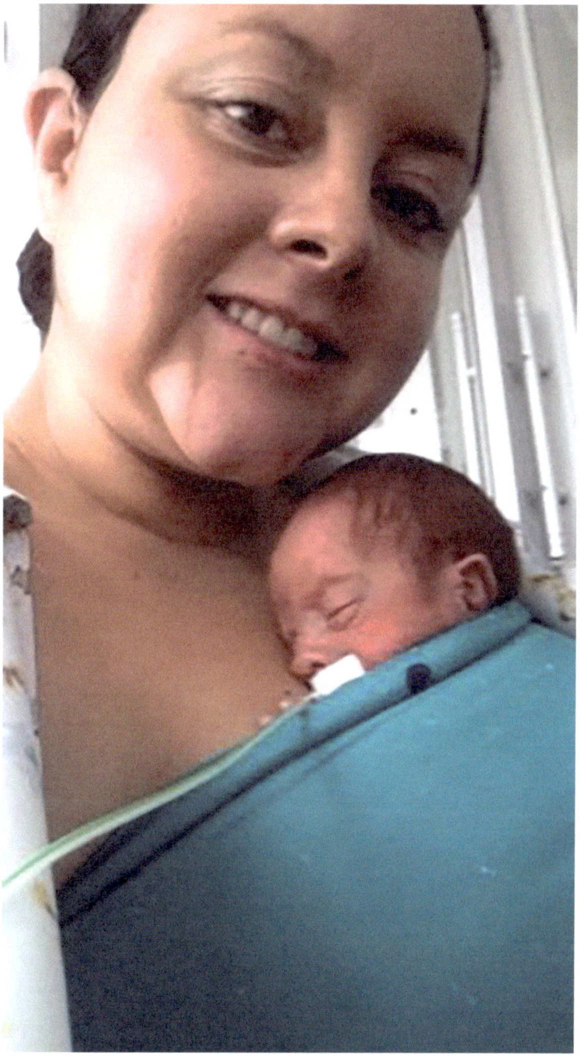

Fig. 8 Mother with Lycra Band KMC holder. (Figure used with permission from Dr. Charpak)

- Blankets or wraps used to secure neonates to their mothers as per local culture as seen in Fig. 11 (These are often not ideal for use 24/7 but are often used for short-duration KMC.).

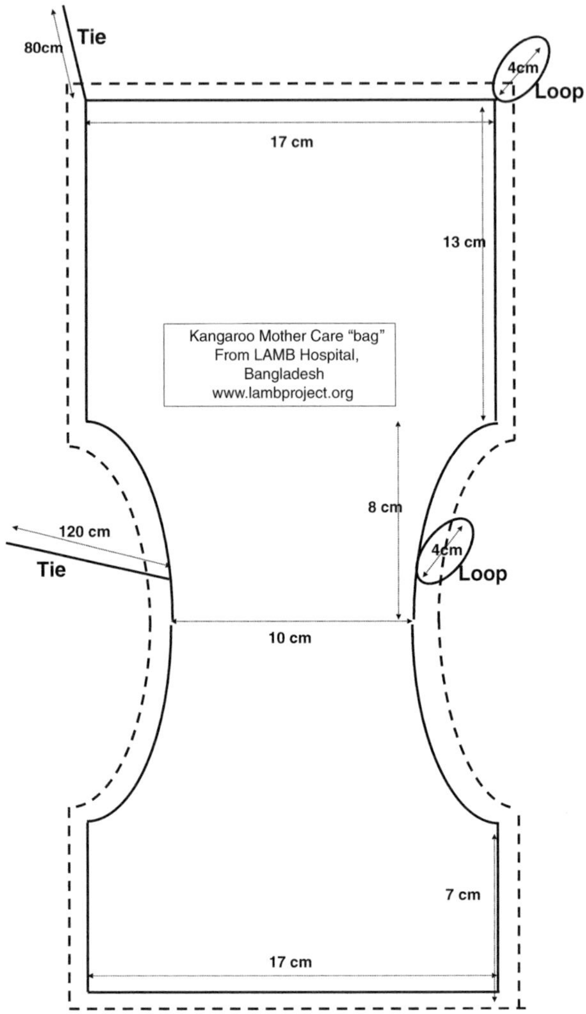

Fig. 9 Pattern for the KMC "bag" from LAMB Hospital, Bangladesh. (Courtesy of Dr. Day)

5.1.1 Complications

Complications are rare when KMC is done properly and parents and caregivers are trained in how to do it correctly. Carefull attention must be paid with IVs and other tubes and lines in KMC as well as possible complications as airway obstruction and exposure to infections such as tuberculosis if mother is early or untreated [9].

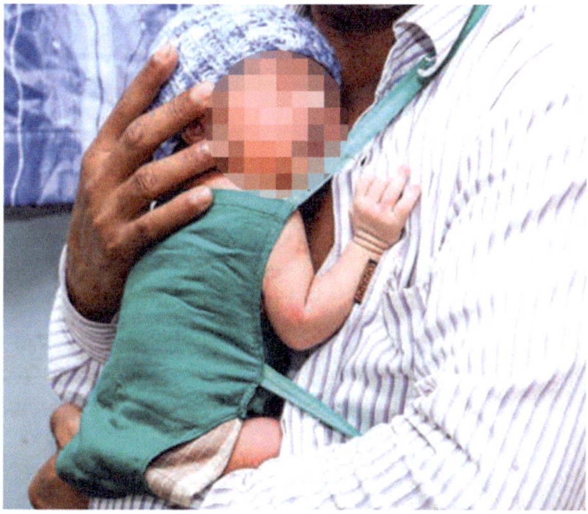

Fig. 10 Baby in Lamb KMC “bag”. (Photo from Lessons from the Ground) (Figure used with permission from Dr. Day)

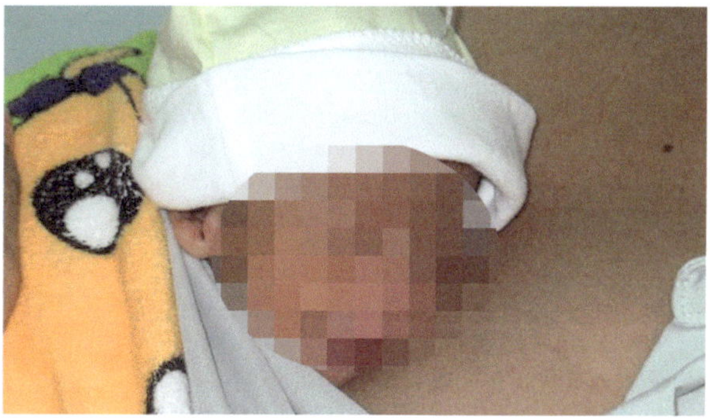

Fig. 11 Baby in blankets and KMC

5.1.2 Case Resolution

The nurse-midwife who comes on that night had been trained in KMC. She placed the infant in a KMC holder that her local church made. She taught the mother to extract her colostrum and to give it every hour through the tube that she installed without removing the baby from its position. She remains cardiorespiratory stable overnight without doing hypoglicemia. In the morning, the mother-infant pair was safely transferred in the KMC position during the journey to the KMC ward in Kampala where she was helped to do KMC for most of the 24-hour period with the baby’s father and grandmother supporting the mother several hours a day. After 2 weeks, she was able to cup and spoon feed and started to feed at the breast. She was discharged home in the KMC to keep her warm on the journey. She continued in KMC until she kicked herself out of KMC (as most babies do when they no longer need KMC) most of the time when they reach 38 weeks of gestational age [10].

References

1. Tools for the successful scale-up of Kangaroo Mother Care (KMC) in health care facilities and communities. 2020 December 10, 2020 [cited 2021 October 21, 2021]; Available from: https://www.who.int/news/item/10-12-2020-tools-for-the-successful-scale-up-of-kangaroo-mother-care-(kmc)-in-health-care-facilities-and-communities.
2. Charpak N. Protocol for the care of low birth weight (LBW) and premature infants with the kangaroo mother care (KMC) method in a low-income setting (no intensive care unit and no parental nutrition. Fundación Canguro: 44 B, 5350, Bogota, Colombia.
3. Lawn JE, et al. 'Kangaroo mother care' to prevent neonatal deaths due to preterm birth complications. Int J Epidemiol. 2010;39(Suppl 1):i144–54.
4. Boundy EO, et al. Kangaroo mother care and neonatal outcomes: a meta-analysis. Pediatrics. 2016;137(1):e20152238.
5. Wang Y, et al. Positive effects of kangaroo mother care on long-term breastfeeding rates, growth, and neurodevelopment in preterm infants. Breastfeed Med. 2021;16(4):282–91.
6. Charpak, N., Tessier, R., Ruiz, J. G., Uriz, F., Hernandez, J. T., Cortes, D., & Montealegre-Pomar, A. Kangaroo mother care had a protective effect on the volume of brain structures in young adults born preterm. Acta Paediatrica 2022 https://doi.org/10.1111/apa.16265
7. Aziz K, et al. Part 5: neonatal resuscitation 2020 American Heart Association guidelines for cardiopulmonary resuscitation and emergency cardiovascular care. Pediatrics. 2021;147(Suppl 1)
8. Foundacion Canguro. [cited 2021 09/01/2021]; Available from: http://fundacioncanguro.co/PFMMC/en/docs/KMCMM/2.%20THE%20KANGAROO%20POSITION.pdfn.
9. Heyns L, et al. Nosocomial transmission of mycobacterium tuberculosis in kangaroo mother care units: a risk in tuberculosis-endemic areas. Acta Paediatr. 2006;95(5):535–9.
10. Montealegre-Pomar A, Charpak N. Individual factors determine how long infants born preterm or with a low birth weight need to be kept in the Kangaroo position. Acta Paediatrica, 2022;111(2):305–6.

Safe Options for Obtaining Blood and Vascular Access in Neonates and Children in a Low-Resource Setting

Zubaida Farouk, Udochukwu M. Diala, and Stephen Oguche

Abbreviations

IV	Intravenous
LMICs	Low- and middle-income countries
TBV	Total blood volume

1 Case Example

A 6-day-old baby girl is brought into your clinic in Nigeria with jaundice of the eyes, palms, and soles. She is found to be febrile to 39 °C. She is still feeding well with a strong normal cry and tone. She needs a sepsis work-up and evaluation of her jaundice. Additionally, she needs intravenous antibiotics. The intern starts to do a femoral venous draw for the labs. The attending consultant shows him other options and discourages femoral venous draws except in extreme emergencies.

Z. Farouk
Department of Paediatrics, Bayero University, Kano, Nigeria

U. M. Diala · S. Oguche (✉)
Department of Paediatrics, University of Jos, Jos, Nigeria
e-mail: oguches@unijos.edu.ng

T. M. Slusher et al. (eds.), *Pediatric Procedural Adaptations for Low-Resource Settings*, https://doi.org/10.1007/978-3-030-99955-1_10

2 Introduction

In the care of sick neonates and children, there is often a need to obtain blood for laboratory investigations to determine the cause of their illness. This makes the need for knowing options for blood drawing in infants and children important. Point-of-care diagnostic equipment or other micro methods for analyzing samples that require small quantities of blood for the tests are often unavailable in low- and middle-income countries (LMICs) [1, 2]. Blood draws usually pose a challenge to health workers without training in this skill [3]. Additionally, it must be noted that infants/children have a small blood volume compared to adults, and therefore care should be taken in the amount/volume of blood obtained at a given time. Venipuncture is the technique of choice for multiple blood sampling as it provides more accurate results and it is less painful than a heel stick [4, 5]. This chapter will discuss vascular access, venipuncture, and heel stick techniques with some adaptations or pearls from these procedures when in a limited resource setting.

Obtaining blood from neonates and children is challenging. Some of the reasons for difficult blood draw in these children are related to the patient, the materials used, or the physician's disposition. It is difficult to obtain blood from small preterm and post-date neonates, dehydrated or chubby infants, infants and children with skin lesion over the anticipated blood draw sites, and neonates or children with bleeding diathesis.

Provider anxiety, exhaustion, hunger, or inexperience can also complicate these situations. In addition, parents may feel uncomfortable watching the procedure. It is important that parents are counseled on realistic expectations and potentially removed from the procedure area if their presence seems likely to complicate an already challenging procedure. This likely depends on cultural norms and provider preference.

3 Indications

Need for laboratory evaluations.

4 Contraindications

Site for venipuncture or heel stick should be evaluated for the following contraindications:

1. Cellulitis or abscess in the skin and soft tissue over blood vessels
2. Evidence of fibrosis of the vein on palpation, usually in a previously thrombosed vein
3. Presence of arteriovenous malformation
4. Hematoma formation at the site

5 Venipuncture

5.1 Equipment/Supplies

The availability of the relevant materials for the blood draw in neonates and children varies, depending on the type of one healthcare facility. The following materials are often required for a venous draw:

1. Clean disposable medical gloves.
2. Tourniquet (giving sets, or disposable gloves are often improvised as tourniquet in low-resource settings).
3. Skin disinfectants (e.g., 70% alcohol swab).
4. Needle and collection/transfer devices (i.e., Vacutainer tube system, hypodermic needle and syringe, intravenous (IV) cannula and syringe, or winged butterfly device with syringe) (Fig. 1 and Table 1). Breaking of the hub off the needle in order to facilitate getting the specimen into the container should be discouraged due to the risk of needle puncture of the clinician obtaining the blood.

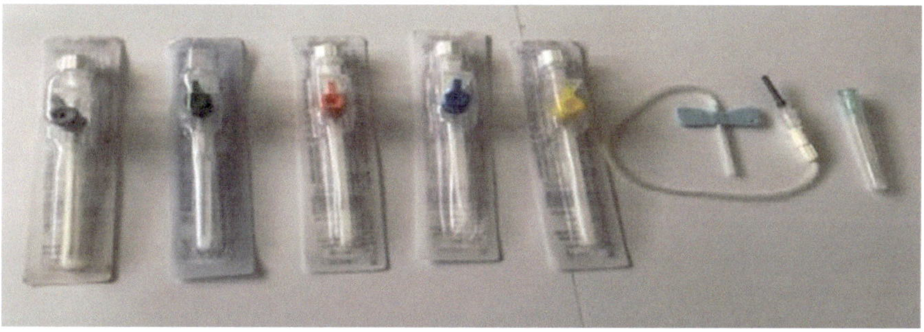

Fig. 1 Cannula and needles used for blood draw. (Figure used with permission from Professor Oguche)

Table 1 Cannula/needle sizes

Color – cannula/needle	Gauge	Age of children
Orange	14G	
White	17G	Uncommon for children
Gray	16G	Uncommon for children
Green	18G	Adolescents
Pink	20G	Adolescents
Blue	22G	Young children, term neonates
Yellow	24G	Small neonates
Violet	26G	Pre-terms
Hypodermic needle	Variable sizes	Any age
Butterfly needle	Variable sizes	Neonates, young children

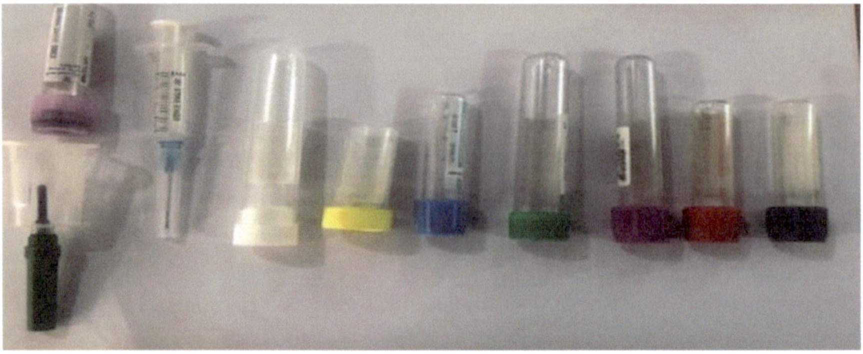

Fig. 2 Color-coded specimen containers. (Figure used with permission from Professor Oguche)

Table 2 Specimen containers and the tests they are used for

Color of container	Anticoagulant content	Laboratory	Test
White	None	Hematology/ chemistry	Serum-based tests
Yellow	Fluoride	Chemistry	Glucose
Blue	Sodium citrate	Hematology	Clotting profile
Green	Lithium/sodium heparin	Hematology	Plasma, whole blood, blood gas
Purple	EDTA	Hematology	Complete blood count
Gray	Fluoride oxalate	Chemistry	Glucose assay
Red	None	Serum	Serum-based tests
Brown	None	Chemistry	Bilirubin

5. For children and infants, a 23 G winged butterfly needle device is preferred to 20–24 G intravenous cannula because of lower risk of sample hemolysis with the former. However, intravenous cannulas are often used especially when intravenous access for treatment is also required.
6. Blood bottles (Fig. 2 and Table 2 show different types of blood sample tubes and their color coding, respectively).
7. Sharps disposal bin (may be homemade from thick plastic bottles such as those used for vegetable oil or heavy cardboard).

6 Technique

6.1 Emotional Support

- Reassure and be empathic to the caregiver/mother.
- Offer breast milk or sucrose (0.012–0.12 g) to mitigate pain after the procedure [6, 7].

- The mother can put the baby in a skin-to-skin contact position to alleviate pain [8].
- For older children, allowing the child to sit in the caregiver's lap may decrease anxiety.
- Distraction can be a helpful technique – engage children in conversation or play [9, 10].
- Avoid raw honey in children under 1 year of age due to the risk of botulism [11].

6.2 *Preparation for Venipuncture*

1. Explain the procedure clearly stating the indication to the caregiver in order to obtain verbal consent. Give age-appropriate information to the child to decrease anxiety.
2. Complete the laboratory request form. It is essential to record all necessary information, for example, date of collection, time of sample collection, patients' name, hospital number, ward, method of collection venous or capillary, and the investigation required.
3. Prepare a tray with the equipment listed above. Select the type of bottle/tube and label it appropriately.
4. Determine the minimum amount of blood required for the investigation(s). Careful considerations should be made to minimize volume of blood drawn at a given time to <1–5% of total blood volume (TBV) [12]. A practical approach to minimize the effect of large volume draws in neonates (>5% of TBV) is to schedule such draws during exchange transfusions or before blood transfusions if indicated and appropriate.
5. Wash hands with soap and water, dry, and then put on nonsterile gloves.
6. Place the infant or child in a position of comfort. For infants, this can be achieved with the swaddling, breastfeeding, or holding the infant in a breastfeeding position by the caregiver/assistant with the limb of interest exposed.
7. The physician should be seated or standing comfortably in a well-lit area. Availability of an assistant is encouraged (could be a caregiver or another healthcare worker).
8. Select the most suitable site of blood draw. This is first determined by the volume of blood required and the type of investigation required, as well as the infant or child's anatomy.
9. For venous blood sampling, it is important to carefully choose the site and prepare the vein for a blood draw. Preparation of the vein includes warming the extremity, applying the tourniquet, rubbing or patting the vein, and cleaning it with antiseptic solution.

    (a) Knowledge of the vascular anatomy (arteries and veins) is crucial for blood draw. In neonates, some of the most utilized sites are the *dorsal metacarpal veins* (dorsum of the hand), *the antecubital veins, and the dorsalis pedis vein* (Fig. 3). *Scalp veins* may also be utilized when needed.

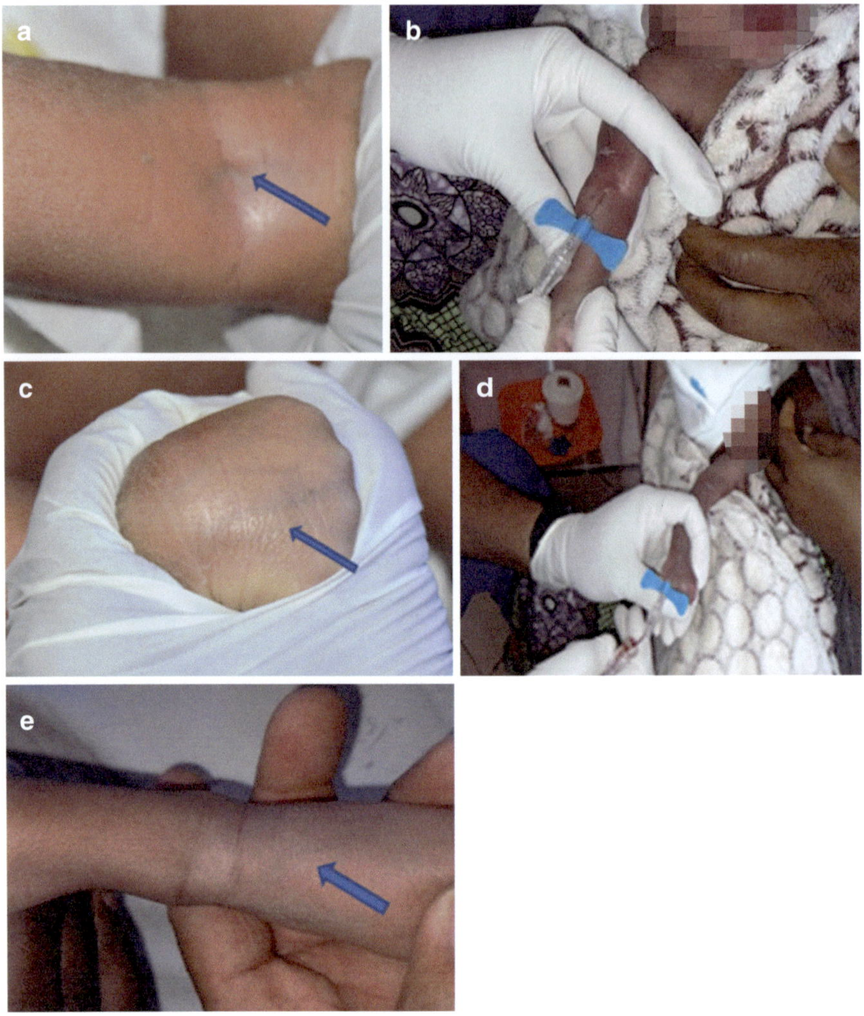

Fig. 3 (**a**) Vein in antecubital fossa. (Figure used with permission from Dr. Farouk). (**b**) Drawing blood from antecubital vein. (Figure used with permission from Dr. Diala). (**c**) Vein in dorsal venous network of the hand. (Figure used with permission from Dr. Farouk). (**d**) Drawing blood from hand vein. (Figure used with permission from Dr. Diala). (**e**) Dorsal pedis vein. (Figure used with permission from Dr. Diala)

(b) Except in emergencies, *blood should not be obtained from femoral vessels* (i.e., "femoral stick") in neonates, infants, and children. There is a rare but real risk of either septic or aseptic necrosis of the femoral head. If an infant or child gets necrosis of the femoral head, they may have permanent damage to the hip making walking difficult or impossible.

(c) When obtaining blood is urgent and the healthcare worker is not able to obtain blood from peripheral veins, a *radial artery draw ("arterial stick")* is generally safer than a femoral stick. If the radial artery is used, assure hemostasis before leaving the patient.
(d) Additionally, the *external jugular vein* is a site that may be appropriate for venous access. Blood can often be drawn from the catheter that is placed in this situation since a larger size catheter is utilized in this procedure than is typically placed in a peripheral vein.

6.3 Procedure for Venipuncture

1. Apply a tourniquet about 6–10 cm proximal to the selected site (except when accessing the external jugular vein). Examples of possible sites are seen in Fig. 3a–d. Gently tapping the vein may "cultivate" the vein to facilitate identification. In light-skinned neonates or children, the veins appear greenish. On palpation, veins are soft and easily refill after being depressed.
2. Clean the skin with disinfectant swabs and allow it to dry for 30 seconds.
3. Apply some traction to the skin a few centimeters distal to the selected site to stabilize the skin with the thumb of the nondominant hand. In neonates and infants, the procedure could be modified by applying gentle pressure proximal to the selected vein using the flexed index finger of the nondominant hand while simultaneously stretching the skin distal to the selected site with the thumb of the same hand (Fig. 3d, e).
4. Introduce the needle with a bevel facing up at an angle of 15–30 degrees (or 10–15 degrees for winged "butterfly" or "scalp vein" needles) until the vein is entered which is signaled by decreased resistance or a popping sensation and observe for backflow of blood into the hub of the needle or a cannula. Once in the vein, reduce the angle further and advance the needle another 3–5 mm into the vein. If an intravenous catheter is used, advance until one reaches the wing or hub and gently withdraw the needle leaving the catheter in place. It is important to avoid placing cannula over joints when intended for administration of intravenous fluids to avoid irregular flow.
5. Once in place, switch hands with your nondominant hand holding the needle or catheter in place and your dominant hand holding the bottle allowing blood to drip into the bottle or pulling the plunger of the syringe until the required volume of blood has been drawn. A second person can assist by pulling the plunger slowly simultaneously while the person doing the procedure accesses the vein.
6. Once sample collection is complete, gently invert the bottle about five to seven times for bottles containing anticoagulants to ensure admixing.
7. Discard sharps into a sharps container.

8. Untie the tourniquet and withdraw the needle applying pressure over the site with a dry swab for about 30 seconds until bleeding stops and to prevent swelling. With arterial access, you may need to hold pressure longer. Taking the needed time to ensure hemostasis often ensures the vein can be used for future draws.
9. Every effort should be made to successfully perform the procedure at the first attempt! Children will hardly cooperate if the first attempt fails and repeat attempts are needed.

7 Heel Puncture/"Heel Stick" Procedure for Neonates and Infants

7.1 Equipment/Supplies (Fig. 4a–c)

- Gloves (Fig. 4a)
- Lancet or size 24G hypodermic needle
- Alcohol swab

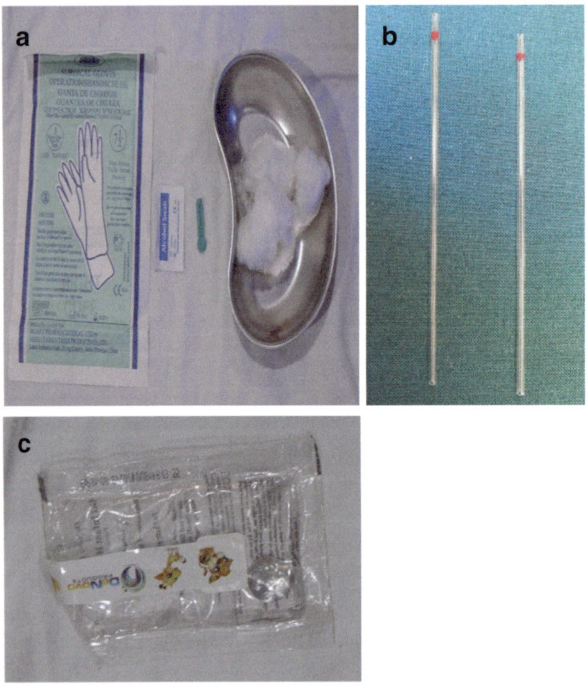

Fig. 4 (**a**) Gloves, alcohol swab, lancet, and dry swab. (Figure used with permission from Dr. Farouk). (**b**) Capillary tubes. (Figure used with permission from Dr. Farouk). (**c**) Warming gel. (Figure used with permission from Dr. Farouk)

- Dry swab (cotton)
- Specimen bottles, capillary tube (Fig. 4b), or microtubes
- Disposal bin for sharps
- Additional light source, e.g., pen torch
- Warming gel (Fig. 4c) or warm cloth (not hot!!!)

7.2 Technique

7.2.1 Preparation for Heel Prick

Follow emotional support and "preparing for venipuncture" steps as described above.

7.2.2 Heel Prick Procedure

1. Hold heel correctly (Fig. 5a) and then select the site for the puncture. Medial and lateral heel is recommended (Fig. 5a–d); avoid the posterior heel (Fig. 5a–d) because the skin to bone distance is shorter and you risk injuring the bone or tendon. Avoid finger prick in the neonate.

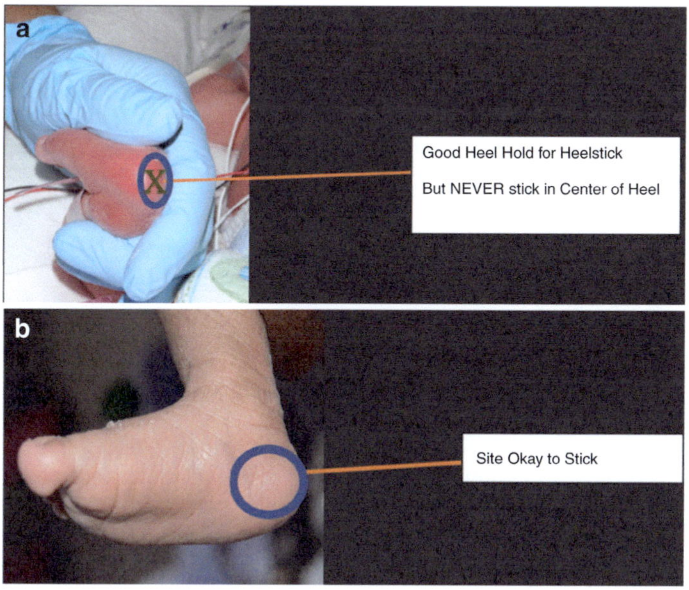

Fig. 5 (**a**) Holding heel correctly (but never sticking in middle of heel). (Figure used with permission from Dr. Farouk). (**b**) Medial heel – proper location for heel stick (Figure used with permission from Dr. Farouk). (**c**) Outside of heel – proper location for heel stick. (Figure used with permission from Dr. Farouk). (**d**) Safe and unsafe areas for heel sticks summarized. (Figure used with permission from Adrian M Slusher)

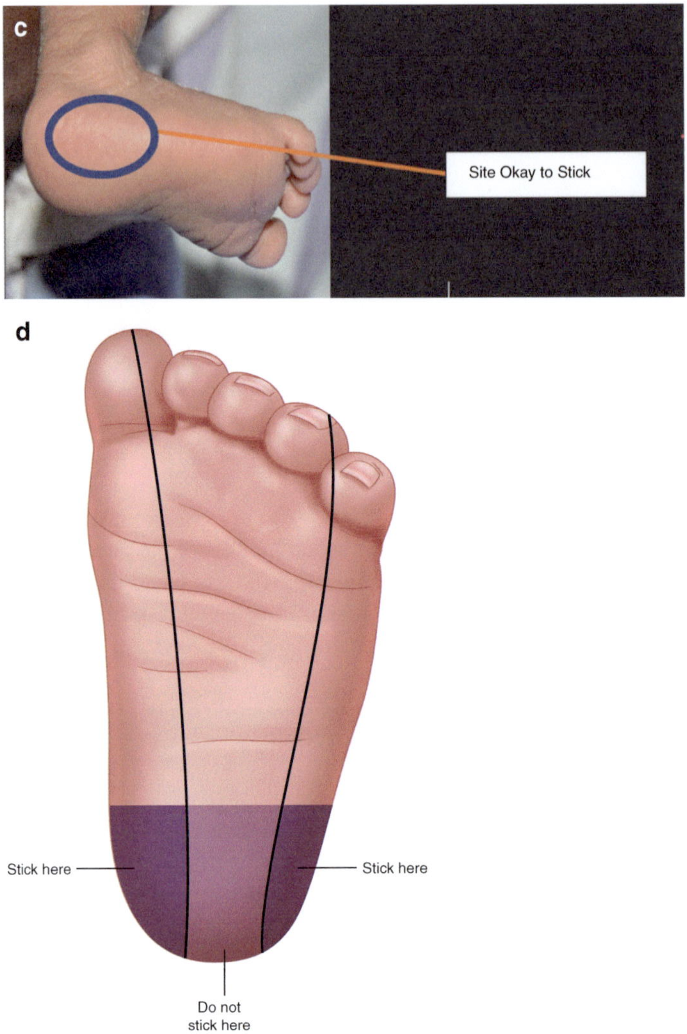

Fig. 5 (continued)

2. You can warm the selected site by applying a warming gel and warm cloth (not hot!) or by gently cupping the heel in your palm and rubbing gently.
3. Select appropriate size lancet/needle (size 20–24G) depending on the amount of blood needed (larger needle for larger volume draw). Do not use surgical blade for the puncture.
4. Clean the selected area with an alcohol swab and allow it to air-dry.
5. Prick the heel with the needle at right angle to the skin by a quick single stroke. The depth should not go beyond 2.4 mm in full-term neonates and 0.85 mm in preterm neonates.

6. Clean off the first drop of blood with a dry cotton swab.
7. While encircling the foot of the neonate in your palm with your fingers and thumbs, milk the blood by gently squeezing the foot intermittently.
8. Collect the blood specimen into the sample bottle/capillary tube.
9. After sampling, apply a dry cotton swab and firmly press to stop the blood flow.
10. Use the lancet single time only.
11. Do not puncture the skin at one site multiple times to avoid skin flora contaminating the sample.
12. Dispose of sharps and swabs in the appropriate bin.
13. Label the sample appropriately with patient name, hospital number, location, and time. It is important to fill in all the patient data correctly.

7.3 Complications

7.3.1 Venipuncture

Blood draws are generally considered safe. Compared to adults, neonates and children have a much lower circulating blood volume; thus, it is important to minimize the volume of blood draws as much as possible. Obtaining more than the necessary amount of blood could endanger the child, especially the small premature infants. Dangers of blood draw include the following:

1. Iatrogenic anemia from large volume blood draws or repeated blood draws [13, 14]
2. Hematoma formation [15]
3. Infection of the vein or overlying skin – cellulitis, phlebitis, and abscess formation
4. Injury to the bones
5. Digital gangrene from arterial vasospasm
6. Allergy to collection equipment, for example, latex
7. Excessive or abnormal bleeding
    - Difficulty with hemostasis resulting from platelet abnormalities, coagulopathy (congenital or acquired), or blood vessel disorders. This may not be known by the provider until the procedure has started.

In the event of abnormal excessive bleeding following venipuncture, do the following:

- Apply firm pressure using gauze and tape or a compression dressing to the site.
- Do the bleeding time for quick assessment of platelet function.
- Transfuse fresh whole blood or platelet concentrate.
- Refer to see pediatrician as soon as possible.

7.3.2 Heel Prick

1. Injury to the posterior tibial artery
2. Osteomyelitis of the calcaneus
3. Injury to the Achilles tendon
4. Hematoma formation
5. Scarring of soft tissues
6. Tissue necrosis

7.4 Case Resolution

Blood is drawn successfully from the dorsum of the hand using a size 24G intravenous cannula which is secured for administration of antibiotics. Bilirubin level is within treatment range and phototherapy is begun. The baby does well and is discharged with negative cultures and falling bilirubin levels on the 11th day of life.

References

1. Katoba J, Kuupiel D, Mashamba-Thompson TP. Toward improving accessibility of point-of-care diagnostic Services for Maternal and Child Health in low- and middle-income countries. Point Care. 2019;18(1):17–25.
2. Buttery JP. Blood cultures in newborns and children: optimising an everyday test. Arch Dis Child Fetal Neonatal Ed. 2002;87(1):F25.
3. WHO. 6, Paediatric and neonatal blood sampling. In WHO guidelines on drawing blood: best practices in phlebotomy. Geneva: World Health Organization; 2010.
4. Ogawa S, et al. Venepuncture is preferable to heel lance for blood sampling in term neonates. Arch Dis Child Fetal Neonatal Ed. 2005;90(5):F432–6.
5. Shah VS, Ohlsson A. Venepuncture versus heel lance for blood sampling in term neonates. Cochrane Database Syst Rev. 2011;2011(10):CD001452.
6. Stevens B, et al. Sucrose for analgesia in newborn infants undergoing painful procedures. Cochrane Database Syst Rev. 2016;7(7):CD001069.
7. Codipietro L, Ceccarelli M, Ponzone A. Breastfeeding or oral sucrose solution in term neonates receiving heel lance: a randomized, controlled trial. Pediatrics. 2008;122(3):e716.
8. Bembich S, et al. Infant analgesia with a combination of breast milk, glucose, or maternal holding. Pediatrics. 2018;142(3):e20173416.
9. Uman LS, et al. Psychological interventions for needle-related procedural pain and distress in children and adolescents. Cochrane Database Syst Rev. 2013;10:CD005179.
10. Cho M-K, Choi M-Y. Effect of distraction intervention for needle-related pain and distress in children: a systematic review and meta-analysis. Int J Environ Res Public Health. 2021;18(17):9159.
11. Abdulla CO, et al. Infant botulism following honey ingestion. BMJ Case Rep. 2012;2012:bcr1120115153.

12. Howie SRC. Blood sample volumes in child health research: review of safe limits. Bull World Health Organ. 2011;89(1):46–53.
13. Jakacka N, Snarski E, Mekuria S. Prevention of iatrogenic anemia in critical and neonatal care. Adv Clin Exp Med. 2016;25(1):191–7.
14. Puia-Dumitrescu M, et al. Patterns of phlebotomy blood loss and transfusions in extremely low birth weight infants. J Perinatol. 2019;39(12):1670–5.
15. Buowari OY. Complications of venepuncture. Adv Biosci Biotech. 2013;4:126–8.

Pediatric Resuscitation Guidelines for Limited-Resource Settings

Bhupinder Reel, Demet Sulemanji, Ndidiamaka L. Musa, and Mark Ralston

Abbreviations

BP	Blood pressure
ETAT	Emergency triage and treatment
ICU	Intensive care unit
IMCI	Integrated management of childhood illnesses
LMICs	Low- and middle-income countries
PALS	Pediatric advanced life support
WBC	White blood count
WHO	World Health Organization

B. Reel
Department of Pediatrics and Child Health, and Paediatric Emergency and Critical Care, University of Nairobi, Nairobi, Kenya

D. Sulemanji
MP Shah Hospital, Critical Care, Nairobi, Kenya

N. L. Musa (✉)
Department of Pediatrics, Division of Critical Care, University of Washington, Seattle, WA, USA
e-mail: Ndidi.Musa@seattlechildrens.org

M. Ralston
Department of Pediatrics, Uniformed Services University of the Health Sciences, Bethesda, MD, USA

T. M. Slusher et al. (eds.), *Pediatric Procedural Adaptations for Low-Resource Settings*, https://doi.org/10.1007/978-3-030-99955-1_11

1 Case

A 4-year-old male with no significant past medical history presents with fever, cough, dyspnea, tachycardia, and cold extremities. He does not have myalgias, malaise, nausea, vomiting, or diarrhea. On examination in the pediatric high acuity unit, the child has as a temperature of 39.2 °C, a weak radial pulse of 148 beats per minute, a respiratory rate of 60 breaths per minute, and an oxygen saturation of 85% on ambient air. He has marked respiratory distress, poor perfusion of his extremities with a capillary refill time of 6–7 seconds, and a Glasgow Coma Scale Score of 9/15. Blood pressure (BP) is not obtained as there are no pediatric blood pressure cuffs. He is assumed to be hypotensive secondary to his prolonged capillary refill and weak peripheral pulses. Laboratory workup shows a hemoglobin of 11.9 g/dL (11.3–14.1 g/dL), WBC count of 19.3 ×10^3/uL (10.9–15.0 × 10^3/uL), neutrophil count of 12.1 × 10^3/uL (1.5–8.5 × 10^3/uL), lymphocyte count of 4.5 × 10^3/uL (2.0–8.0 × 10^3/uL), and platelet count of 155 × 10^9/L (150–400 × 10^9/L). The chest radiograph reveals a left lower lobe opacification. Oxygen saturations on a non-rebreather mask increase to 92% with minimal improvement in his work of breathing and retractions.

An intravenous (IV) line is attempted, so that IV fluid replacement and broad-spectrum antibiotics can be administered. After several unsuccessful attempts at the IV, an intraosseous line is placed in the right tibia. A Ringer's lactate fluid infusion of 20 ml/kg is given over 30 minutes followed by maintenance IV fluid rehydration. Frequent reassessment of the child is planned to monitor the child's progress. He is given a working diagnosis of severe pneumonia with septic shock.

2 Introduction

In 2019, the estimate of global annual deaths in children under the age of 5 was 5.1 million, or 38 deaths per 1000 live births. Nearly all (99%) of mortality under the age of 5 occurs in low- and middle-income countries (LMICs), predominantly in sub-Saharan Africa where 1 in every 13 children dies before their fifth birthday. Children in need of emergency care often do not reach even the basic healthcare facilities. The majority of pediatric deaths occur outside hospitals. About 50% of deaths of children admitted to the hospital occur within 24 hours of admission.

Existing management guidelines for children with emergency conditions, as taught in a variety of current pediatric life support courses, are mostly applicable to high-income countries (HICs) with a different disease range and access to the full spectrum of acute care management resources. For this reason, these standardized courses lack universal applicability despite their universal acceptance. A revised curriculum with evidence-based application to limited-resource settings would expand the potential for reducing pediatric mortality worldwide.

This chapter provides a broad case-based discussion of selected pediatric emergency conditions with attention to the context of disease range and level-specific resources in low- and middle-income countries (LMICs). Discussion includes contextualized management guidelines to create a framework for realistic approaches to common emergency scenarios. A critical care case is discussed with different characteristics and through alternative scenarios with variable resource availability. Appropriate management options are streamlined and recommended depending on the available resources. Consistent with other chapters in this book, these guidelines should be utilized by healthcare providers with existing experience in caring for acutely ill children, and this chapter alone would be insufficient education for a non-healthcare provider.

3 Case Continuation in Healthcare Settings with No Availability of Intensive Care

The patient was kept in the acute care unit (which is the best staffed unit in many hospitals without ICU availability). Over the next 2 hours, his heart rate slowly increased to 168 beats per minute and capillary refill time remained at 4–5 seconds with weak peripheral and central pulses. He continued to have significant respiratory distress, and on a spot check (there is only one pulse oximeter for the entire unit), his oxygen saturation was 84–86% on 2LPM of oxygen via nasal cannula (he was not placed on face mask due to the need for high flow rates and limited oxygen supply). His Glasgow Coma Scale Score decreased to 6/15, prompting delivery of another fluid infusion of 10 mL/kg administered over 30 minutes. On repeat examination, by the nurse, he was noted to be cyanotic appearing and pulses could no longer be palpated.

Cardiopulmonary resuscitation was initiated using PALS guidelines [1]. *The provider recognized that the child was malnourished and therefore estimated the weight rather than using the Broselow tape* [2]. *Return of spontaneous circulation was achieved in 5 minutes. Pulses remained weak but palpable and the child had a respiratory rate of 35 breaths per minute, albeit shallow with an oxygen saturation of 90% on 4LPM with a nasal cannula. Parents were informed about the initial management and need for further advanced care requiring transfer to a tertiary care center. The closest tertiary care facility was 6 hours away by road. Transport was arranged in the morning.*

Survival Tips

- When calculating drug doses in a resuscitation, a Broselow tape cannot be used with malnourished children as it may significantly overestimate doses.
- In the absence of intraosseous needles, a 16- or 18-gauge needle can be used for IO access. See chapter "Intraosseous Line Placement for Medical Therapy in a Low-Resource Setting" on modified IO options.

- Continuous monitoring of vital signs would be ideal, but lack of availability of bedside monitors requires greater reliance on constant re-evaluation often conducted by nursing staff.
- With fluid bolus administration, fluids should be stopped with any sign of fluid overload in this setting.
- Check for hypoglycemia if possible. Alternatively treatment for hypoglycemia should be considered in children with altered mental status if unable to check the blood sugar level.

4 Case Management Discussion

4.1 Non-ICU Setting

If the child had a normal blood pressure, maintenance fluids would be started but bolus fluid therapy should be avoided [3]. The presence of hypotension/decompensated shock in this case warranted the use of isotonic buffered crystalloid, preferably Ringer's lactate, 10–20 mL/kg boluses (up to 40 mL/kg in first hour) titrated to therapeutic end-points and discontinued if signs of fluid overload develop [4]. Re-evaluation for signs of fluid overload should be frequent in this setting due to concern of increased mortality with fluid boluses as demonstrated in the FEAST trial and now also incorporated into PALS [1, 3].

Many guidelines in LMICs recommend lower total fluids and slower infusions than those in HICs including the recently updated pediatric ETAT guidelines [5]. These guidelines recommend that children with *all* signs of shock – defined as having cold extremities, capillary refill more than 3 seconds, and a weak, fast pulse – should receive a 10–20 ml/kg fluid bolus of isotonic crystalloid over 30–60 minutes. They should be reassessed frequently and only be given additional fluid boluses (10 mL/kg over 30 minutes) if still in shock. A fluid bolus should be stopped if there is evidence of fluid overload (crackles on lung exam, new hepatomegaly, worsening respiratory status) or cardiac failure. One clinical method of determining fluid overload in addition to listening for crackles or rales is for the clinician to put their hand below the liver as the bolus is being given and stop fluid if liver size is increasing. Although results are mixed and more studies are needed, point-of-care ultrasound may be used to determine volume status. This is especially helpful in LMICs where access to central venous pressure monitoring may be limited [6].

The rest of the treatment of septic shock should be adhered to as closely as possible (LMIC or HIC):

1. Empiric broad-spectrum antimicrobial therapy should be commenced as soon as possible, ideally within an hour of recognition of a child with septic shock [7].
2. Blood cultures should be obtained prior to therapy, as recommended, as long as this does not delay antibiotic administration. Narrowing or stopping antibiotic therapy should be based on culture results/sensitivities if possible and clinical improvement [4, 8].

3. Red blood cell transfusion should be reserved for children with hemoglobin concentrations of less than 7 g/dL in a hemodynamically stable child. However, the child in shock and severe anemia (hemoglobin <5 g/dL) should receive a blood transfusion as soon as possible and receive maintenance intravenous fluids [9]. There is no current suggested hemoglobin threshold for critically ill children with unstable septic shock [4].

Very careful consideration should be given prior to any fluid resuscitation in *children with severe acute malnutrition*. Any fluids given should be given judiciously and more slowly than in other scenarios. Children *with shock and severe acute malnutrition* should receive 10–15 mL/kg of intravenous fluids over the first hour with frequent reassessment. The child who does not improve should be given a 10 ml/kg blood transfusion over 3–4 hours [9]. Once hemodynamic stability is achieved, children should transition to receiving fluid through either oral or nasogastric routes (avoiding IVF as much as possible).

Shock due to hypovolemia from gastroenteritis or other causes of dehydration should be treated per appropriate World Health Organization (WHO) guidelines as reviewed in chapter "Oral Rehydration Therapy in a Low-Resource Setting" on ORS. Fluid resuscitation is much more liberal in this setting based on degree of dehydration and ongoing losses.

Depending on the resources available, each hospital will need to decide when advanced resuscitation is possible, feasible, and appropriate. When resuscitating a pediatric patient, an infant or child with a heart rate ≥60 beats per minute with absent or inadequate breathing would be given one rescue breath every 2–3 seconds (20–30 breaths per minute) [10]. A child without a pulse or a symptomatic child who has a heart rate <60 beats per minute and signs of poor perfusion would require immediate initiation of CPR. High-quality CPR is essential, if CPR is to be administered. Details of standard resuscitation are beyond the scope of this book; for algorithms, consult ETAT or PALS [1, 11].

Survival Tips

- Many pediatric emergency departments lack the appropriate sized blood pressure cuffs for accurate monitoring; therefore, the evaluation of clinical markers of cardiac output, such as tachycardia, peripheral perfusion, and capillary refill, is valuable.
- Immediate availability of RBCs, or other blood products, may not be possible in LMIC even if indicated.
- Fluid resuscitation in limited-resource settings and patients with severe acute malnutrition requires frequent reexamination for fluid overload.
- Resuscitation should be guided by the resources that are available in each hospital and per in-country guidelines. Most pediatric codes start with respiratory failure; therefore, providing appropriate rescue breaths can be lifesaving even in locations where more advanced resuscitation is not feasible.

4.2 Referral and Transport Considerations

As a general rule, a referral to a location with ICU capacity should be made, if possible, whenever local capabilities are exceeded. Time is of the essence in referring and transferring critically ill or injured children to an appropriate facility of higher capability. It is important to initiate both lifesaving treatment at the referring location (instead of deferring treatment until the child reaches the referral facility) and referral arrangements as soon as possible. Without these plans in place, the child may not survive the transport or hospitalization at the referral facility. Referral indications for critically ill or injured children by emergency condition include:

- *Respiratory*: hypoxemia, bag-mask ventilation, severe upper airway obstruction, severe asthma, very severe pneumonia, pulmonary edema, and tension pneumothorax
- *Circulatory*: severe dehydration, hypotension, septic shock, anaphylaxis, neurogenic shock, arrhythmia, congestive heart failure, and central cyanosis
- *Neurological*: GCS score ≤12, meningitis, encephalitis/cerebral malaria, seizure, increased ICP, and stroke
- *Other*: severe malnutrition, hypothermia, severe infection (i.e., viral, bacterial, malaria, fungal), severe trauma (including severe burns), severe anemia, jaundice, severe hypoglycemia, and toxin

A referral note needs to be written to the referral facility to communicate specific information about the patient including the type of treatment received at the referring location. The referral note should include the following information: date, referring location, referring practitioner, accepting practitioner (i.e., at referral facility), patient name, patient age, weight, emergency condition, last vital signs, fluids (volume, date, time), medications (dose, date, time), and laboratory results.

4.3 Transport

The following checklist of equipment and monitoring (Table 1) can make it possible to transport critically ill children in a basic ambulance. Ideally, transport should be performed by an anesthetist or an intensivist. If this is not possible, a healthcare provider with airway skills and ability to manage hemodynamic changes is required. Ideally, when able, the airway should be well secured, the position of any endotracheal tube must be confirmed, and circulation stabilized prior to transport of the child.

Table 1 Transport considerations and equipment in limited-resource settings

Considerations
Stabilize patient Airway protection if required Adequate intravenous access
Discuss the case and estimated time of arrival with the referral facility
Equipment
Full oxygen tank and reserve to last duration of transport
Monitoring: Pulse oximetry, blood pressure. If available – *ETCO*$_2$, *cardiac monitoring*
Ambu-bag with appropriate size face mask
Non-rebreather mask – If sufficient O_2 available to run at 10–15LPM
Endotracheal tubes (spare size of current tube and a size smaller) – If available
Laryngoscope with appropriate size blades – If available
Portable suction with appropriate size suction catheters – If available
Defibrillator – If available
Transport ventilator – If available, can transport on bubble CPAP in appropriate patients
Resuscitation drugs – Isotonic fluids, dextrose, pain/sedation meds, epinephrine

Survival Tips

- In low-resource settings, ground transportation is often completed by non-critical care ambulances.
- Table 1 contents are not always readily available for transport of a critically ill child. It is likely that transport will be performed with pulse oximetry as the sole monitor while child is manually ventilated by bag-mask with 100% oxygen.
- Monitoring the saturations together with waveform and pulse rate cautiously throughout the transport is essential. The transport physician must carefully monitor for appropriate chest rise to ensure the location and patency of the endotracheal tube.
- Availability of reserve oxygen should be ensured as transport may be delayed by traffic, government stops, ambulance breakdowns, severe weather conditions, etc. Oxygen tank gauge must be in working order prior to transport.
- It is unlikely to have the equipment to blend oxygen as would be required for congenital heart disease or neonates.
- At least two viable intravenous lines should be obtained prior to transport and appropriate sedation provided. Sedation may need to be provided via intermittent boluses of sedatives due to the lack of infusion pumps.

5 Case Continuation in Healthcare Settings with Availability of Intensive Care

The patient was moved to the pediatric intensive care unit in the capitol city. This hospital has the capability to support patients with mechanical ventilation, perform dialysis, and administer vasopressors. They had an appropriate size BP cuff, which showed the child's BP was 55/20 (32) mmHg. Another Ringer's lactate fluid bolus of 20 ml/kg was given with some improvement in perfusion with a capillary refill time of 4–5 secs; however, BP was still low at 70/40. An epinephrine (adrenaline) infusion was started peripherally at 0.03mcg/kg/min. He was immediately intubated and placed on a ventilator. Mechanical ventilation was initiated with a peak inspiratory pressure of 15 cm of water, positive end-expiratory pressure of 5 cm of water, a fraction of inspired oxygen (FiO_2) of 0.70, and a mean airway pressure of 13 cm of water, resulting in a partial pressure of arterial oxygen (PaO_2) of 110 mm Hg and a partial pressure of arterial carbon dioxide ($PaCO_2$) of 37 mm Hg. Lung protective ventilation strategies were implemented, targeting a tidal volume of 6 mL/kg and reducing fraction of inspired oxygen (FiO_2), in order to keep the oxygen saturations above 92%. A central line was placed. Both epinephrine and norepinephrine infusions were moved to the central venous catheter and titrated to 0.15mcg/kg/min and 0.1mcg/kg/min, respectively, achieving a BP (systolic/diastolic (mean)) of 83/41 (59) mmHg. A few hours later, he acutely worsened, dropping his oxygen saturations to 70% without improvement despite bagging with 100% FiO_2. You listened to his chest and noted that he had no breath sound on the right side of his chest. You performed a rapid point-of-care ultrasound and noted that he had no sliding signs on his right chest. You emergently aspirated the chest and got a large amount of air. Because he was on mechanical ventilation, you placed a chest tube (chapter "Modified Chest Drainage System for Use in a Low-Resource Settings"). He immediately improved with an increase in his oxygen saturations to 94%. Over the coming 72 hours, his peripheral perfusion improved again with a capillary refill time of 2–3 seconds, urine output improved, and you were able to wean his vasopressors off. On hospital day 4, you were able to wean the patient to extubation. You expect this patient to remain stable as he recovers over the next few weeks.

6 Case Discussion

6.1 ICU Setting

In any situation where ICU capacity and resources are available, the latest surviving pediatric sepsis guidelines, acute life support resuscitation guidelines, as well as ongoing critical care management – including managing ventilator, fluids, vasopressors, sedation and analgesia, etc. – should be followed as close as possible, with

Table 2 High-risk vital signs for children [20]

Age	Heart rate (bpm)	Respiratory rate (bpm)	SBP estimate (5th %ile)	SBP estimates	Temperature (C)
0–1mo	<110 or >170	<30 or >60	= 2 (× age) + 70	<60	<35.5 or >37.4
1–12mo	<100 or >160	<25 or >55		<70	<36 or >38
>1–2yo	<100 or >150	<25 or >45		<80	
>2–7yo	<75 or >140	<20 or >30		<90	
>7–12yo	<60 or >120	<15 or >25			
>12yo	<50 or >130	<10 or >28			

adaptations per in-country guidelines and protocols. Many guidelines for management of shock in low-resource setting recommend slower boluses and less total fluids than guidelines from high-resource settings.

Surviving sepsis guidelines recommend that fluids be carefully titrated in 10–20 mL/kg boluses up to 40–60 mL/kg in the first hour for patients with hypotensive shock (Table 2) [4]. However, summarizing other studies [12, 13], the latest pediatric advanced life support (PALS) guidelines noted that patients with septic shock receiving higher volumes faster were more likely to need mechanical ventilation and have worse oxygenation [1]. Total volume should be titrated to therapeutic end-points and discontinued if the child develops signs of fluid overload [4]. Epinephrine or norepinephrine should be started in the presence of fluid-refractory shock, or when fluid resuscitation leads to the development of signs of fluid overload such as hepatomegaly or crackles [14]. A mean arterial pressure that is appropriate for child's age should be targeted [4, 15]. Hydrocortisone (dose 2 mg/kg IV/IO, maximum dose 100 mg) should be considered if shock is fluid-refractory and catecholamine-resistant or if suspected/proven adrenal insufficiency is present [4]. Enteral feeding within 48 hours in a stepwise manner could be administered via a nasogastric tube [16, 17].

Point-of-care ultrasound is rapidly becoming more affordable and available in LMICs. It can be extremely helpful in diagnosing and managing many urgent and emergent conditions in the ICU. It has the ability to be used to rapidly diagnosis pneumothoraxes, pericardial tamponade, pneumonia, and pulmonary edema, as well as allow the experienced providers to estimate cardiac function [18, 19].

6.2 *Medication Preparation/Dosing Chart*

Emergency Drug Calculator – Evelina London. https://www.evelinalondon.nhs.uk/resources/our-services/hospital/south-thames-retrieval-service/Drug-calculators/emergency-drug-calculator.pdf.

7 Summary

This case is provided as an example of how pediatric resuscitation (e.g., acute management of septic shock) in a resource-limited setting must be modified based on available resources and local protocols. General principles of pediatric care and resuscitation are the same in any setting and can improve mortality if adhered to. It is also important to know when there are differences in protocols or management guidelines specific to a population or disease pattern (e.g., effect of malnutrition on guidelines/weight-based protocols). Careful consideration of fluid resuscitation, vasopressor management, antibiotic administration, and respiratory support is essential. Consideration of early transport/transfer and resources needed for travel will aid in reducing mortality.

8 Case Resolution

The child was appropriately treated per local sepsis guidelines with fluids, vasopressors, mechanical ventilation, and antibiotics. He improved over the course of the next 2 weeks and was discharged to home without disability.

9 For Further Reading

1. World Health Organization. Guideline: Updates on the management of severe acute malnutrition in infants and children. Geneva, World Health Organization; 2013. Available at: https://www.who.int/publications/i/item/9789241506328. Accessed on March 10, 2021.
2. Fleming S, Thompson M, Stevens R, Heneghan C, et al. Normal ranges of heart rate and respiratory rate in children from birth to 18 years of age: a systematic review of observational studies. Lancet. 2011;377(9770):1011–8. https://doi.org/10.1016/S0140-6736(10)62226-X. PMID: 21411136.
3. Haque IU, Zaritsky AL. Analysis of the evidence for the lower limit of systolic and mean arterial pressure in children. Pediatr Crit Care Med. 2007;8(2):138–44. https://doi.org/10.1097/01.PCC.0000257039.32593.DC. PMID: 17273118.
4. Hazinski MF. Children are different. In: Nursing Care of the Critically Ill Child. 3rd ed. Mosby; 2013. p. 1–18, copyright Elsevier.
5. World Health Organization. Integrated Management of Childhood Illness: distance learning course: Module 4 Diarrhoea. Geneva: WHO Press; 2014.
6. Guarino A, Albano F, Ashkenazi S, Gendrel D, Hoekstra JH, Shamir R, et al. European Society for Paediatric Gastroenterology, Hepatology, and Nutrition/ European Society for Paediatric Infection Diseases evidence-based guidelines

for the management of acute gastroenteritis in children in Europe. J Pediatr Gastroenterol Nutr 2008;46:S81.

7. Gorelick MH, Shaw KN, Murphy KO. Validity and reliability of clinical signs in the diagnosis of dehydration in children. Pediatrics 1997;99:E6.
8. Steiner MJ, DeWalt DA, Byerley JS. Is this child dehydrated? JAMA 2004;291: 2746.
9. Guideline: Assessing and Managing Children at Primary Health-Care Facilities to Prevent Overweight and Obesity in the Context of the Double Burden of Malnutrition: Updates for the Integrated Management of Childhood Illness (IMCI). Geneva: World Health Organization 2017.
10. Khilnani P, Singhi S, Lodha R, Santhanam I, Sachdev A, Chugh K, et al. Pediatric Sepsis Guidelines: summary for resource-limited countries. Indian J Crit Care Med 2010;14:41.
11. Akech SO, Karisa J, Nakamya P, Boga M, Maitland K. Phase II trial of isotonic fluid resuscitation in Kenyan children with severe malnutrition and hypovolaemia. BMC Pediatr 2010;10:71.
12. APLS – Management of Status Epilepticus Algorithm. Advanced Paediatric Life Support: The Practical Approach 6th Edition', 2017.
13. Kander V, Wilmshurst JM. Training doctors in basic EEG: analysis of a learning tool relevant to resource-limited settings. Epileptic Disord. 2015;17(1):58–66; quiz 66. https://doi.org/10.1684/epd.2015.0729. PMID: 25711247.
14. Kochanek PM, Tasker RC, Bell MJ, Adelson PD, Carney N, et al. Management of pediatric severe traumatic brain injury: 2019 consensus and guidelines-based algorithm for first and second tier therapies. Pediatr Crit Care Med. 2019;20(3):269–79. https://doi.org/10.1097/PCC.0000000000001737. PMID: 30830015.
15. Kochanek PM, Tasker RC, Carney N, Totten AM, Adelson PD, et al. Guidelines for the Management of Pediatric Severe Traumatic Brain Injury, Third Edition: Update of the Brain Trauma Foundation Guidelines, Executive Summary. Neurosurgery. 2019;84(6):1169–78. https://doi.org/10.1093/neuros/nyz051. PMID: 30822776.
16. Chesnut RM, Temkin N, Carney N, Dikmen S, Rondina C, et al. Global Neurotrauma Research Group. A trial of intracranial-pressure monitoring in traumatic brain injury. N Engl J Med. 2012;367(26):2471–81. https://doi.org/10.1056/NEJMoa1207363. Epub 2012 Dec 12. Erratum in: N Engl J Med. 2013 Dec 19;369(25):2465. PMID: 23234472; PMCID: PMC3565432.
17. Nathanson MH, Andrzejowski J, Dinsmore J, Eynon CA, Ferguson K, et al. Guidelines for safe transfer of the brain-injured patient: trauma and stroke, 2019: Guidelines from the Association of Anaesthetists and the Neuro Anaesthesia and Critical Care Society. Anaesthesia. 2020;75(2):234–46. https://doi.org/10.1111/anae.14866.

References

1. Topjian AA, et al. Part 4: pediatric basic and advanced life support: 2020 American Heart Association guidelines for cardiopulmonary resuscitation and emergency cardiovascular care. Circulation. 2020;142(16_suppl_2):S469–523.
2. Clark MC, et al. Accuracy of the Broselow tape in South Sudan, "the hungriest place on earth". Acad Emerg Med. 2016;23(1):21–8.
3. Maitland K, et al. Mortality after fluid bolus in African children with severe infection. N Engl J Med. 2011;364(26):2483–95.
4. Weiss SL, et al. Surviving sepsis campaign international guidelines for the Management of Septic Shock and Sepsis-Associated Organ Dysfunction in children. Pediatr Crit Care Med. 2020;21(2):e52–e106.
5. WHO. Guideline: updates on paediatric emergency triage, assessment and treatment: care of critically-ill children. Geneva: World Health Organization; 2016.
6. Modi P, et al. Accuracy of inferior vena cava ultrasound for predicting dehydration in children with acute diarrhea in resource-limited settings. PLoS One. 2016;11(1):e0146859.
7. Weiss SL, et al. Delayed antimicrobial therapy increases mortality and organ dysfunction duration in pediatric sepsis. Crit Care Med. 2014;42(11):2409–17.
8. Klatte JM. Pediatric antimicrobial stewardship programs: current perspectives. Pediatric Health Med Ther. 2020;11:245–55.
9. WHO. Pocket book of hospital care for children: Second edition, Guidelines for the management of common childhood illnesses. W.H. Organization, editor. World Health Organization; 2013. p. 473.
10. Sutton RM, et al. Ventilation rates and pediatric in-hospital cardiac arrest survival outcomes. Crit Care Med. 2019;47(11):1627–36.
11. WHO. Emergency Triage Assessment and Treatment (ETAT), manual for participants. Geneva: Child Health and Development, Maternal, Newborn, Child and Adolescent Health, and Ageing, World Health Organization; 2005. p. 78.
12. Sankar J, et al. Fluid bolus over 15-20 versus 5-10 minutes each in the first hour of resuscitation in children with septic shock: a randomized controlled trial. Pediatr Crit Care Med. 2017;18(10):e435–45.
13. Inwald DP, et al. Restricted fluid bolus volume in early septic shock: results of the fluids in shock pilot trial. Arch Dis Child. 2019;104(5):426–31.
14. Davis AL, et al. American College of Critical Care Medicine Clinical Practice Parameters for hemodynamic support of pediatric and neonatal septic shock. Crit Care Med. 2017;45(6):1061–93.
15. Lamontagne F, et al. Pooled analysis of higher versus lower blood pressure targets for vasopressor therapy septic and vasodilatory shock. Intensive Care Med. 2018;44(1):12–21.
16. Prakash V, Parameswaran N, Biswal N. Early versus late enteral feeding in critically ill children: a randomized controlled trial. Intensive Care Med. 2016;42(3):481–2.
17. Hamilton S, et al. A stepwise enteral nutrition algorithm for critically ill children helps achieve nutrient delivery goals*. Pediatr Crit Care Med. 2014;15(7):583–9.
18. Fentress M, et al. Point-of-care ultrasound in resource-limited settings: common applications. South Med J. 2018;111(7):424–33.
19. Balk DS, et al. Lung ultrasound compared to chest X-ray for diagnosis of pediatric pneumonia: a meta-analysis. Pediatr Pulmonol. 2018;53(8):1130–9.
20. Khan A, Rice B, Acker P. Developing emergency triage Systems in Cambodia. Cureus. 2020;12(10):e11233.

Oral Rehydration Therapy in a Low-Resource Setting

Cynthia Howard and Daniel A. Gbadero

Abbreviations

IVF	Intravenous fluids
ORS	Oral rehydration salts
ORT	Oral rehydration therapy
ReSoMal	Rehydration Solution for Malnutrition
SSS	Sugar-salt solution
UNICEF	United Nations Children's Fund
WHO	World Health Organization

1 Case Example 1

Ade is a 4-year-old boy recovering from measles in Ogbomoso, Nigeria. His appetite is poor and every effort to cajole him to eat anything is followed by vomiting with each bout of measly cough. Stools are frequent and watery. Parents bring him to the clinic due to decreased urine output. On examination his vital signs are normal including his capillary refill. He is alert and thirsty. Mucous membranes are dry. On examination he appears to be mildly dehydrated. The nurse, who is caring for him, reassures the family and Ade, while offering him ORS to drink in small sips to prevent vomiting.

C. Howard (✉)
Division of Hospital Medicine, University of Minnesota, Minneapolis, MN, USA
e-mail: drcindy@umn.edu

D. A. Gbadero
Department of Paediatrics, Bowen University, Ogbomoso, Nigeria

T. M. Slusher et al. (eds.), *Pediatric Procedural Adaptations for Low-Resource Settings*, https://doi.org/10.1007/978-3-030-99955-1_12

2 Introduction

Oral rehydration therapy (ORT), the use of the oral rehydration salt (ORS) solution to restore fluid and electrolyte balance resulting from fluid loss, is the key treatment for dehydration [1]. ORS actively stimulates the intestinal sodium/glucose transporter, SGLT1, to induce fluid absorption from the intestines [2]. Developed out of desperation, in a unique World Health Organization (WHO)/United Nations Children's Fund (UNICEF) collaboration, ORS has saved millions of children from morbidity and mortality secondary to diarrhea and dehydration [3]. ORS is a simple combination of salt, sugar, and water which, if necessary, can be made at home [4]. ORT is a simple, inexpensive, effective remedy that makes use of ORS to treat children and people with vomiting and diarrhea. It is a noninvasive alternative to intravenous fluids (IVF) except when severe dehydration with shock is present [5, 6]. Literature has shown that moderate dehydration can be treated as successfully with ORT and is the recommended treatment for moderate dehydration [7, 8]. In a systematic review by Hartling et al., only 4% of children treated with ORT required intravenous fluids [9]. While ORT is probably the most cost-beneficial scientific discovery of the twentieth century, many healthcare providers do not use it [7, 8]. This conforms with a Yoruba adage that says, "A free remedy often goes unused." Many more lives, from newborn to grandparent, could be saved by timely use of ORS in the treatment of vomiting and diarrhea regardless of the cause.

2.1 Oral Rehydration Salt Solution

In 1978, the standard WHO/UNICEF ORS (311 mmol/L) was approved for use to prevent and treat children with dehydration. Hypernatremia secondary to the high osmolality of the solution was observed resulting with the introduction of a reduced osmolality ORS (245 mmol/L) (Table 1) a few years later [10]. In a systematic review of randomized controlled trials by Houston et al. [11], stool output volume, diarrhea duration, and time to rehydration were better with reduced osmolality ORS compared with the standard WHO sodium ORS. The use of standard ORS

Table 1 Compositions of oral rehydration fluids

	Reduced osmolality ORS (mmol/L)	ReSoMal (mmol/L)
Glucose	75	125
Sodium	75	45
Potassium	20	40
Citrate	10	7
Chloride	65	76
Osmolality	245	300

(311 mmol/L) is no longer recommended [12]. The quantity of potassium chloride remains the same in the standard and reduced osmolality ORS because of the importance of potassium to replenish loss from diarrhea.

2.2 ReSoMal

In 2002, *Re*hydration *So*lution for *Mal*nutrition (ReSoMal) was created as an ORS to specifically address both dehydration and micronutrient deficiency in malnourished children. Severely malnourished children are prone to hyponatremia. The composition of ReSoMal is noted in Table 1. ReSoMal is strongly recommended by WHO in severely malnourished children with dehydration [11]. There was no difference in rehydration failure rate between ReSoMal and the standard and reduced osmolality ORS, though studies have shown more children on ReSoMal developing hyponatremia and hyponatremic seizures [11]. Because of the increased risk of hyponatremic seizures, investigators have questioned whether it is the ideal solution for children with SAM and recommend further study in African children [11]. Care should be taken when using ReSoMal to watch closely for hyponatremia and consider currently recommended reduced osmolality ORS with added potassium and other electrolytes/minerals if indicated if hyponatremia develops or worsens other on ReSoMal.

2.3 Ongoing Refinement of ORS

Despite the undeniable success of ORS, barriers to broader and more consistent use of ORS persist [5, 6]. This is believed, in part, to be because the reduction in stool output with the reduced osmolality ORS is often too subtle to perceive. Efforts to refine and improve ORS are ongoing. Zinc has been shown to reduce the duration and severity of diarrheal episodes and prevent future episodes [13]. Zinc sulfate is being considered as the latest addition to the ORS. The lifesaving properties, safety, and cost-effectiveness of ORS and zinc supplementation for treatment of diarrhea have been well-demonstrated.

2.4 Cost of Not Using ORS

IVF therapy in LMICs may prove significantly more expensive than an average family finance can accommodate. In resource-limited settings, with a paucity of trained staff to provide care for children in very busy emergency rooms, it often proves challenging for nursing to attend too many dehydrated children. It takes extra time and skill to secure IV lines in dehydrated children, in addition to time necessary for mixing fluid components. Additionally, adequately monitoring delivery of IVF can proved difficult in a busy hospital setting with limited healthcare workers. Administering IVF in resource-poor settings can be dangerous when a large volume of fluids runs inadvertently fast from IVF bags (not burettes or on pumps) with risk of causing cardiorespiratory compromise due to fluid overload. And perhaps even more importantly, even in high-income countries, ORT is appropriate for the management of the majority of children with mild to moderate dehydration.

3 Indications

- Prevention of dehydration in patients with poor oral intake or increased fluid losses. Vomiting is not a contraindication to ORT.
- Treatment of dehydration.

4 Contraindications

There are only a few absolute contraindications to using ORT for preventing and correcting dehydration.

- Acute surgical abdomen
- Shock or hemodynamic instability with poor gastrointestinal perfusion
  - *Once shock has been corrected, patients can safely be given ORS even while they continue to receive IVF therapy which is not an absolute contraindication to ORT.*
- Intractable or uncontrolled vomiting (such as that associated with a bowel obstruction)
- Altered mental status, if unable to pass nasogastric tube
  - *Comatose patients with dehydration could be given modified ORT by passing a nasogastric tube and feeding ORS to them in measured volumes through the tube.*

5 Equipment/Supplies

- Cup
- Spoon
- Nasogastric tube (NGT)
- ORS packets, ReSoMal, or homemade salt-sugar solution (SSS)

5.1 *Homemade Salt-Sugar Solution*

- Table salt
- Sugar
- Clean drinkable water

6 Technique

6.1 *Homemade Recipe*

The homemade salt-sugar solution (SSS) is a rehydration solution that can be produced in all homes regardless of the level of social status and affluence (Fig. 1). It is composed of approximately *2.6 grams of table salt* and *27 grams of sugar* dissolved in *1 liter of clean water*. SSS gives approximately 86 mmol/L of salt and 116 mmol/L of sugar but can vary dramatically depending on the recipe used. Caregivers in low-resource settings may not have access to accurately weigh the components for SSS. An alternative to weighing these ingredients is to use the nearly universally available *teaspoon* for measurements. The solution is made of *8 level-teaspoonful of granulated sugar* (three cubes of sugar) and *1/2 level-teaspoonful of table salt* added to *1 liter of clean water* [14]. Some recipes call for only 6 level teaspoons of granulated sugar

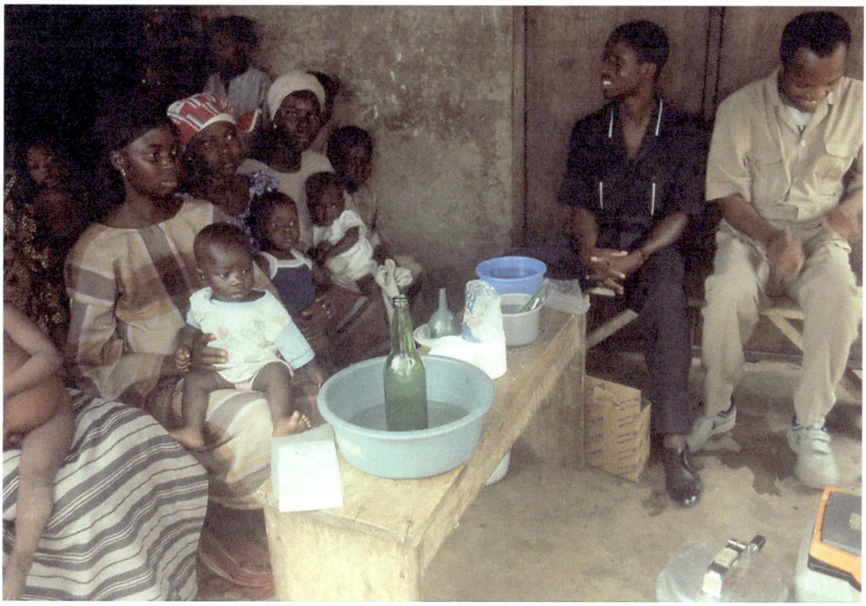

Fig. 1 Making ORS in clinic. (Figure used with permission from Dr. Howard)

instead of 8 teaspoons [15]. It is also advisable to ask the parents to *encourage foods containing potassium* such as oranges/orange juice or bananas. Parents are being taught how to make homemade ORS in Fig. 1.

A mistake to be avoided while making SSS is that of swapping the measurements of sugar and salt resulting in hypernatremic solution. Ask the parents to taste the solution before giving it to the child as a safeguard against swapping the sugar and salt. While this solution does work, in general, it is preferred to use the ORS packets if they are available due to the other components and accurate osmolality. WHO guidelines state that a range of osmolality is safe, from 245 to 310 mmol/L, with a range of higher and lower sodium and glucose contents as well [5].

7 Instructions for Use

Oral rehydration therapy can be administered most effectively based on the treatment plans outlined in the World Health Organization Pocketbook of Hospital Care for Children, 13th edition "Diarrhea Treatment Plans." There are three plans (A, B, C) that can be chosen from based on the clinical status of the child [5].

- *No signs of dehydration (<5%) → Plan A*: home treatment.
- *Some signs of dehydration (5–10%) → Plan B*: ORS administered in the clinic with reassessment for admission or discharge home.
- *Severe signs of dehydration (>10%) → Plan C*: admission and intravenous fluids (IVF) – *described in Case Example 2.*

7.1 Determine Level of Dehydration

The volume of ORS to administer to a child is determined mainly by the degree of dehydration of the patient. Degree of dehydration (mild, moderate, or severe or no, some severe if using the WHO classification) can be determined by the patients' weight, or physical exam.

If the recent ideal weight of the patient is known, the current weight may be subtracted from the ideal weight to determine the percentage of dehydration. For example, if the weight is 10 kg as measured on attending the healthy baby clinic and the child arrives with diarrhea the following day with a weight of 9.5 kg the percentage weight loss is calculated as follows:

$$\text{Percentage wt.loss} = \text{difference in weight}\left(0.5\,\text{kg}\right) / \text{real weight}\left(10\,\text{kg}\right) \times 100 = 5\%$$

It is important that during physical examination, care is taken to observe and document the signs of dehydration in patients. Please note that percentage numbers assigned to each category of dehydration in infants, that is, 5%, 10%, and 15% for mild, moderate, and severe dehydration, respectively, are different for older children

Table 2 Physical exam findings and level of dehydration

Physical exam findings and level of dehydration			
	Mild	Moderate	Severe
Mental status	Alert	Lethargic	Obtunded
Anterior Fontanelle	Flat	Flat to sunken	Sunken
Eyes	Normal	Normal	Sunken
Mouth	Moist	Dry	Parched
Skin turgor	Normal	Sluggish	Tenting
Heart rate	Normal	Increased	Increased
Capillary refill	Normal	2–3 seconds	>3 seconds
Pulses	Easily palpated	Palpated	Thready to absent
Blood pressure	Normal	Borderline to normal	Decreased
Tears	Normal	Decreased	Absent

Adapted from World Health Organization. The Treatment of diarrhoea: a manual for physicians and other senior health workers [5]

who are assigned the percentages of 3%, 6%, and 9%, respectively, for mild, moderate and severe dehydration. This is since the proportion of body water in infants is much higher than in older children.

Careful physical examination also helps both to determine the level of dehydration (Table 2) of patients and exclude the presence of an acute surgical abdomen.

Urine output may also be used to determine state of hydration. Oliguria indicates severe dehydration.

Most children in the mildly dehydrated group can safely be treated on an ambulatory basis. The volume of ORS needed for rehydration should be calculated to take care of deficit, maintenance, and ongoing losses.

7.2 *Treatment Plan A and B*

The caregiver is instructed to give ORS frequently at a calculated volume per unit time. Those with mild and moderate dehydration not requiring admission should be placed on ORT and observed in the clinic before they are allowed to go home if they tolerate ORS well. Cup and spoon should be used to administer ORS to younger children. A guide which we have found useful for our patients is using different spoon sizes to give calculated ORS at a spoon per 1–2 minutes while the child is awake.

Practically, ORS volume for rehydrating children per minute varies from 2 ml for term newborns to 15 ml for full-grown adolescents. Table 3 provides some estimated volumes for amount to give in the first 4 hours [16]. For those on observation, the patient and parent should be comfortably located in an ORS space in the clinic for 2–4 hours. After the allotted time, the child is evaluated for ORS tolerance and improvement to determine whether the child should be discharged, have ongoing observation, or be admitted to the hospital. If frequent stooling or persistent

Table 3 Fluid replacement or treatment recommendations per Center for Disease Control and Prevention

Fluid replacement or treatment recommendations				
Dehydration type	Treatment recommendation	Administration method		
Severe dehydration	Intravenous Ringer's lactate or, if not available, normal saline and ORS as outlined in the guidance above	Administer as follows:		
		Age <1 year	Timeframe	Total volume
			0–60 min	30 ml/kg[a]
			60 min–6 h	70 ml/kg
			6 h–24 h	100 ml/kg
		Administer as follows:		
		Age≥1 year	Timeframe	Total volume
			0–30 min	30 ml/kg[a]
			30 min–3 h	70 ml/kg
Some dehydration	Oral rehydration solution	*Administer in first 4 hours*:		
		Age all ages	Volume of ORS	
			75 ml/kg in first 4 hours. Then reassess, and if patient still shows signs of dehydration, repeat. If not, use ORS to replace ongoing diarrheal losses using the treatment plan for no dehydration below. Patients do not need IV fluids, but need close monitoring during the first 4 hours	
No dehydration	*Oral rehydration solution*	*Administer after each loose stool*:		
		Age	Volume of ORS	
		<2 years	50–100 ml	
		2–9 years	100–200 ml	
		≥10 years	As much as patient wants	

[a] Repeat once if radial pulse is still very weak or not detectable

vomiting, or the child is without significant improvement, the child should be admitted for further observation and consideration for nasogastric tube or intravenous fluid (IVF) therapy if evidence of shock (Case Example 2). Continue ORT along with the IVFs, decreasing the volume and increasing the times between spoons of ORT until tolerance is achieved. For example, in a toddler who is still vomiting, consider decreasing from 1 teaspoon every 1–2 minutes to 3/4 teaspoon every 3–5 minutes.

There is no benefit to be gained by giving ORS rapidly. In fact, rapid administration can be counterproductive by causing distention of the stomach and vomiting, which discourages parents and suggests that ORT does not work. Slow administration allows for glucose-enhanced absorption of sodium and water, which takes place in the intestines and the stomach. If the volume of ORS absorbable per unit time is not exceeded, the possibility of vomiting by patients is reduced to the barest minimum [5].

While using ORS to rehydrate patients, it is okay to give additional potable water in small volumes to patients if they are thirsty and express desire to drink. Breastfeeding infants on ORT should also be permitted to breastfeed on demand.

8 Case 1 Resolution

Ade meets criteria for WHO ORT plan B initially. Ade's parents agree to offer him sips (5 ml) of ORS (WHO packet) every 2 minutes in the waiting room. Within 2 hours, he urinates and eats 1/2 of a banana without vomiting. He is transitioned to WHO ORT plan A. Parents are given recipe for homemade ORS should they use all their ORS packets. He returns home and on follow-up the next day he appears well-hydrated with moist mucus membranes. ORT is stopped and parents are advised to continue feeding Ade a well-balanced diet of fruits, vegetables, grains, and protein.

9 Case Example 2

Ayo, an 8-month-old, previously healthy female infant presents to the acute care unit in Ibadan, Nigeria, with her parents whose chief complaint is diarrhea for 3 days. Her parents decided to bring her for medical attention due to lack of production of identifiable urine for at least 12 hours and refusal to drink. In addition, she was vomiting occasionally and had felt "hot to touch." No blood has been noted in the stool or the vomit. Her immunization shots are up to date except for the rotavirus vaccine. It is of note that Ayo was weaned from breastfeeding at 6 months of age at which time she refused breastfeeding despite her mother's efforts to continue. Her diet now is primarily corn pap mixed with formula milk, when available and some adult diet eaten in the family which the mother is trying to introduce to her. No one else in the household is ill, although an 18-month-old cousin visited the hospital 5 days earlier with diarrhea. No prior weight is available.

On physical examination, she has a temperature of 38°C (100°F), respiratory rate of 50 bpm, heart rate of 140 bpm, and blood pressure of 68/35 mmHg. Her weight is 6 kg and her height is 67 cm with Wt/Ht < 2 SD. She appears sleepy and lethargic. No tears are formed when she cries. Her anterior fontanelle is open and sunken. She has slightly sunken eyes and dry mucus membranes. She has a normal respiratory exam apart from increased respiratory rate and she is tachycardic with weak pulses and capillary refill of 4 seconds. She has tenting of her skin.

Her labs reveal a hemoglobin of 11.5 g/dl, negative malaria smear, and serum glucose of 3.3 mmol/L (60 mg/dl).

She is diagnosed with:

1. *Acute diarrheal disease*
2. *Severe (>10%) dehydration*
3. *Hypoglycemia*
4. *Malnutrition specifically wasting*

She is treated with a bolus of 12 ml of 12.5% dextrose. Ayo opens her eyes but refuses to drink. No NGT is available. WHO plan C is started with administration of IVF based on her calculated fluid requirement.

Her fluid requirement for 24 hours is calculated thus:

- *Estimated ongoing losses: 5 ml/kg per stool/emesis.*
- *Total fluid requirement for 24 hours is about 1200 mL plus additional fluids for ongoing stools and emesis as above.*
- *The total volume divided into three parts. 0–60 minutes 30mL/kg or 180 mLs; 60 minutes–6 hours 70 mL/kg or 420 mLs; 6–24 hours 100 mLs/kg or 600 mLs.*
- *The first portion of 180 ml fluid is given as Ringer's lactate solution given in 60 minutes. As the child improves and is eager to drink, the remaining fluid is administered as reduced osmolality ORS (ReSolMol) 420 mL or about 84 mL/hour from 60 minutes through 6 hours with the final 600 mL being given over the reminder of the 24 hours or about 33 mL/hour. In addition she is given 30 mL each time she passes diarrheal stool or vomits. She is monitored closely for any evidence of over-hydration and ongoing looses which would change total amount of fluid given. (In this scenario ie when a child is both hypovolemic and hypoglycemic, some clinicians will give D5 lactated ringers or D5 normal saline as the initial bolus of IVF's instead of giving the bolus of dextrose and fluids separately. In either methods glucose must be rechecked to assure that the child is now normoglycemic. If possible the serum sodium should also be followed with change to the standard reduced osmolality ORS if she becomes hyponatremic.*
- *After her shock resolves the child is permitted to drink water and eat food on request to alleviate her thirst and hunger. If she were still breastfeeding this would be continued as well.*

9.1 Treatment Plan C

Reassessment of the patient's hydration status must be regularly done to ensure that the hydration plan is effective. Attention to mental status and urine output is particularly important markers of success or failure. One of the common reasons for unsuccessful treatment is the inability or oversight in replacing ongoing losses. Records must be strictly kept of fluid input and output along with the vital signs in addition to recording daily weights of patients on admission. Estimated volumes of vomitus, stools, and urine must be recorded to aid review process and ability to calculate accurately the fluid balance with each review to determine whether patients are making good progress. Regular evaluations of patients must be undertaken at the end of each period for which fluid was calculated to ensure that the patient is responding appropriately.

10 Complications

- Electrolyte imbalance (hyponatremia, hypoglycemia, hypernatremia)
- Emesis
- Aspiration

11 Conclusion

In summary, ORS is effective for preventing and correcting dehydration in all ages. It has proved the saving grace of many children and their families. ORS is an important remedy for preventing dehydration as well as for replacing lost fluids and electrolytes in children with acute diarrhea. On a short-term basis, the classic WHO oral rehydration solution, and its modified forms, can be used in all patients including those who are severely malnourished, and the salt-sugar solution (SSS) works effectively to prevent and correct severe dehydration, hypoglycemia, electrolyte imbalance, acute kidney injury, malnutrition, and death that often result from poorly treated acute diarrheal episodes.

As a simple and highly effective remedy is available in ORT for preventing and correcting dehydration, all efforts must be made to assure that parents and health-care providers are knowledgeable about ORS and the appropriate use of ORS. Widespread acceptance of ORS as an effective treatment to prevent and treat dehydration will further reduce the morbidity and mortality resulting from diarrhea and dehydration.

12 Case 2 Resolution

Her glucose normalizes on recheck at 1 hour. Her vomiting decreases and resolves at 6 hours. After 24 hours Ayo is adequately hydrated. She continues to receive her daily requirement of fluid with a bland diet, orange juice, and occasional drinks of water to satisfy her thirst until she is discharged home 3 days after admission when diarrhea has resolved. She is transitioned to a high-protein meal fortified with milk, eggs, and ground fish meals. Ayo is given vitamin A 100,000 units to be repeated a week later, vitamin B 5 ml daily for a month, and zinc supplement 20 mg daily for 2 weeks. She is followed regularly for the next 7 months. Her malnutrition resolves. At 15 months she is thriving and developing normally.

13 For Further Reading

1. Firima E, Forsberg B. Knowledge and recommendation of oral rehydration solution and zinc for management of childhood diarrhoea among patent and proprietary medicine vendors in Port Harcourt, Nigeria. https://doi.org/10.29392/001c.12252.
2. Blum LS, Oria PA, Olson CK, Breiman RF, Pavani K. Ram examining the use of oral rehydration salts and other oral rehydration therapy for childhood diarrhea in Kenya. Am J Trop Med Hyg. 2011;85(6):1126–33. https://doi.org/10.4269/ajtmh.2011.11-0171.
3. Nalin DR, Cash RA. 50 years of oral rehydration therapy: the solution is still simple. Lancet. 2018;392(10147):536–8. This provides a great 50 years overview about the history of ORS as well as recent advancements and changes to the formulation.
4. Black R, Fontaine O, Lamberti L, Bhan M, Huicho L, El Arifeen S, Masanja H, Walker CF, Mengestu TK, Pearson L, Young M, Orobaton N, Chu Y, Jackson B, Bateman M, Walker N, Merson M. Drivers of the reduction in childhood diarrhea mortality 1980–2015 and interventions to eliminate preventable diarrhea deaths by 2030.
5. Black RE, Morris, Bryce J. Where and why are 10 million dying every year. Lancet 2003;361: 2226–34.
6. GBD Diarrhoea Diseases Collaborators, C. et al. Estimates of global, regional and national morbidity, mortality and aetiologies of diarrhea diseases: a systemic analysis for the Global Burden of Diseases Study 2015. Lancet Infect Dis. 2014;17:909–48.
7. Barnett E, Parashar HD, Tate JE. Global impact of Rotavirus vaccination on diarrhoea hospitalizations and deaths among children <5 years old: 2006–2019. J Infect Dis. 2020. https://doi.org/10.1093/Infdis/Jiaa089.

References

1. Ofei SY, Fuchs GJ 3rd. Principles and practice of Oral rehydration. Curr Gastroenterol Rep. 2019;21(12):67.
2. Chen L, Tuo B, Dong H. Regulation of intestinal glucose absorption by ion channels and transporters. Nutrients. 2016;8(1):43.
3. Hirschhorn N. The treatment of acute diarrhea in children. An historical and physiological perspective. Am J Clin Nutr. 1980;33(3):637–63.
4. Binder HJ, et al. Oral rehydration therapy in the second decade of the twenty-first century. Curr Gastroenterol Rep. 2014;16(3):376.
5. WHO. The treatment of diarrhoea: a manual for physicians and other senior health workers, 4th rev. World Health Organization; 2005.

6. Boschi-Pinto C, Velebit L, Shibuya K. Estimating child mortality due to diarrhoea in developing countries. Bull World Health Organ. 2008;86(9):710–7.
7. Spandorfer PR, et al. Oral versus intravenous rehydration of moderately dehydrated children: a randomized, controlled trial. Pediatrics. 2005;115(2):295–301.
8. Hartman S, et al. Gastroenteritis in children. Am Fam Physician. 2019;99(3):159–65.
9. Hartling L, et al. Oral versus intravenous rehydration for treating dehydration due to gastroenteritis in children. Cochrane Database Syst Rev. 2006;3:CD004390.
10. WHO. Oral rehydration salts production of the new ORS. World Health Organization; 2006.
11. Houston KA, Gibb JG, Maitland K. Oral rehydration of malnourished children with diarrhoea and dehydration: a systematic review. Wellcome Open Res. 2017;2:66.
12. Santosham M, et al. A double-blind clinical trial comparing World Health Organization oral rehydration solution with a reduced osmolarity solution containing equal amounts of sodium and glucose. J Pediatr. 1996;128(1):45–51.
13. Walker CL, Black RE. Zinc for the treatment of diarrhoea: effect on diarrhoea morbidity, mortality and incidence of future episodes. Int J Epidemiol. 2010;39(Suppl 1):i63–9.
14. Dippenaar H, Joubert G, Nel R, Bantobetse ML, Opawole AA, Roshen KS. Homemade sugar-salt solution for oral rehydration: knowledge of mothers and caregivers. SA Fam Pract. 2005;47(2):51–3.
15. Focus of Diarrhea, Dehydration and Rehydration. [cited 2021 10/27/2021]; Available from: rehydrate.org.
16. CDC. Rehydration therapy. [2020 October 2, 2020 11/16/2021]; Available from: https://www.cdc.gov/cholera/treatment/rehydration-therapy.html.

Malnutrition: Practical Approaches to Feeding a Severely Malnourished Child in a Low-Resource Setting

Lindsey Cooper and Victor Musiime

Abbreviations

RUTF Ready to use Therapeutic Food
WHO World Health Organization

1 Case Example

A 4-year-old child presents to your outlying health facility in the Democratic Republic of Congo with whole-body edema and anemia with no appetite. He seems very small. You are not accustomed to seeing this and do not have many resources. He tests positive for malaria. You are looking for practical ways to prepare therapeutic milk and calculate calories. You are also looking for advice on whether you should place a nasogastric tube.

L. Cooper (✉)
Centre Medicale Evangelique-Nyankunde, Democratic Republic of Congo, Department of Pediatrics, Nyankunde, Democratic Republic of Congo

V. Musiime
Makerere University, Department of Paediatrics and Child Health, Kampala, Uganda

Joint Clinical Research Centre, Kampala, Uganda

T. M. Slusher et al. (eds.), *Pediatric Procedural Adaptations for Low-Resource Settings*, https://doi.org/10.1007/978-3-030-99955-1_13

2 Introduction

Malnutrition in children under 5 years is very prevalent in low- to middle-income countries. One out of four children in low- to middle-income countries is underweight. The risk of death increases tenfold with the most severely malnourished children compared to well-nourished children [1]. It is critical for the practitioner to know the basics of re-feeding a malnourished child, perhaps in a lower resource setting.

The goal of this chapter is to give practical information on working with re-feeding protocols in the stabilization and rehabilitation phases with malnourished children, in the inpatient setting and on discharge or as an outpatient. Regarding stabilization, this chapter addresses how to use therapeutic milk (F75/F100) and ready-to-use therapeutic feeds (RUTF), how to calculate daily caloric needs, and when/how to transition to complementary foods. In regard to rehabilitation, it addresses practical complementary foods, follow-up and recovery foods, and practical cooking and feeding advice. There is a short section that addresses failure to thrive in babies less than six (6) months of life. Management of the malnourished child is a very extensive topic and includes treating concurrent infections and specific deficiencies. This chapter only deals with the very basics of feeding a malnourished child. Whereas overweight and obesity are a form of malnutrition, this chapter focuses on undernutrition.

The goal of this chapter is not to discuss detailed diagnosis and management of malnutrition. Please refer to the WHO Ten Steps for Management of Malnutrition (Fig. 1) or other similar in-country protocols when caring for children with malnutrition. These children often present with a host of problems such as hypothermia, electrolyte imbalances, infection, etc. Feeding is only one piece of their treatment.

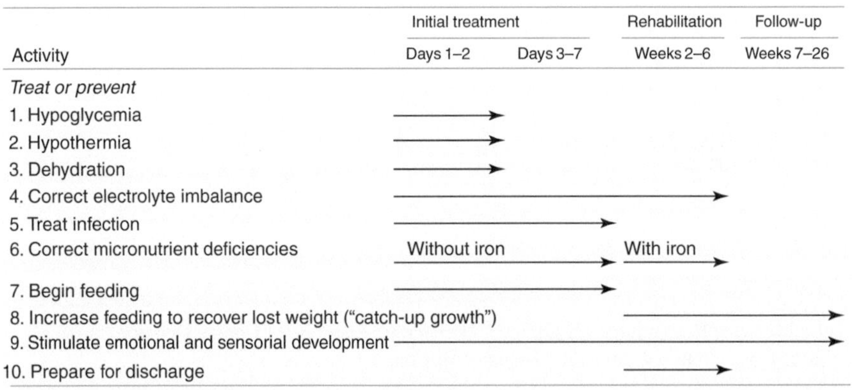

Fig. 1 World Health Organization's 10-step plan for the management of severe acute malnutrition [2]

See Fig. 1 that shows one long-standing guide for the management of these children [2]. Another resource is the WHO pocketbook for Care of Hospitalized Children which is currently being updated [3].

2.1 Indications for Inpatient Re-feeding

If a child has severe edema or falls in the standard deviation −3 weight for height or has medical complications he should be hospitalized and treated for severe malnutrition. The goal of the initial stabilization phase is to meet the child's basic metabolic needs without overwhelming the body systems. The goal is to reduce edema, treat concurrent infections, correct electrolyte imbalances, and gain an appetite. The initial stage of re-feeding is done with a formula called F75 and calories are kept at 100 kcal/kg/day.

If the child passes an appetite test with RUTF, he enters the second phase with the goal of weight gain. Calories are increased to 130 kcal/kg/day. The current WHO recommendation is to wait until the child achieves the standard deviation of −2 weight/height standard and has resolution of edema for 2 weeks prior to discharge to an appropriate outpatient nutrition program.

3 Contraindications

There are no contraindications to admitting a child for inpatient re-feeding therapy.

4 Equipment

4.1 Stabilization Phase: Therapeutic Milk: F75/F100

The initial phase of inpatient nutritional treatment is based on a low-protein milk known as F75. Children are started on F75 with the goal of restoring metabolic homeostasis, prior to changing to F100 or RUTF for catch-up growth. The majority of calories in F75 come from carbohydrates, including sucrose, lactose, and maltodextrin. Malabsorption can occur in the stabilization phase leading to osmotic diarrhea. Zinc supplements are recommended to assist in absorption.

The current World Health Organization guidelines suggest transitioning from F75 directly to RUTF like Plumpy Nut if the child's appetite is preserved and they pass the 'appetite test' [4, 5]. A successful appetite test is considered the ability to consume at least 50% of RUTF such as Plumpy Nut. If children fail the 'appetite test' it is recommended to proceed with F100 and make a slower transition [5–7].

F75 obtained its' name due to the concentration of the milk: 75 kcal and 0.9 g protein/100 cc; F100 contains 100 kcal and 2.9 g protein/100 cc.

4.2 Rehabilitation Phase

4.2.1 Complimentary and Transition Foods

Following the stabilization phase (usually 1–2 weeks), children begin the rehabilitation phase with the goal of replenishing nutrient stories and attaining a healthy weight gain. During a hospitalization, children wean to complimentary foods such as fortified porridge and Plumpy Nut. The focus is on providing a diet with high energy density. There are reduced amounts of water to avoid early satiety.

Fortified porridge may consist of ground mixes of soy/corn/rice/peanut/sorghum, or other grains. Ready-to-use therapeutic food (RUTF)/Plumpy Nut® is a cereal-based preparation that has a similar nutrient composition as F100.

The goal in the rehabilitation phase is to provide at least 150 kcal/kg/day macronutrient foods and 4 g protein/kg/day. This transition to recovery foods should begin in the inpatient setting to ensure success.

Children should receive an average of five (5) meals/day and snacks with high energy content. As a practical point, families need to be encouraged to cook foods early in the day that can be used throughout the day. In many cultures the main meal is consumed in the evening, so the change to an earlier cooking schedule needs to be reinforced. Also, in many parts of the world, charcoal and wood are used as fuel sources which are available in limited quantity. Beans are often a good plant protein choice as they are durable and can be easily reheated. Families can be encouraged to roast nuts, prepare eggs as ready-made protein-rich snacks.

Protein-rich foods consist of eggs, nuts, beans, meats, certain green leafy vegetables, etc. The suggested protein intake should be 12% of the daily energy consumption. Meat products are rich in micronutrients and low in anti-nutrients and are needed in the diet in addition to plant proteins. Anti-nutrients such as phytates or tannins are compounds in plant-based foods that bind nutrients of other positively charged minerals (calcium, magnesium, and iron). Phytates are found in certain vegetables, and tannins in black tea and dark sorghum. Roasting, malting, and fermenting can reduce the content of phytates before consumption. The so-called 'meat factor' allows for greater absorption of iron from plant-based sources.

Fat consumption should be 35–50% of daily calories. Essential fatty acids are crucial in skin health. Carbohydrates should make up to 60% of daily calorie intake.

Recipes for good mixed meals for more specifics on examples for well-balanced recovery foods [8] (Table 1). Other recipes are provided here, compliments of Dr. Ife Ojo (West Africa recipe) and Dr. Eyovwherhi Ibiyeye (Table 2).

4.2.2 Other Situations: Children Younger Than 6 Months

Recent research shows that malnutrition in the first 6 months of life is fairly prevalent, reaching up to 30% in some countries and 15% in lower-income countries. The WHO doubles this prevalence of malnutrition in children <6 months [4]. The goal in children <6 months of life should always be to return to exclusive breastfeeding

Table 1 Recipes for good mixed meals (each meal fulfills 1/3 daily energy, protein, iron, and Vitamin A needs)

Ingredients		Food preparation directions
Example from East Africa (maize + groundnuts + spinach meal)		Make porridge with maize flour. Pound groundnuts and add to porridge. Before serving, add the raw egg and cook for a few minutes. Fry onion and tomato for flavor, add spinach.
Thick maize porridge	4½ tablespoons (140 g)	
Groundnut paste	1 tablespoon (15 g)	
Egg	One (30 g)	
Spinach	Handful of leaves (20 g)	
Example from India (chapati + dhal + carrot/ amaranthus meal)		Cook lentils with spices. Add carrot and ghee when dhal is nearly ready. Serve with chapati and steamed amaranthus.
Chapati	Half (50 g)	
Dhal (cooked)	1 tablespoon	
Carrot	Half (25 g)	
Amaranthus	Handful (30 g)	
Ghee	1 teaspoon (5 g)	
Milk	1/2 cup (50 g)	
Example from South America (rice + beans + liver)		Boil the beans with onions and spices until soft. Add potato and continue cooking. Cook liver and add to stew. Mash potato, beans, and liver with well-cooked rice a little margarine.
Rice	3 tablespoons (84 g)	
Bean and potato stew	1 tablespoon (30 g)	
Liver	1/2 tablespoon (15 g)	
Margarine	1 teaspoon (5 g)	
Example from Syria, Middle East (rice + lentils + yoghurt)		Fry onions and add spices. Boil lentils until soft. Cook rice and add rice and lentils and liquid to the onions. Simmer and serve with yogurt.
Cooked rice	3 tablespoons (84 g)	
Lentils	1.5 tablespoons (30 g)	
Oil	1 teaspoon (5 g)	
Yoghurt	3 tablespoons (50 g)	
Orange	½ (50 g)	
Fry onions and add spices. Boil lentils until soft. Cook rice and add rice and lentils and liquid to the onions. Simmer and serve with yogurt.		
Example from West Africa (lentils + beans + crayfish *Tom Brown recipe:*		Wash outer layer off beans Mix all ingredients and roast and grind to paste Take a desired quantity of powder for a meal. Boil and stir for 5–10 minutes (like Ogi)
Groundnuts roasted	1 cup	
Guinea corn.	4 cups	
Millet.	2 cups	
Maize	4 cups	
Beans	½ cup	
Crayfish.	½ cup	

From "Complimentary Feeding: Family Foods for Breastfed Children", WHO, 2000 [8]. West Africa, which is compliments of Dr. Ife Ojo

Table 2 Other examples of good meals (compliments of Eyovwherhi Ibiyeye)

Ingredients	Preparation
Guinea corn, crayfish, date syrup and soybeans flour Guinea corn and maize powder: 4 tablespoons (60 g) Soybeans powder: 2 tablespoons (30 g) Blended crayfish: 1 tablespoon (15 g) Date syrup: 1 tablespoon (15 ml)	Mix the guinea corn water with a little quantity of water to make a paste, Add already boiling water to the paste, add the soybeans powder and blended crayfish allow to cook for 5 minutes. Serve into a plate and add the date syrup
Cowpea, fresh maize, onion, chili pepper, palm oil, and crayfish Cowpea: 1 cup Fresh maize: 2 medium cob Med sized onion: 1 Chili pepper: 1 Palm oil: 2 tablespoons (30 ml) Crayfish: 2 tablespoons blended (30 g) Salt: Pinch	Remove the maize from the cob, while beans is already cooking. When the beans is half cooked, add the maize, the medium chopped onion, blended chili pepper, and palm oil. Add the pinch of salt, allow to cook until it is very tender add the crayfish cook for another 3 minutes. Serve on a plate for baby
Guinea corn, millet, groundnut, soybean flour, date syrup Guinea corn and millet powder: 4 tablespoons (60 g) Soybean powder: 2 tablespoons (30 g) Date syrup: 1 tablespoon (15 ml)	Mix guinea corn and millet flour into a thick paste, measure 2 cups of water into a pot bring to boil, pour the paste into the boiling water, allow to cook until it is smooth and consistent texture, add the Soybeans powder, allow to cook for 3 minutes. Serve into a plate and add the date syrup serve to baby
Yam porridge, spinach, onion, pepper, palm oil, crayfish, and boiled egg Yam: 100 g Onion: 1 medium Chili pepper: 1 Palm oil: 3 tablespoons (45 ml) Crayfish: 2 tablespoons (30 g) Egg: 1 boiled Spinach: as desired	Slice the peeled yam into small cuts place into a pot, add the pepper, onion, and palm oil. Allow to cook until the water is almost completely dry, mash the yam using the ladle, add a pinch of salt, pounded spinach, and blended crayfish cover the pot with the lid to retain nutrients in the spinach cook for 2 minutes. Serve to baby with the boiled egg
Ewedu or okro and yam flour or cassava flour **2 cups yam/cassava flour** Grated okro/ewedu: 50 g Chili pepper: 1 Palm oil: 2 teaspoons (10 ml) Fermented locust beans: 1 tablespoon (15 g) Salt: pinch Mashed fish: 50 g	To prepare yam flour (Amala), mix the 2 cups with little quantity of water to make a paste, boil 500 ml of water in a pot, add the paste, use the ladle to stir until it turns brown in color and it forms a soft pudding. To prepare soup, add a little quantity of water to the ewedu/okro, add the pepper, pinch of salt, palm oil, and locust beans. Lastly, add the mashed fish, allow everything to cook for 7 minutes, serve into a plate for baby, alongside the amala

whenever possible. The WHO recommends using human milk followed by infant formula, F-75, and diluted F-100 (1:1.5 ratio formula to water). A medical work-up should be done to look for organic causes of malnutrition, such as Hirschsprung's disease or milk-protein allergy.

First foods should be introduced after 6 months of life, such as porridge and pureed vegetables.

Table 3 Calculating caloric needs in stabilization and rehabilitation phases

Goals	Example: child weighing 10 kg	Calculation of kcal to volume in cc	Cc/feed (cc/#feeds per day)
Stabilization phase: F75@ 100 kcal/kg/day and up to 135 kcal/kg/day	100 kcal/kg/day × 10 kg = 1000 kcal/day	1000 kcal × 100 cc/75 kcal (concentration of F75) = 1333 cc/day	1333 cc F75/6feeds =222 cc/feed
Rehabilitation phase: Transition to F100 or ready-to-use therapeutic food 150–200 kcal/kg/day	150 kcal/kg/day × 10 kg = 1500 kcal/day	1500 kcal × 100 cc/100 kcal (concentration of F100) = 1500 cc/jour	1500 cc (1500 kcal) of F100/6 feeds = 250 cc/feed OR 500 kcal (1 packet plumpy nut) × 3

5 Technique/Goals

The goal of the initial stabilization phase is to meet the child's basic metabolic needs without overwhelming the body systems. The goal is to reduce edema, treat concurrent infections, correct electrolyte imbalances, and gain an appetite. The initial stage of re-feeding is done with a formula called F75 and calories are kept at 100 kcal/kg/day.

If the child passes an appetite test with RUTF, he enters the rehabilitation phase with the goal of weight gain (Table 3). Calories are increased to 130–150 kcal/kg/day. The current WHO recommendation is to wait until the child achieves the standard deviation of −2 weight/height standard and has resolution of edema for 2 weeks prior to discharge to an appropriate outpatient nutrition program.

6 Instructions for Use

Sometimes the commercial formulation of F75 and F100 is not available or programmatic support ends. It is necessary that hospitals and clinics have the ability to reformulate therapeutic milk. This can be done with dried whole milk or fresh cow's milk and microvitamins can be replaced separately.

It is possible to reconstitute F75 and F100 from locally available ingredients! Dried whole milk or fresh cow's milk can be used to make the milk, which is a great option as it does not require cooking facilities. Using the recipe listed below follow these general steps (Table 4) for exact quantities):

- Mix the milk powder and sugar together in 1 L measuring container [9].
- Add oil to make a paste.
- Add mineral mix and then add boiled, cooled water up to 1000 ml.
- Whisk vigorously.

Table 4 Recipes for F75 and F100

Alternatives	Ingredient	Amount of F-75	Amount of F-100
Re-constitute with dried whole milk	Dried whole milk	35 g	110 g
	Sugar	100 g	50 g
	Vegetable oil	20 g	30 g
	Mineral mix (ORS)	20 ml	20 ml
	Water to make 1000 ml	1000 ml	1000 ml
Make with fresh cow's milk	Fresh cow's milk or full cream long-life milk	300 ml	880 ml
	Sugar	100 g	75 g
	Vegetable oil	20 g	20 g
	Mineral mix (ORS)	20 ml	20 ml
	Water to make 1000 ml	1000 ml	1000 ml

6.1 Discharge from an Inpatient Facility

There are basic principles for discharge from an inpatient re-feeding program. In general, this includes reduced body edema, a good appetite, increased activity, resolve of medical complications, and the ability to be discharged to community-based care. It is recommended to achieve a weight-height z-score of >−2 and MUAC >125 mm whenever possible. It has been recommended to have had resolve of edema for more than 2 weeks, especially if there is a long history of malnutrition. It may not always be possible to base discharge on long-standing resolve of edema, but it is a conservative approach. It is absolutely critical to have good outpatient follow-up, daily initially and then weekly for several months. If there is a concern for food insecurity in the home, prolonged inpatient therapy or daily outpatient supplementation may be indicated. Alternative home placement may need to be considered [5, 10].

7 Complications/Troubleshooting

See resources on management of severe acute malnutrition for details on diagnosis, prevention, and management of re-feeding syndrome [5]. As noted in the introduction, these children are at risk for severe fluid and electrolyte, mineral, vitamin deficits, and imbalances both acutely with SAM and with re-feeding, i.e., hypernatremia, hypokalemia, hypomagnesemia, hypophosphatemia, fluid overload, etc. Additionally, they are at increased risk for infections, anemia, neurodevelopmental delay, and a host of other problems. If after a child passes into the rehabilitation phase and develops complications such as a poor appetite or poor weight gain, he should receive therapeutic milk again. Even during the rehabilitation phase consider all possible medical complications which can impact appetite, namely anemia and infectious diseases such as tuberculosis.

8 Case Resolution

The child tests positive for severe malaria and is treated with artemisin. He starts on F75 (100 kcal/kg/day) and makes rapid progress in his appetite for a few days, but then has regression. His edema remains and you decide to check his hemoglobin, finding it to be 5 g/dl. After receiving blood transfusion given slowly in repeated small aliquots of 5 ml/kg, his edema improves and he is able to transition to F100. After 2 weeks he shows interest in solid foods and transitions to Plumpy Nut and fortified porridge. He achieves the SD-1 and is discharged to outpatient therapy.

References

1. Lenters LM, et al. Treatment of severe and moderate acute malnutrition in low- and middle-income settings: a systematic review, meta-analysis and Delphi process. BMC Public Health. 2013;13(Suppl 3):S23.
2. Black RE, et al. Reproductive, maternal, newborn, and child health: key messages of this volume. In: Black RE, et al., editors. Reproductive, maternal, newborn, and child health: disease control priorities, vol. 2. 3rd ed. Washington: World Bank; 2016.
3. WHO. Pocket book of hospital care for children: guidelines for the management of common childhood illnesses. 2nd ed. Geneva: World Health Organization; 2013.
4. Kerac M, et al. Prevalence of wasting among under 6-month-old infants in developing countries and implications of new case definitions using WHO growth standards: a secondary data analysis. Arch Dis Child. 2011;96(11):1008–13.
5. WHO. Guideline: updates on the management of severe acute malnutrition in infants and children. Geneva: World Health Organization; 2013.
6. Lanyero B, et al. Transition from F-75 to ready-to-use therapeutic food in children with severe acute malnutrition, an observational study in Uganda. Nutr J. 2017;16(1):52.
7. WHO. Training course on the management of severe malnutrition. Genava: World Health Organization; 2002.
8. WHO. Complementary feeding family foods for breasged children. Genava: World Health Organization; 2000.
9. Ashworth A, Khanum S, Jackson A, Schofield C. Guidelines for the inpatient treatment of severely malnourished children/ Ann Ashworth U' [et al.]. Appendix 5. https://apps.who.int/iris/handle/10665/42724; 2003.
10. Fox D, Erbele P, Philip F. Textbook of global child health. 2nd ed. Chapter 22. Malnutrition. USA: American Academy of Pediatrics; 2015.

Intraosseous Line Placement for Medical Therapy in a Low-Resource Setting

Beatrice Odongkara and Venice Omona

Abbreviation

IO Intraosseous

1 Case Example

An 8-month-old female infant is admitted to a pediatric acute care unit in Uganda with a one-week history of fever, vomiting, and diarrhea. On admission, she had generalized weakness and failure to breastfeed with a declining level of consciousness. On your examination, she appears to have good nutritional status, but is unresponsive (coma), with hyperpyrexia to 39.5 °C, hepatosplenomegaly, and severe palmar and mucous membranes pallor. Malaria rapid diagnostic test is positive, and microscopy shows two plus malaria parasites. Hemoglobin is 3.7 g/dl. The presentation is consistent with a diagnosis of severe malaria anemia. Intravenous access is unsuccessful after several attempts, therefore intraosseous (IO) access is deemed appropriate but no commercial IO needles are available. You wonder what other options are available.

B. Odongkara (✉)
Department of Paediatrics and Child Health Gulu, Gulu University, Gulu, Uganda

V. Omona
Department of Paediatrics and Child Health, Gulu University, Gulu, Uganda

Department of Paediatrics and Child Health, St Mary's Hospital Lacor, Gulu, Uganda

T. M. Slusher et al. (eds.), *Pediatric Procedural Adaptations for Low-Resource Settings*, https://doi.org/10.1007/978-3-030-99955-1_14

2 Introduction

Intraosseous (IO) access is the placement of a needle through the bone into the medullary space to provide lifesaving treatment to critically ill patients, when peripheral intravenous vascular access has failed or is unattainable [1, 2]. IO access may be used in all age groups with an acceptable safety profile, and is increasingly being used by physicians, clinicians, nurses, and paramedics [3–6]. IO access is meant to be used temporarily for initial treatment, and volume expansion. It should be removed as soon as venous access is obtained or replaced within 24 to 48 hours, if vascular access remains problematic, to avoid infection risks [7]. There are many commercialized IO devices available in the market today; however, in resource-limited settings, access to these devices is limited or unavailable. Several routinely available needles can be used to obtain IO access. These include but are not limited to sturdy needles that do not bend when accessing the bone, needles with a stylet (lumbar puncture or bone marrow biopsy needles). When needles with stylets are not available, we use readily available needles from blood giving set, 5 ml or more syringes, or a 14–18G hypodermic needle for intravenous access (Fig. 1).

3 Indications

- Failed venous access after two or more attempts in an emergency for resuscitation
- Need for rapid access for lifesaving treatment administration

Fig. 1 Commonly used IO access sites in the lower limbs in low resource settings. (Figure used with permission from Christine Ajonye Howard)

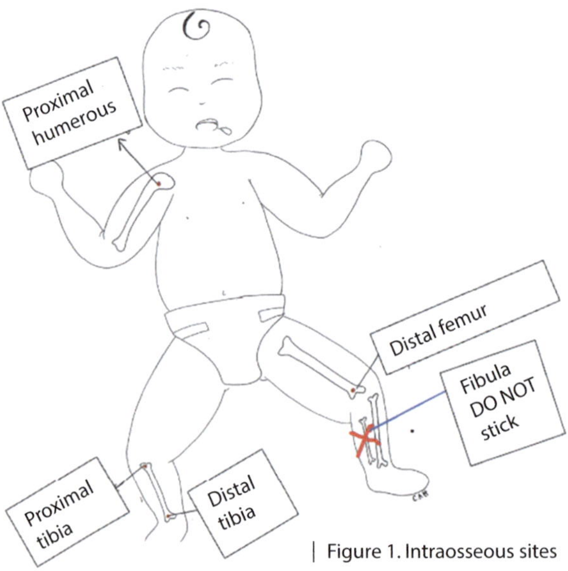

4 Contraindications

IO access is contraindicated when the integrity of the bone to be accessed is compromised by infections (osteomyelitis), fractures, osteogenesis imperfect or a previous IO or attempts within 48 hours on the same bone. Other relative contraindications include burns or infections (cellulitis) at the access site.

5 Equipment/Supplies

In resource-limited settings, access to standard commercialized devices for IO placement is limited. A low-cost, non-commercialized IO access device can be easily fashioned.

- Needle options: spinal/lumbar needle or bone marrow needle, 14–18G hypodermic needle (14–16G needles are often found in a blood giving set), and needles from 5– 20 ml syringes
- 5–20 ml syringes (any size can be used, 10 ml syringe is ideal)
- Antiseptic solution – to cleanse the skin
- Gauze – to help secure the device
- Tape ("plaster") – to secure the device
- Saline fluids (to flush)
- Clean or sterile medical gloves
- Optional: lidocaine or another local anesthetic (generally not needed/used), needle cap and scissors/razor

6 Technique and Instructions for Use

6.1 Preparation

Aseptic technique and infection control principles must be adhered to. Local anesthesia is optional.

6.2 Placement of IO

1. Identify the appropriate site (Fig. 1) [1, 7].
   (a) Proximal tibia: Anteromedial surface, 2–3 cm below the tibial tuberosity
   (b) Distal tibia: Proximal to the medial malleolus
   (c) Distal femur: Midline, 2–3 cm above the external condyle

2. Optional step: At this point, the operator can choose to use the needle cap to fashion a needle guard to help prevent placing the needle too deep. Approximate the distance from the overlying skin and subcutaneous tissue to the middle of the bone (in cm). Then take the needle cap and cut off the just measured depth (cm) from the distal end of the needle cap. Put the needle back in the cap. The needle will protrude through the cut needle cap the distance that has been approximated (Fig. 2) to appropriately enter the bone.
3. Position the bone for easy access. For a tibial approach, a small roll under the knee and leg can be helpful. *Never place your hand behind the insertion site on the patient's extremity when placing the needle. You can go through the bone and into your own hand.*
4. Wear clean or sterile gloves. Clean the skin with antiseptic.
5. Connect the syringe to the sterile needle as seen in Fig. 3. This step will be skipped if using a needle with a stylet.
6. Place the sterile needle (with syringe and optional cap guard attached) perpendicular to the skin over the chosen bone insertion site (Fig. 4b).
7. Push the needle through the skin to the bone surface. At this point, the needle tip should be at the bone cortex.
8. Maintain a firm pressure perpendicularly to the bone. Twist the needle with a quarter turn back and forth while applying pressure to advance the needle into the bone. When a sudden give/decrease in resistance is felt, the needle should be in the medullary space. Be careful not to advance after this point as you can go through the back of the bone. The needle should stand up on its own at this point if it is in the correct position (Fig. 4c). Blood may be seen coming back through the needle, though sometimes because it is in the bone marrow space there may not be backflow.
9. Attempt to draw back – you may or may not be able to obtain labs/blood flow. If you have back flow you can obtain blood for culture or blood chemistry. Blood cultures obtained from the bone marrow space are typically very high yield.

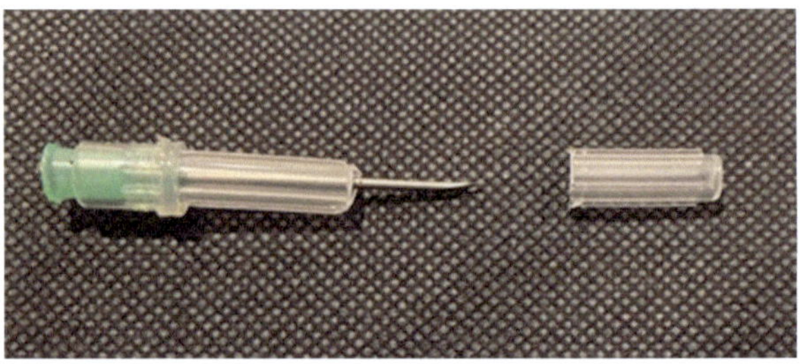

Fig. 2 Needle with cut cap guard

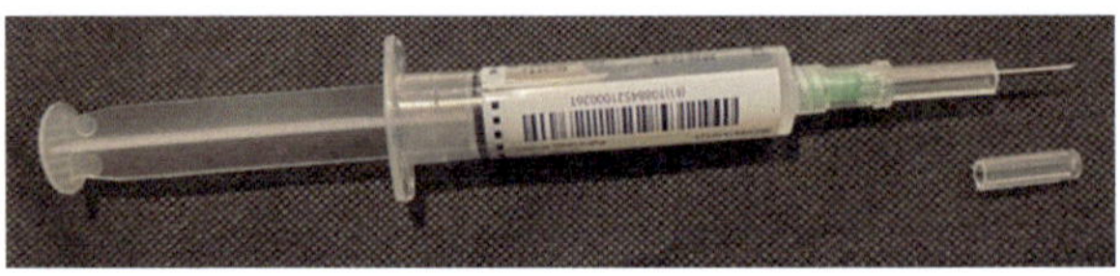

Fig. 3 Needle (with cap guard) attached to syringe

a Supplies for IO

1. Sterile gloves
2. Drape or inside paper of sterile gloves
3. Cleaning solution
4. 14, 16, or 18-guage needles with cap
5. Way to secure IO
6. Syringe
7. Clean or sterile scissors

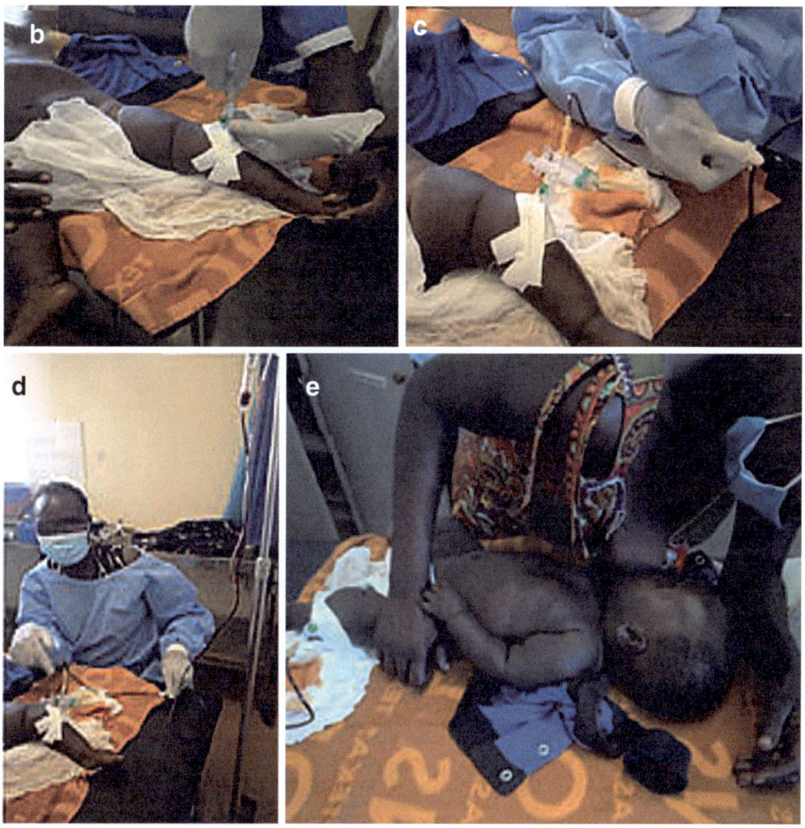

Fig. 4 (**a**–**e**) Steps for intraosseous placement and use. (**a**) Basic equipment. (**b**) Access and flushing. (**c**, **d**) Transfusion. (**e**) Breastfeeding during transfusion after gaining consciousness

10. You may flush with 0.5–1 ml of lidocaine to reduce pain during injection, but this is not typically used.
11. Flush the needle with 2–10 ml of normal saline. It should flush easily if it is in the correct position. Feel behind and around the site for any signs of swelling, which would indicate that the needle tip is not in the bone appropriately (either a through and through insertion or partial entry into the bone medullary cavity).
12. If the needle is not in the correct position or infiltrates, it should be removed and any additional attempts at IO placement should be in a different bone.

13. Secure the needle with tape/plaster. There are many ways to secure the IO, but 2 good options for securement include:
    (a) Bolster the sides with bulky gauze or pieces of torn sheets or cotton made into rolls and then tape it to the child (Fig. 5)
    (b) Use an empty tape roll and secure it to the child's leg leaving the needle free then securing the IV tubing to the child's leg (Fig. 6)

Be sure that if a needle cap guard was used, that it is not pushing down too hard on the overlying skin to cause a wound.

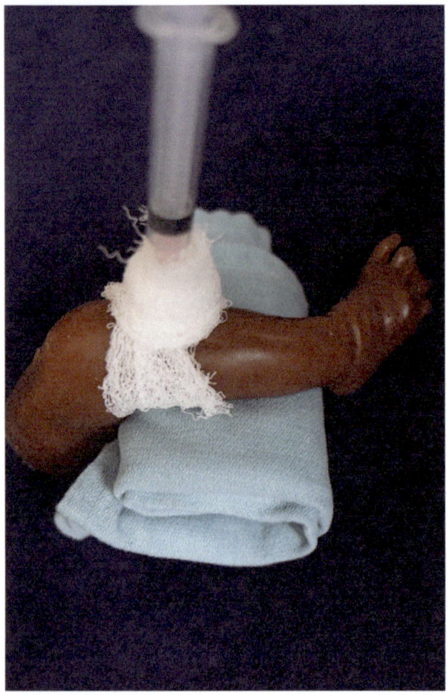

Fig. 5 Bolstered IO

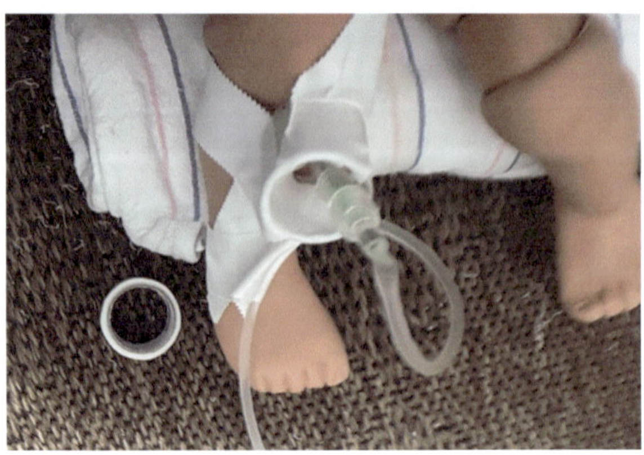

Fig. 6 IO with tape roll securement

14. Administration of any fluid (including blood) through an IO must be given using a pump, pressure bag or manually administered with bolus syringes (Fig. 4c, d). Passive flow with gravity alone will not likely be possible with an IO.
15. Document date and time of placement.
16. Remove the interosseous needle as soon as venous access has been achieved. Discourage use beyond 24 hours.

7 Complications

Complications of IO access include failure to enter the bone cavity or through and through penetration of the bone resulting in extravasation or sub-periosteal infusion [1]. Rarely osteomyelitis, cellulitis, epiphyseal/growth plate injury, skin necrosis, compartment syndrome, fat and bone microemboli have also all been reported. Pain with the initial flush is relatively common and additional pain with ongoing infusion has been reported. These complications can be minimized by optimal placement technique and prompt removal once additional access has been obtained or access is no longer needed.

8 Case Resolution

*An IO was successfully placed using an 18G hypodermic needle. The child was given a 5 ml/kg lactated ringers bolus over 30 minutes while awaiting blood to arrive. Blood transfusion was given through the IO. The child's mental status improved with transfusion and she was able to breastfeed (*Fig. 4e*). Additional IV access was obtained, and the IO was removed after 4 hours when the blood transfusion had been completed. The child was treated for severe malaria anemia and recovered fully. Throughout the child's stay in the acute care unit, the IO site was evaluated and showed no signs of overlying skin infection.*

References

1. Rosenberg H, Cheung WJ. Intraosseous access. CMAJ. 2013;185(5):E238.
2. Luck RP, Haines C, Mull CC. Intraosseous access. J Emerg Med. 2010;39(4):468–75.
3. Fisher R, Prosser D. Intraosseous access in infant resuscitation. Arch Dis Child. 2000;83(1):87.
4. Fiorito BA, et al. Intraosseous access in the setting of pediatric critical care transport. Pediatr Crit Care Med. 2005;6(1):50–3.
5. Fenwick R. Intraosseous approach to vascular access in adult resuscitation. Emerg Nurse. 2010;18(4):22–5.
6. DeBoer S, et al. Intraosseous insights: tips and tricks. Air Med J. 2020;39(2):137–9.
7. Dornhofer P, Kellar JZ. Intraosseous vascular access. In: StatPearls. Treasure Island: StatPearls Publishing LLC; 2021.

Intravenous Fluid Administration Without Programmable Infusion Pumps in a Low-Resource Setting

Ifelayo Ojo, Kayode Bamigbola, Alaba Ogunsiji, and Viviane Leuche

Abbreviations

cc	Cubic centimeter
gtts	Drops
IV	Intravenous
IVF	Intravenous fluids
LMICs	Low- and middle-income countries
mL	milliliter

1 Case Example

An 8-year-old previously healthy male presented with a 2-day history of intestinal obstruction due to intussusception, which required intestinal resection and anastomosis. He is currently admitted to the pediatric surgical ward for post-operative

I. Ojo (✉)
Department of Pediatrics, Global Pediatrics Program, University of Minnesota, Minneapolis, MN, USA

Department of Pediatrics, Hennepin Healthcare, Minneapolis, MN, USA
e-mail: iojo@umn.edu

K. Bamigbola
Department of Surgery, Federal Medical Centre, Ondo, Nigeria

A. Ogunsiji
Intensive Treatment Unit, Epsom and St. Heller University Hospital, NHS Trust, Carshalton, UK

V. Leuche
Department of Pediatrics, Division of Emergency Medicine, Global Pediatrics Program, University of Minnesota, Minneapolis, MN, USA
e-mail: tchon002@umn.edu

T. M. Slusher et al. (eds.), *Pediatric Procedural Adaptations for Low-Resource Settings*, https://doi.org/10.1007/978-3-030-99955-1_15

recovery and needs to receive intravenous (IV) fluids for hydration while awaiting return of bowel function. The child's weight is 32 kilograms.

Using the "100–50-20 rule", maintenance fluids is calculated as 1740mLs in 24 hours or approximately 72mLs per hour using the "4–2-1 rule."

You are working in a rural medical center without a programmable IV infusion pump and you have been given a 500 mL bag of 5% Dextrose in Normal Saline and a standard intravenous fluid administration set. An infusion pump is a programmable medical device electronically or battery powered that is used to deliver fluids, medicine, or nutrients into a patient [1]. *Intravenous fluid administration sets consist of a perforator, drop counting chamber, tubing, precision flow regulator, and distal connector* [2]. *How are you going to give the fluids?*

2 Introduction

Delivery of intravenous fluids is an important treatment modality for many patients and disease processes. Incorrect volumes and rates of delivered fluid can result in fluid overload or dehydration. Many high-income settings have programable pumps to deliver fluids. In contrast, in many resource-limited settings, the rate must be manually adjusted and drip counting utilized to deliver appropriate fluid volumes. This chapter reviews the supplies needed for manual delivery of intravenous fluid, a description of the three main types of intravenous fluid administration sets, and how to adjust the sets to deliver the precise volume of fluid desired.

3 Indications

Understanding how to deliver precise volumes of fluid at specified rates is necessary for any fluid or medication delivered via drip without a programable pump or desire to deliver by gravity.

3.1 Supplies Needed for Manual Delivery of Intravenous Fluid (Figures under Section Discussed)

1. Intravenous fluid (IVF) administration set also known as infusion or "giving set" (Figs. 1, 2, and 3)
2. Stopwatch or timepiece with time in seconds
3. Intravenous fluid pole (drip stand or other methods of suspending the IVF bag or bottle)
4. A small cup to drip fluid into if drops (gtts) per mL are not known
5. A syringe that can accurately measure 1 mL, ideally a 1 mL syringe

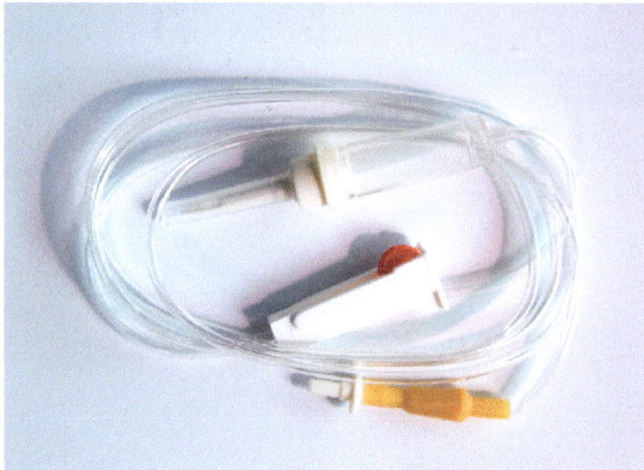

Fig. 1 IV fluid giving set

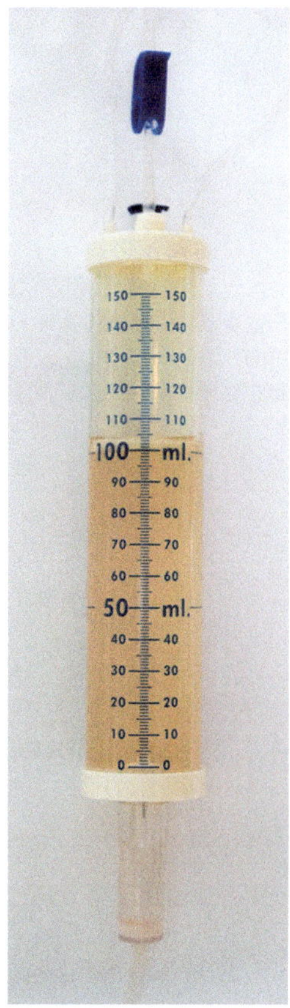

Fig. 2 Microdrip solution giving with a set volume control chamber

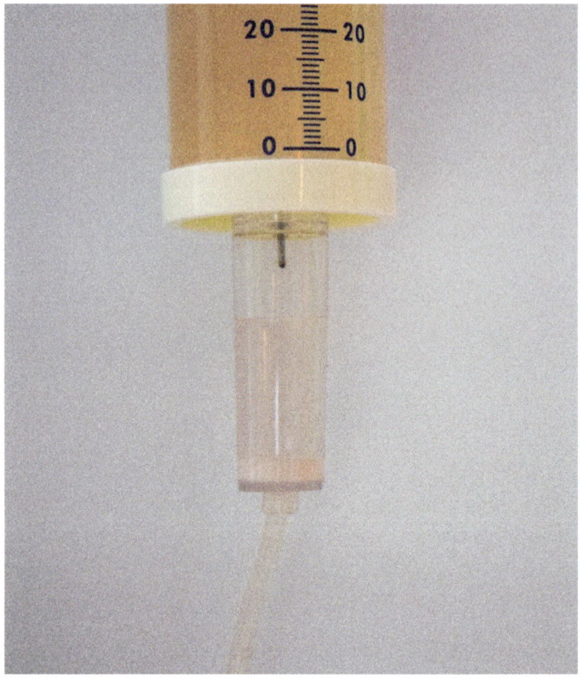

Fig. 3 Drip chamber for microdrip solution giving set

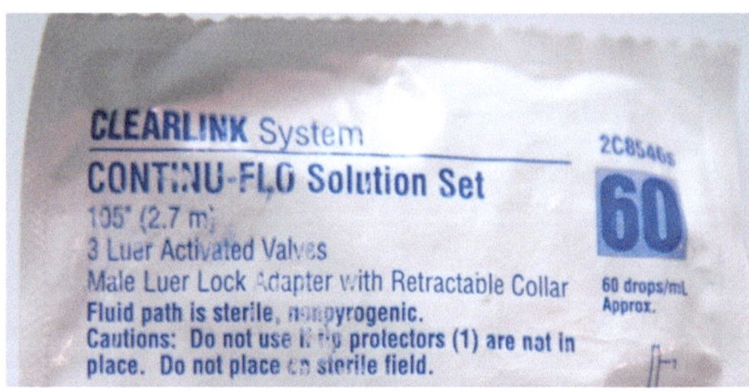

Fig. 4 Example of microdrip solution giving set

4 Types of Intravenous Fluid Administration Sets

There are three main types:

(a) Standard IV fluid administration set (Fig. 1)
(b) Microdrip infusion set (Figs. 2, 3, and 4)
(c) Blood transfusion set (Figs. 5, 6, and 7)

Table 1 shows the number of drops that constitute a milliliter (also known as drop factor) as well as drop factor constant for the three common fluid administration sets.

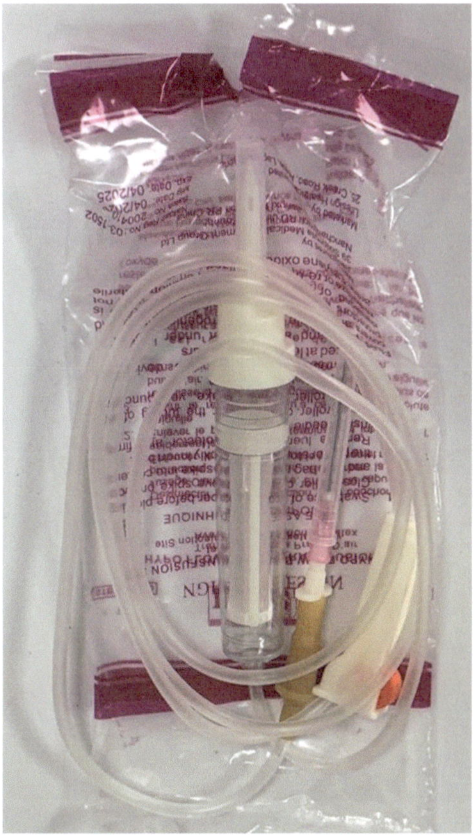

Fig. 5 Blood transfusion giving set at 15 drops (gtts) per mL

5 Standard IV Fluid Administration Set

According to UNICEF, this is a "sterile single use device used for parenteral administration of infusions (IV fluids) by gravity" [2]. The drop counting or drip chamber is considered a macro-drip delivery chamber and in many LMICs is calibrated at 20 drops (gtts) per milliliter (Table 1). It is not intended for administration of blood or blood products.

It is composed of the following parts:

1. A sharp piercing perforator with a protective cap.
2. An air inlet with integrated bacteriological filter.
3. A transparent drop counting or drip chamber calibrated at 20 drops (gtts)/mL.
4. Transparent tubing with injection site (or Y-injection port), and distal connector preferably Luer Lock connector.
5. Precision flow regulator: smooth roller clamp for adjusting the rate of fluid flow into the drop counting chamber.

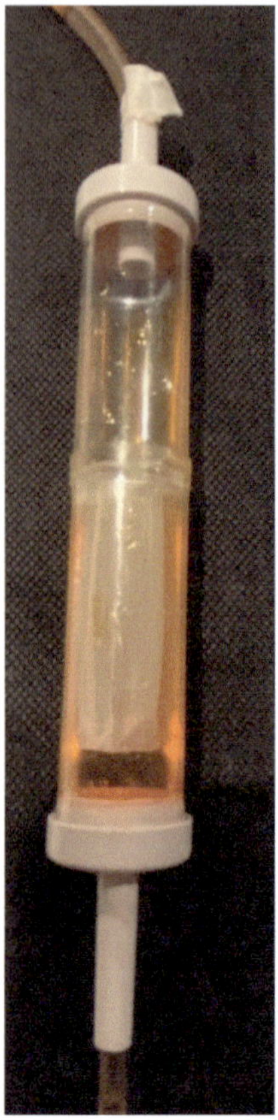

Fig. 6 Blood transfusion set showing filter

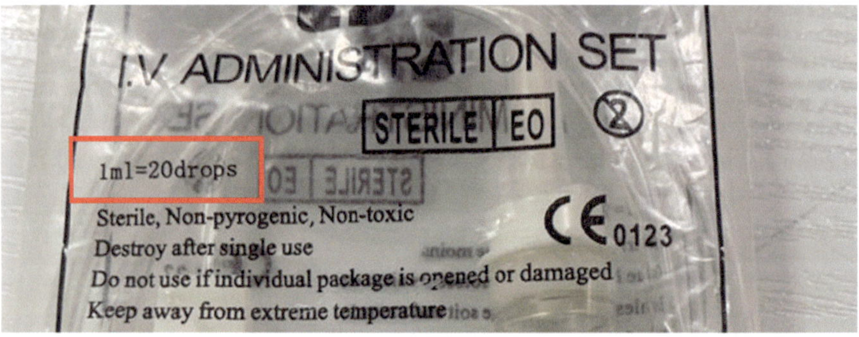

Fig. 7 IV fluid giving set from Nigeria with number of drops per milliliter highlighted

Table 1 Drop per milliliter and drip factor constant

Fluid administration set	Number of drops per milliliter (drop factor)	Drop factor constant
IV fluid administration set	20 drops (gtts)/mL	3
Microdrip infusion set	60 drops (gtts)/mL	1
Blood transfusion set	15 drops (gtts)/mL	4

6 Microdrip Infusion Set with Volume Control Chamber

Microdrip solution giving sets (Figs. 2, 3, and 4) are used for delivering more precise, smaller volume fluids or medications intravenously. They are commonly used in neonatal intensive care units and pediatric intensive care units. Many also have the advantage of having a volume control chamber where a set volume of fluid can be measured out of a larger IV fluid bag (e.g., Soluset/Buretrol set can usually hold a maximum of 100 to 150 mL of fluids). The microdrip infusion set may sometimes consist of only the microdrip chamber which can be recognized by the tiny wire in the drip chamber and the tiny drops. The microdrip chamber is calibrated to deliver 60 drops (gtts) per milliliter (Table 1).

The microdrip infusion set is typically made up of the following components:

1. A hollow plastic perforator located at the proximal end of the infusion set for connection to the infusion bottle or bag.
2. An air inlet incorporated into the perforator and fitted with an air filter (bacteriological filter).
3. A transparent plastic graduated chamber with capacity of approximately 100–150 ml, connected to the perforator by a 15 cm tube.
4. Automatic shut off valve, to prevent air from entering the drop-counting chamber and/or the tube after the pre-determined volume of fluid in the plastic graduated chamber is complete.
5. A drop-counting chamber containing a metal tube which is located under the graduated chamber and calibrated at 60 drops (gtts)/ml.
6. Precision flow regulator: smooth roller clamp for adjusting the rate of fluid flow into the drop-counting chamber.
7. An injection portal made of plastic and fitted with rubber.

6.1 Blood Transfusion Set

Device Components Blood transfusion sets (Fig. 5) contain similar components as the standard IV fluid administration set except that it contains a filter (Fig. 6) in the drop-counting or drip chamber to keep blood clots from being transfused into a patient. The standard calibration of the drip chamber in a blood giving set is 15 drops per mL (Table 1). **However, some blood giving sets are 20 drops (gtts) per mL. If in doubt, drop 15 or 20 drops into a cup and verify how many mL's are in the cup.**

7 Instructions for Calculating the Drip Rate for a Giving Set

7.1 How to Calculate Drip Rate for any Fluid Administration Set

- Step 1: Determine the number of drops needed to obtain 1 milliliter from the set (Fig. 7). This is usually called the drop or drip factor (Table 1).

  Note: If the number of drops (gtts) per milliliter or drop factor is not stated on the packaging, the drop factor can be calculated as follows: (a) Release 20 drops of fluid into a small cup. Then, measure the volume of fluid in the cup with a small syringe (1–5 mL syringe). If the syringe contains approximately 1 mL then the giving set is a 20 drops (gtts)/mL giving set. If the syringe contains approximately 2 mL then the giving set is a 10 drops (gtts)/mL giving set, etc.
- Step 2: Calculate the volume of fluid to be infused into the patient every hour in milliliters; then divide by 60 minutes to determine the volume you need to deliver per minute.
- Step 3: Convert the volume of fluid per minute to drops per minute by multiplying the volume of fluid (in milliliters) per minute above by the number of drops, which constitute 1 mL for the fluid administration set being utilized (i.e., Multiply answer from step 1 by step 2).
- Step 4: Close the precision flow regulator on the fluid administration set.
- Step 5: Spike the IV fluid (Figs. 8a and b) or blood bag with the perforator from the fluid administration set. Ensure sterile surface on the IV fluid bag tubing to be spiked with the perforator. Clean gloves are to be worn for the procedure, and sterile surfaces should not be contaminated.
- Step 6: Hang up the IV fluid or blood bag on an IV pole.
- Step 7: Prime the drop counting or drip chamber (Fig. 9) by squeezing the chamber gently to generate negative pressure and allow for entry of fluid from the bag into the chamber. Fill the drop counting chamber to about one-third capacity. Note: for the micro drip chamber, ensure there is sufficient space between the primer fluid collected in the chamber and the narrow metal tubing to clearly visualize the drops.
- Step 8: Prime the fluid administration tubing by opening the precision flow regulator to release fluid through the connector into a waste bag or cup. Ensure there are no bubbles in the tubing, except the air-fluid level within the drop counting chamber. Then close the precision flow regulator.

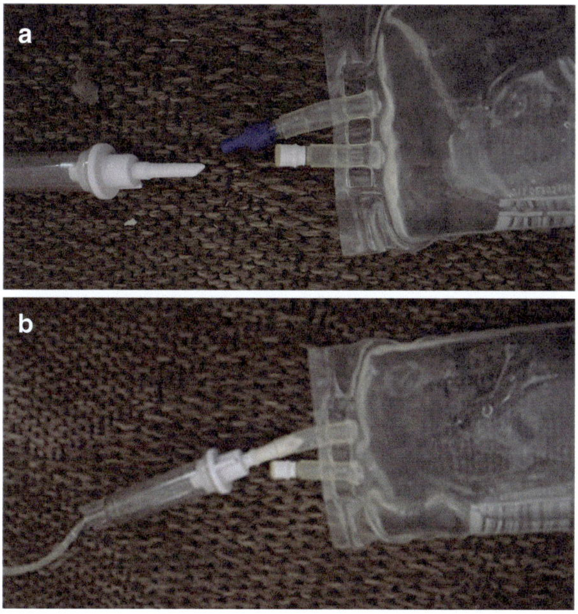

Fig. 8 (**a**): IVF bag ready to be spiked. (**b**): IVF bag spiked

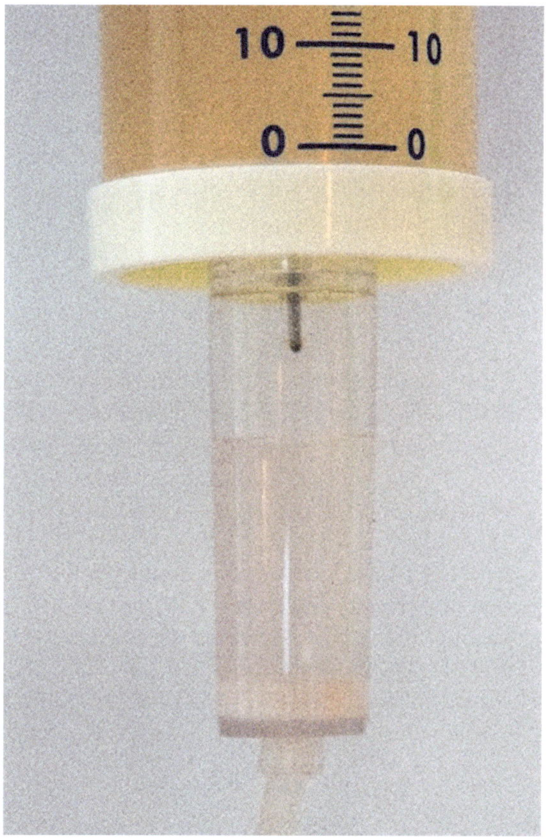

Fig. 9 Drip chamber primed

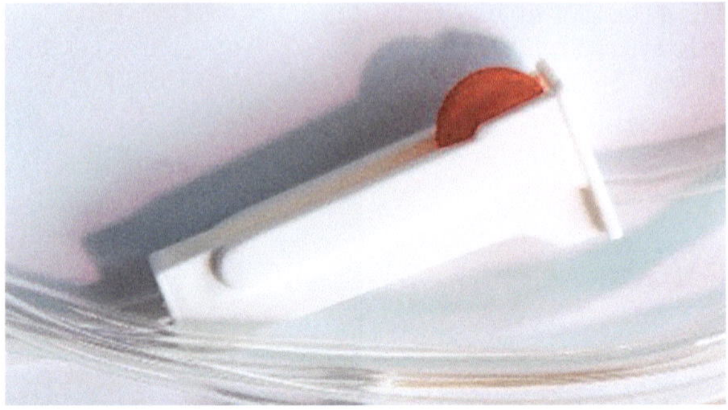

Fig. 10 Precision flow regulator

- Step 9: Connect the fluid administration set to patient's IV cannula or port, while ensuring that the patient has their infusion site resting on a comfortable surface and that there are no kinks in the tubing of the fluid administration set.
- Step 10: Slowly reopen the precision flow regulator (Fig. 10) and watch the drop counting chamber for rate of flow of fluid from fluid bag.
- Step 11: Divide the number of drops you plan to deliver in a minute by 4 and gently regulate the number of drops going through drop counting chamber for 15 seconds using the precision flow regulator and stopwatch. When the approximate rate of flow is achieved, count the number of drops being delivered for a full minute to ensure it corresponds with the calculated number of drops desired from Step 3 above.
- Step 12: Plan to recheck the rate of flow of fluid from drop counting chamber every 2 hours to confirm the fluid is being delivered at the appropriate rate. Also, the bag of IV fluid should be checked to ensure that the approximate volume infused and volume remaining is appropriate.

7.2 Patient Safety Measures

1. Only administer intravenous fluids when a patient's gastrointestinal system cannot be utilized, or would not achieve desired effect (for instance, fluid resuscitation in shock, intestinal obstruction, post-operative ileus, inability to take oral fluids). Reconsider indication and continued need for IV fluids at least two times every day. Enteral hydration and nutrition is safer than, and as effective as intravenous [3, 4].
2. Calculate number of drops per minute for the ordered fluid volume per hour with bedside nurse and request that the rate of fluid per hour and equivalent number of drops per minute be written on a sticker or tape that is placed on the IV fluid bag for easy verification.
3. Provide expected volume of IV fluid to be infused every 4–6 hours as a part of your order. This serves as a way for the bedside nurse to double check that

appropriate volume of fluids is being delivered. For instance, with the case illustration above, the goal is for the patient to receive 72mLs per hour or about 300 mL every 4 hours. If the order is written both hourly and Q4 hourly to include the expected volume in 4 hours, the bedside nurse would reassess the amount of fluid left in the bag of IV fluids at 4 hours and determine whether the right volume has been infused. The bedside nurse can slow down the rate if the fluid appears to be going down faster than the aimed rate of administration, or increase the rate if the rate of infusion is slower than expected.

4. Recheck or request drop counting chamber be inspected every 2 hours to confirm that number of drops per minute is same as the drop count that was originally set. Patient positioning affects drop rate as the fluid is flowing by gravity. Factors such as laying on the limb with the intravenous cannula, flexion of adjacent joint, or moving the extremity where the IV cannula is placed to a more dependent position may slow down the rate of flow, while extension of the adjacent joint may increase the rate.
5. Consider using a microdrip administration set for all neonatal/small infant infusions and when possible for all pediatric infusions. Use a micro drip set for infusion of medications where careful titration is important such as vasopressors and insulin, or patients that require less than 40 mL/hour of IV fluids. The microdrip chamber should be filled with just enough fluid for a 4 hours period to reduce the risk of fluid overload compared with when a larger IV fluid bag 500 mL or 1000 mL is utilized. When available, use a volume control chamber for any drip requiring precise amounts of drugs or fluids. When using a microdrip giving set mL/hour is equal to drops per minutes. If a neonate requires 10 mL per hour of fluids and you are using a micro drip giving set they would get 10 drips (gets) per minute.

8 Complications

- Inappropriate rate/volume of fluid delivered causing fluid overload, dehydration, or incorrect dose of medication

9 Case Resolution (with Calculation)

Recall the patient/situation: Using the 100–50-20 rule, maintenance fluids were calculated as 1740mLs in 24 hours or approximately 72mLs per hour using the 4–2-1 rule. You have been given a 500 mL bag of 5% Dextrose in Normal Saline and a standard intravenous fluid administration set. Following the directions above you follow the steps outlined in Table 2.

Table 2 Steps to calculate drip rate and case illustration

Steps	Example
Step 1: Determine number of drops per milliliter for standard IV fluid administration set	20 drops/mL
Step 2: **Divide** volume of fluid to be infused per hour in milliliters **by** 60 minutes to determine the volume to deliver per minute	$\frac{72\,\text{mLs}}{1\,\text{hour}} \times \frac{1\,\text{hour}}{60\,\text{mins}} = 1.2\,\text{mL / min}$
Step 3: Convert the volume of fluid per minute to drops per minute by **multiplying** the volume of fluid (in milliliters) per minute **and** the number of drops which constitute 1 mL for the fluid administration set being utilized i.e. step 1 x step 2	$\frac{1.2\,\text{mL}}{1\,\text{min}} \times \frac{20\,drops(\text{gtts})}{1\,\text{mL}} = 24\,drops(\text{gtts}) / \text{min}$
An alternative long hand calculation is	For the 20 drops (gtts)/mL giving set $\frac{72\,\text{mLs}}{1\,\text{hr}} \times \frac{20\,\text{gtts}}{1\,\text{ml}} = \frac{1440\,\text{gtts}}{1\,\text{hr}}$ OR $\frac{1440\,\text{gtts}}{60\,\text{minutes}} = 24\,\text{drops}(\text{gtts}) / \text{minutes}$
Quick work around for steps 1 through 3 above: Divide 60 minutes by the drip factor (number of drops/mL) to get the "drop factor constant"	Drop factor constant for standard IV fluid administration set (20 drops/mL) $\frac{60\,\text{mins}}{20\,\text{drops}(\text{gtts}) / \text{mL}} = 3$ For simplicity of calculation, the drop factor constant is 3 i.e. in this example you 72 mL/hour. If you divide 72 by your drip factor of 3 you get 24 drops per minute or 6 drops (gtts) every 15 seconds
Perform steps 4 through 10	
Step 11: Divide the number of drops you plan to deliver in a minute by 4 – Which will give you the number of drops for a 15 seconds period. Gently regulate the number of drops going through the drop counting chamber for 15 seconds using the precision flow regulator and stopwatch. When the desired drop rate is achieved, count the number of drops being delivered for a full minute to ensure it corresponds with the calculated number of drops desired from step 3 above	24 gtts/min ÷ 4 = 6 drops (gtts) every 15 seconds

10 Case Resolution

You appropriately calculate the fluid rate, adjust the precision regulator, and the patient receives the appropriate fluid volume for the next three days. His bowel function returns and he is advanced on an appropriate oral hydration plan.

References

1. What is an infusion pump? 2017 May 5, 2021; Available from: https://www.fda.gov/medical-devices/infusion-pumps/what-infusion-pump.
2. Infusion giving set,sterile,s.u. May 5, 2021; Available from: https://supply.unicef.org/s0531991.html.
3. Hartling L, et al. Oral versus intravenous rehydration for treating dehydration due to gastroenteritis in children. Cochrane Database Syst Rev. 2006;3:CD004390.
4. Simpson JN, Teach SJ. Pediatric rapid fluid resuscitation. Curr Opin Pediatr. 2011;23(3):286–92.

Mixing Intravenous Fluids in a Low-Resource Setting

Bose O. Toma, Akinyemi O. D. Ofakunrin, and Caroline E. Jasada

Abbreviations

D10W	10% Dextrose in Water
D12.5W	12.5% Dextrose in Water
D5 ½ NS	5% Dextrose in ½ (0.45%) Saline
D5LR	5% Dextrose in Ringer's Lactate
D5NS	5% Dextrose Saline
IVFs	Intravenous fluids
LMICs	Low- and middle-income countries
LR	Lactated Ringer's
NICU	Neonatal Intensive Care Unit
NPO	Nil per os
NSS	Normal saline solution

1 Case Scenario 1

A four-hour-old macrosomic infant with birth weight of 4 kg was delivered to a 21-year-old primiparous mother who had no antenatal care and presumed gestational diabetes is brought to your Neonatal Intensive Care Unit (NICU) in Jos, Nigeria. She was born via an emergency cesarean section following a prolonged

B. O. Toma (✉) · A. O. D. Ofakunrin · C. E. Jasada
Department of Paediatrics, Jos University, Jos, Nigeria

T. M. Slusher et al. (eds.), *Pediatric Procedural Adaptations for Low-Resource Settings*, https://doi.org/10.1007/978-3-030-99955-1_16

labor. She required bag mask ventilation for one minute in the delivery room due to asphyxia. You note that the baby is lethargic and has twitching of the face two hours after admission to the NICU. You diagnose her as a large for gestational age infant of a diabetic mother. You do a bedside blood glucose which results as 23 mg/dL (1.3 mmol/l) and send a confirmatory sample to the lab. You determine that Dextrose 10% (D10W) is emergently indicated but have no D10W. You do have vials of Dextrose 50% (D50W). How can you make D10W? You suspect this infant will also need maintenance intravenous fluids (IVFs) due to the inability to eat immediately and will need to mix/reconstitute these as well due to your limited choices of available IVFs.

2 Introduction

Fluid therapy is an important component of pediatric care in the emergency department and among hospitalized infants and children. Prompt and appropriate fluid administration improves the outcome and reduces mortality in children [1]. Whenever there is a significant depletion of water and electrolytes in the body, dehydration occurs. Infants and young children are quite sensitive to mild degrees of dehydration with resultant increased morbidity and mortality. Intravenous fluids are required when the infant/child is unable to take enteral fluid such as breastmilk or oral rehydration fluid for any reason or when oral rehydration has failed.

Depending on the indication for intravenous fluid therapy, different compositions of fluids are needed to ensure adequate and appropriate treatment. In high-resource settings, the various fluid compositions are generally easily available and ready to use. This is not the case in LMICs where various solute concentrations of fluid may have to be constituted using available intravenous fluids.

Additionally, higher concentrations dextrose containing fluid (such as D50W) run the risk of causing small veins to infiltrate, causing hyperglycemia with rebound hypoglycemia or the extremely rare risk of causing an intracranial hemorrhage in neonates due to rapid hyperosmolar fluid infusion [2]. High concentration dextrose infusions must be diluted prior to administration.

This chapter describes how desired compositions of intravenous fluids can be obtained by mixing the available fluids when commercial intravenous fluids with the correct composition are not available. These compositions are generally approximate as noted.

3 Indications

Need for intravenous fluid that is not currently available. Some of the commonly requested intravenous fluid compositions are:

5% Dextrose in Ringer's Lactate (D5LR)
5% Dextrose in Darrow's solution

5% Dextrose Saline (D5NS)
5% Dextrose in ½ (0.45%) Saline (D5 ½ NS)
10% Dextrose in Water (D10W)
12.5% Dextrose in Water (D12.5W)

4 Equipment/Supplies

10 mL, 20 mL, or 50 mL syringes (depending on availability)
Wide bore needles (18–22 gauge)
Sterile gloves
Disposing pan/waste bin
Tray
D50W
D10W (if available)
Sterile water for injection *or*
500 ml normal saline solution (NSS) (0.9%)
Potassium (if indicated)

5 Technique

1. Assemble the items on the tray in a clean procedure room, fluids must be mixed with aseptic technique.
2. Wash hands and put on sterile (ideally) or clean gloves.
3. Inspect fluid bags to ensure there are no leaks.
4. Clean fluid bags with methylated spirits (also known as alcohol or similar cleaning solution).
5. Use a wide bore needle as conduit at the exit points of both bags to be mixed. (These needles are generally left in place taking care that they do not touch any surfaces.)
6. Draw fluid from the bag or vial (i.e., D50W) (Figs. 1 and 2) in the needed amount (Table 1) and inject into the appropriate base solution bag (Tables 1 and 2) [i.e., lactated Ringer's (LR), sterile water, normal saline (NSS)].
7. Mix fluids thoroughly. The most effective method of mixing solutions in plastic infusion bags is to grasp the bag by its two ends and rapidly invert it twice [3].
8. Waste fluids are discarded in a waste pan.
9. The needles are then taken out and the bags sealed with a plaster.
10. Label reconstituted fluids immediately (Fig. 3).
11. Once fluid bags have been punctured, they should be used or discarded within 24 hours.

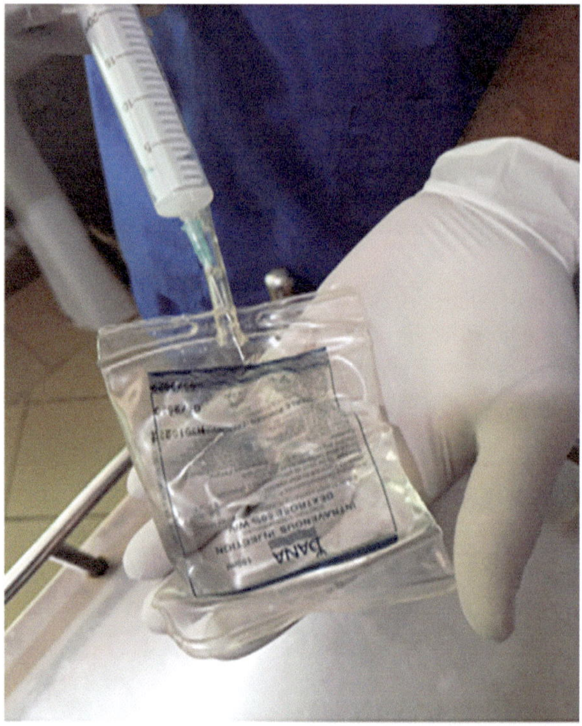

Fig. 1 50% Dextrose infusion being withdrawn

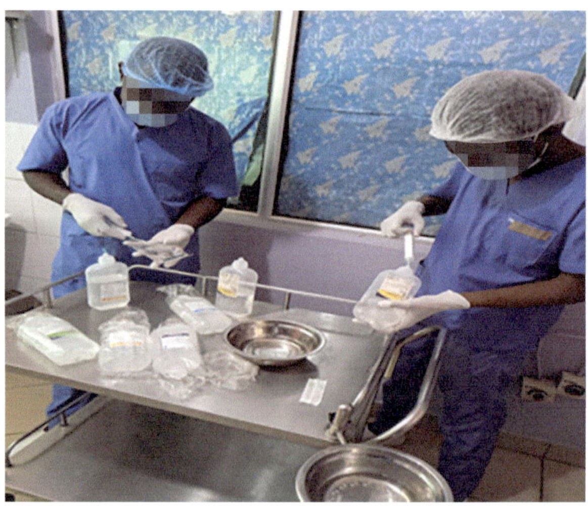

Fig. 2 Fluid reconstitution ongoing

Table 1 Instructions for reconstituting fluids

Desired fluid composition (approximate)	Starting base fluid	Additional fluid needed	Mix instructions	Final volume and approximate concentration[a]	Other comments
D10 W (bolus) in syringes	Sterile water for injection OR Normal saline (NS/NSS)	D50W	2 mL of D50W + 8 mL of NS or sterile water for injection	=10 mL of D10W If mixed in NS/NSS would be D10 ~¾ NSS/NS	*D10W* =10 g of dextrose in 100 mL of fluids [a]Always use D10W in neonates/infants *D50W* =50 g of dextrose in 100 mL of fluids =5 g of dextrose in 10 mL of fluids or =0.5 g of glucose in 1 mL of fluids
D25W bolus in syringe	Sterile water for injection OR NS	D50W	25 mL of D50W + 25 mL of sterile water for injection (or 25 mL of NS)	=50 mL of D25W (or 50 mL of D25 ½ NSS)	[a]D25 should not be bolused in neonates or infants
D10W for infusion	D5W (500 mL)	D50W	450 mL D5W (remove 50 mL from the base (D5W) bag/bottle) + 50 mL of D50W	=500 mL of D10W	
D12.5 W in 500 ml bag/bottle for infusion	D5W (500 mL)	D50W	425 mL D5W (remove 75 mL from the 500 ml D5W bag) + 75 ml D50W	=500 mL of D12.5 W	
D15W in 500 ml bag/bottle for infusion	D5W (500 mL)	D50W	400 mL D5W (remove 100 mL from the 500 ml D5W bag) + 100 ml D50W	=500 mL of D15W	Can only use with central access, such as a UVC or central line

(continued)

Table 1 (continued)

Desired fluid composition (approximate)	Starting base fluid	Additional fluid needed	Mix instructions	Final volume and approximate concentration[a]	Other comments
D5 ¼ NS in 500 ml bag/ bottle for infusion	D5W (500 mL)	NS	320 mL D5 W (remove 180 mL from the 500 mL bag) + 150 ml NS + 30 ml D50W	=500 mL of ~D5 1/4 NS	Hypotonic fluid. Generally used only for neonates on days 3–7 of life, although D10 1/4NS more commonly used
D10 ¼ NS in 500 ml bag/ bottle for infusion	D5W (500 mL)	NS	350 mL D5W (remove 150 mL from the 500 mL bag) + 150 mL NS + 75 ml D50W	=500 mL of ~D10 1/4 NS	Commonly used in neonates on days 3–7 of life if no TPN available
D5 ½ NS in 500 ml bag/ bottle for infusion	D5W (500 mL)	NS	200 mL D5W (remove 280 mL from the 500 mL bag of D5W) + 250 mL NS + 30 mL D50W	=500 mL ~D5 1/2 NS	
D5 NS in 500 ml bag/bottle for infusion	NS (500 mL)	D50W	450 mL NS (remove 50 mL from the 500 mL bag) + 50 mL D50W	=500 mL of ~D5NS	
D10 NS in 500 ml bag/ bottle for infusion	D5NS (500 mL) See above	D50W	450 mL D5NS (remove 50 mL from the 500 mL bag) + 50 mL D50W	=500 mL of D10NS	

D5 LR or Hartman's	LR or Hartman's (500 mL)	D50W	450 mL LR/Hartman's (remove 50 mL from the 500 mL bag) + 50 mL D50W	=500 mL of ~D5 LR or ~D5 Hartman's	
D10 LR or Hartman's	D5LR or D5 Hartman's	D50W	450 mL D5LR or D5Hartman's (remove 50 mL from the 500 mL bag) + 50 mL D50W	=500 mL of ~D10 LR or ~D10 Hartman's	
D5 Darrow's solution	Darrow's solution	D50W	450 mL Darrow's (remove 100 mL from the 500 mL bag) + 50 mL D50W	=500 mL of ~ D5 Darrow's solution	If using Darrow's solution, do not add potassium
D10 Darrow's solution	D5 Darrow's solution	D50W	450 mL D5 Darrow's (remove 50 mL from the 500 mL bag) + 50 mL D50W	=500 mL of ~D10 Darrow's solution	If using Darrow's solution do not add potassium
D5 NS + 10 mEq/L KCL	D5 NS	KCL (check concentration)	500 mL D5NS + 5 mEq KCL (verify the concentration to figure out the mL needed)	=500 mL of D5 NS + 10 mEq/L KCl	The same mixing instructions can be used to add potassium to the other base solutions
D5 NS + 20 mEq/L KCl	D5 NS	KCL (check concentration)	500 mL D5NS + 10 mEq KCL (verify the concentration to figure out the mL needed)	=500 mL of D5 NS + 20 mEq/L KCL	The same mixing instructions can be used to add potassium to the other base solutions

Thank you to Dr. Jessica Jantzer Hennepin Healthcare Pediatric Pharmacist Minneapolis, MN, USA for her help with this table

[a]Concentrations are approximate for electrolytes and glucose in the final solution unless a known exact mEq is added to the solution

D = Dextrose, KCL = Potassium Chloride, NS = Normal Saline, RL = Ringers Lactate, W = Water

Table 2 Electrolyte concentration of commercially available fluids

IV fluid	Na (meq/L)	Cl (mEq/L)	K (mEq/L)	Lactate (mEq/L)	Ca (mEq/L)	mOsm/L
Lactated Ringer's	131	109	4	28	2.7	273
Hartman's	131	111	5	29	2.0	255
Darrow's	121	103	35	53	–	312
Normal saline	154	154	–	–	–	308

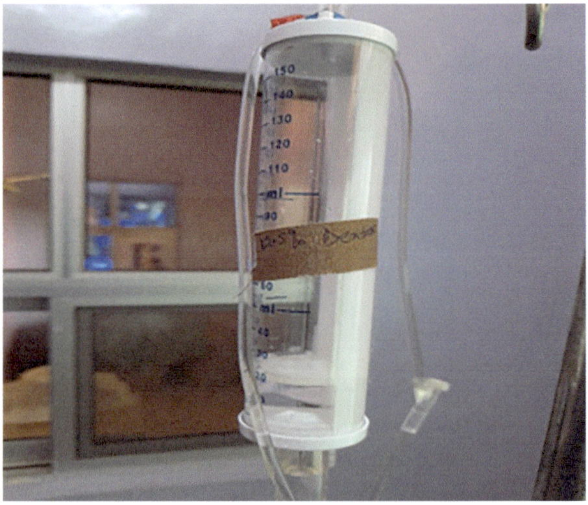

Fig. 3 Reconstituted Dextrose solution appropriately labeled

5.1 Potassium

Potassium is not usually added unless the infant/child is going to be nil per os (NPO) for an extended period. For neonates, if needed, potassium may be added to the fluids at about 3 days of life. In older infants and children who are NPO and are voiding at least 1–2 mL/kg/hour, consider adding potassium for routine maintenance IVF. If the child is eating or taking ORS (which include potassium), potassium should not generally be added to the IVF. Potassium-rich foods such as oranges/orange juice and bananas can be used to replenish potassium stores if the child is able to take oral fluids/foods.

If potassium is added generally add only 10 mEq/L of potassium chloride (KCL) are added for neonates and 20 mEq/L of KCL for infants and children beyond the neonatal period. Due to the dangers associated with hyperkalemia and potential for error in hand mixing and calculations, 2 healthcare workers should verify the amount being added and document, they have checked and verified that the correct amount is being added/has been added.

5.2 *Other Electrolytes*

It is generally best to give calcium as a slow bolus when the child has symptomatic hypocalcemia. If calcium is given using peripheral IV, always use calcium gluconate and assure the IV is patent due to risk of extravasation injury with severe burns. Give bolus over 10 minutes minimum and monitor the heart rate for bradycardia. If the heart rate drops, stop the bolus until the child's heart rate is normal and then resume at a slower rate. If giving calcium through a central line, it can be added to the fluid but consult a pharmacist or drug book for additional details on the amount to add to fluids, fluids calcium is compatible with and other important details. Calcium gluconate should not be added together with sodium bicarbonate in the same IVF as this can react together and precipitate as calcium carbonate. Whenever possible give phosphorus orally. Magnesium generally best given as a separate infusion of 25 mg/kg up to 2 g over 30 minutes to 2 hours depending on the indication for which it is being given. Consult pharmacist or drug book for additional details on these and other additives.

6 Complications/Risks

- Infection (aseptic technique is imperative when making the fluids)
- Electrolyte imbalance (appropriate calculation and mixing is essential, with double checks, if possible, especially if adding potassium or electrolytes to the fluids)

7 Case Resolution

You calculated the bolus dose of glucose needed to treat hypoglycemia using the known formula of 2–4 mL/kg of D10W. Following the above mixing chart, you make D10W with D50W and sterile water for injection. After given the bolus D10W slowly, her serum glucose level was rechecked and was noted to have corrected to 3 mmol/l (54 mg/dL). Using the mixing instructions above, you make D10W for infusion using D5W and D50W. You start her on an infusion of the D10W at maintenance, and her glucose on repeat check on day 2 of life was 18 mmol/l (72 mg/dL). On day 3 of life, she was beginning to take expressed breastmilk. She was transitioned to D10 ¼ NS (mixed from D5W, NS, and D50W) without potassium as she was beginning to take feeds. She was gradually weaned off fluids and was doing well at discharge at one week of life.

References

Martin K, Weiss SL. Initial resuscitation and management of pediatric septic shock. Minerva Pediatr. 2015;67(2):141–58.
Rozance PJ, Hay WW. Neonatal hyperglycemia. NeoReviews. 2010;11(11):e632.
Deardorff DL, Schmidt CN, Wiley RA. Effect of preparation techniques on mixing of additives in intravenous fluids in nonrigid containers. Hosp Pharm. 1993;28(4):306. 309–10, 312–3

Further Reading

Adamkin DH. Committee on fetus and newborn. Postnatal glucose homeostasis in late-preterm and term infants. Pediatrics. 2011;127(3):575–9.
De Leon DD, Stanley CA. Congenital hypoglycemia disorders: new aspects of etiology, diagnosis, treatment and outcomes: highlights of the proceedings of the congenital hypoglycemia disorders symposium, Philadelphia April 2016. Pediatr Diabetes. 2017;18(1):3–9. https://doi.org/10.1111/pedi.12453. Epub 2016 Oct 18. PMID: 27753189; PMCID: PMC5473026.
Kliegman R. Nelson textbook of pediatrics. 21st ed. Philadelphia: Elsevier; 2020.

Respiratory Equipment Adaptations in a Low-Resource Setting

Brinda Desai and Zubin Shah

Abbreviations

LMICs	Low- and middle-income countries
MDI	Metered dose inhaler
NPA	Nasal pharyngeal airway

1 Spacer for a Metered Dose Inhaler

1.1 Case Example

A 4-year-old patient presents to the clinic with their parents in Tanzania. The child has reactive airway disease and has been having increasing wheezing throughout the day. The parents are concerned that he may not be getting the full medication dose. He struggles with coordination of using the metered dose inhaler (MDI). He has difficulty with creating a tight seal around the inhaler. The clinician recommends the use of "spacer" to more effectively deliver the medication; however, a commercial spacer is not available/not affordable. The clinician

B. Desai (✉)
Division of Pulmonary, Critical Care, and Sleep Medicine, University of California San Diego, San Diego, CA, USA
e-mail: bjdesai@health.ucsd.edu

Z. Shah
Division of Neonatology, Nationwide Children's Hospital, Columbus, OH, USA
e-mail: Zubin.Shah@nationwidechildrens.org

T. M. Slusher et al. (eds.), *Pediatric Procedural Adaptations for Low-Resource Settings*, https://doi.org/10.1007/978-3-030-99955-1_17

explains how to make a "do-it-yourself" spacer which will still provide improved medication delivery and a roughly equivalent clinical benefit to a high-cost commercial spacer.

1.2 Introduction

Proper use of a metered dose inhaler (MDI) is essential for the management of pediatric asthma. The use of a spacer with an MDI is the preferred method for administering bronchodilators in asthma therapy. A spacer is a tube placed between the patient and the MDI. It enhances the proper delivery of the medication to the lungs. In addition, a spacer reduces the deposition of the medication inside the mouth and thus decreases local side effects such as thrush and dysphonia. Unfortunately, studies estimate more than half of children who use MDIs without such devices gain little to no clinical benefit from their MDIs due to incorrect inhaler technique [1]. Improper inhaler use can have serious implications in the management of asthma including increased exacerbations, emergency room visits, and overall increased healthcare utilization. A challenge in optimal asthma management in low- and middle-income countries (LMICs) can be the high cost and lack of availability of commercial spacers [2]. Outcomes with nebulizers are not significantly better than those delivered by MDIs with spacers [2]. Dosing for albuterol given with a spacer in children is generally 4 to 10 puffs every twenty minutes based on weight and severity of asthma. In emergency situations, in a monitored healthcare facility, it may be given as 1–2 puff often as every 30 to 60 seconds for a brief time in a child with a severe asthma exacerbation [3].
Below we provide an outline of how to create a spacer for an MDI. A similar design has been described in an article in the Lancet in 1999 by Zar et al. [4] and is also included in a Cochrane review from 2008 [2]. There are two sets of instructions: one for a simple spacer for older children who can create a seal with their mouth around the spacer and another for infants or uncooperative patients who cannot create a seal with their mouth.

1.2.1 Indications

Indications for a spacer include routine use of MDIs and use of MDIs during an asthma exacerbation.

1.2.2 Equipment (Fig. 1)

- Plastic Bottle (empty 16 to 20 ounce water bottle, soda bottle, any malleable water bottle).
- Scissors or scalpel.

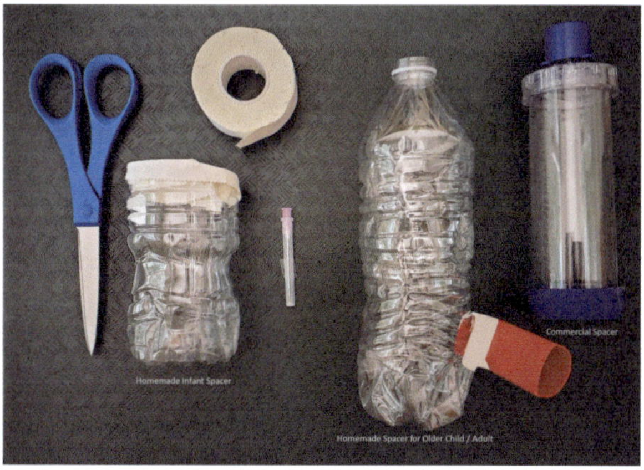

Fig. 1 Supplies for and pictures of homemade spacers and commercial spacers

- Hypodermic needle (any gauge, i.e., 18G, 20G) or nail.
- Durable tape and/or superglue (i.e., duct tape, masking tape).

1.2.3 Technique

Please refer to the sugarprep website for a detailed video on the procedure: https://sugarprep.org/videos/#Spacer_MDI [5]

SPACER FOR MDI (for patients able to create a seal with their mouth around the spacer):

1. Obtain a clean 16-20 oz. (500–600 mL) plastic bottle. Remove the cap.
2. Cut a hole for the mouthpiece of the MDI in the plastic bottle. This hole can be on (1) the bottom of the bottle or (2) on the side, near the bottom of bottle. The hole should be large enough to fit the mouthpiece of the MDI, but as fitted as possible to the mouthpiece.
3. Insert the mouthpiece of the MDI into the hole that was just created (Fig. 2).
4. Tape or superglue the mouthpiece of the MDI to the bottle around the point of insertion. This will seal the MDI to the spacer to prevent the medication from leaking around any gaps in the plastic (Fig. 3).
5. Create two pinholes with a needle or small nail on each side of the bottle at the opposite end from where the MDI is secured. These holes will serve as a pressure release valve, allowing a small amount of air to enter during inhalation and prevent the bottle from collapsing due to a suction effect.

The equipment is now ready to use. Have patient create a seal with their mouth around the mouthpiece of the bottle/spacer and follow instructions for MDI use (Fig. 4). Instructions for use are below.

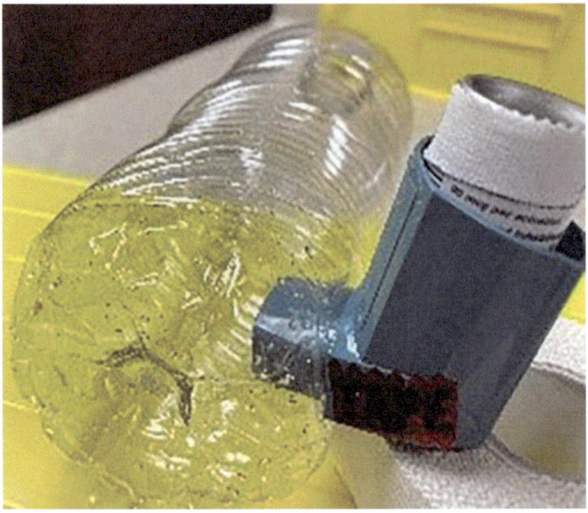

Fig. 2 Plastic bottle with hole with MDI inserted. (Figure used with permission from Dr. Tina Slusher)

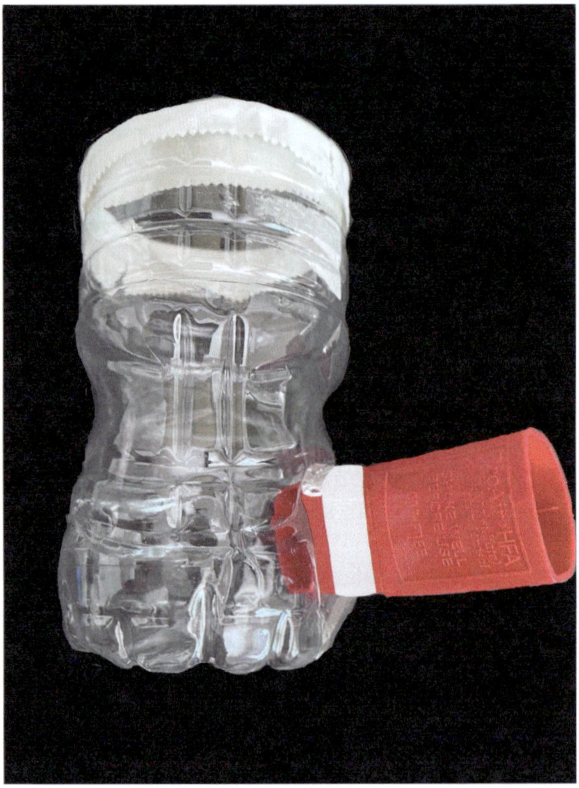

Fig. 3 MDI Infant taped in place. (Figure used with permission from Dr. Tina Slusher)

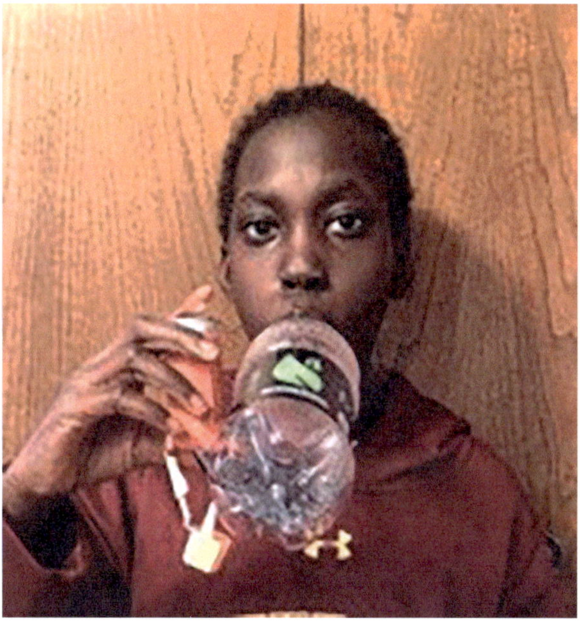

Fig. 4 Spacer ready for use. (Figure used with permission from Drs. Cynthia Howard and Tina Slusher)

Spacer for MDI with "Mask"

1. Follow steps 1–4 above.
2. Cut across the diameter of the bottle to remove the bottle neck (cut as close to the bottom of the bottle neck as possible). This will create an opening that should fit over the mouth and nose of your patient. It is imperative that the area cut across the bottle is big enough to cover both the nose and mouth of your patient during medication administration.
3. Place a layer of tape over the cut plastic edge in order to smooth out any rough edges that could injure the patient. This edge will be placed over the mouth and nose of the patient to function similarly to a facemask.

The spacer now is ready to use. Remember that the opening area must fit over the mouth and nose of the patient (Fig. 5).

1.2.4 Instructions for Use

Instruct the child/family on the number and frequency of medication puffs to use at home. Guidelines will vary based on the child's weight, severity of asthma exacerbation, medication, and the location of care (home, clinic, emergency room, hospital).

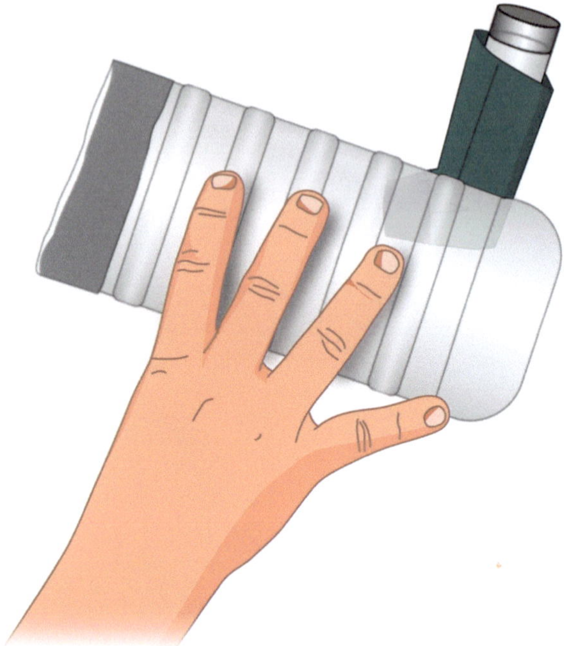

Fig. 5 Finished product. Spacer with "mask" for MDI

General recommendations for albuterol/salbutamol MDI: [6].

Weight (in kg)	Number of puffs	Interval at home	Interval in clinic/hospital
5–10	4	3–4 times/day	Every 20 minutes in clinic or hospital
10–20	6	3–4 times/day	Every 20 minutes in clinic or hospital
>20	8	3–4 times/day	Every 20 minutes in clinic or hospital

[a]The frequency and dosage can be adjusted in an observed clinical situation as needed by a clinician

Spacer Care Replace the bottle with a clean bottle weekly if possible. When not possible to replace, remove the MDI and clean the bottle with mild soapy water. Rinse with clean water and allow to air dry before replacing the MDI.

1.2.5 Complications

There is a very low risk of complications in general. One could consider the possibility of

- Inadequate delivery of medication (too much medication on plastic bottle, or medication not delivered due to leak)
- Skin injury (edges of bottle not covered appropriately)

1.3 Case Resolution

A spacer was made for the family using the above-described technique and use of the spacer reviewed. The child returned home with improved medication delivery using the MDI with spacer.

2 Nasopharyngeal Airway

2.1 Case Example

You are on rounds on the pediatric ward of a Nepali hospital when a nurse from the labor and delivery ward enters. She explains that a 19-year-old woman without full prenatal care just delivered a full-term baby. The infant has signs of respiratory distress despite initial steps of resuscitation including repositioning the infant's neck into the "sniffing position" and nasal bulb suctioning. The healthcare provider notes stridor from the hallway as they approach the infant's room. On arrival they find a crying infant in mild respiratory distress. The infant has suprasternal retractions and inspiratory stridor. They note that lifting the infants jaw provides transient improvement in the stridor. Deep suctioning with a catheter does not help improve the infant's distress. On closer examination, they observe that the infant has a small jaw and recessed chin. Opening the mouth reveals a small U-shaped cleft palate. Breath sounds are clear and equal bilaterally. The infant is diagnosed with Pierre Robin Sequence with micro- and retrognathia causing downward displacement of the tongue into the posterior oropharynx, leading to upper airway obstruction. The clinical team recognizes that they need a device (such as a nasopharyngeal airway) to overcome the area of obstruction and maintain upper airway patency.

2.2 Introduction

A nasopharyngeal airway (NPA) can be used to improve upper airway patency. A NPA, also commonly referred to as a "nasal trumpet", is a long and thin flexible tube that can be inserted into the nasal passageway in order to bypass an obstruction at the level of the nose, nasopharynx, or base of the tongue. Commercial NPAs come in a variety of sizes. The goal is to position the NPA beyond the base of the tongue but above the epiglottis [7]. By relieving upper airway obstruction, the NPA may allow for adequate air entry and effective ventilation of the patient.

2.2.1 Indications

The placement of an NPA may be indicated when the nares and nasopharynx is obstructed by anatomical narrowing, septal deviation, or secretions requiring frequent nasotracheal suctioning. Other indications include oropharyngeal obstruction due to conditions such as micrognathia, retrognathia, glossoptosis, macroglossia, or limited mouth opening (as with syngnathia). Patients with upper airway obstruction due to hypotonia (i.e., infant with peripartum magnesium exposure) or post-operative swelling (i.e., adenoidectomy, tonsillectomy, maxillofacial surgery) are also ideal candidates for temporary placement of an NPA.

2.2.2 Contraindications

Contraindications to NPA placement include basilar skull fracture, nasal bridge trauma, septal trauma, and frontal sinus trauma [8]. Relative contraindications include coagulopathy, thrombocytopenia, and minor nasal trauma.
Overall, the NPA is advantageous due to its simplicity and ease of use in a wide array of clinical scenarios.

2.2.3 Equipment

- Medical gloves (nitrile, rubber, etc.) – ideal
- Flexible hollow tubing (urinary catheter, respiratory tubing, etc.) or an endotracheal tube
- Lubricant (e.g., water-based jelly)
- Scissors/razor blade
- Marker/pen
- Medical tape

Bag valve ask (optional)

2.2.4 Technique

Fashioning an NPA from a Flexible Tube

Though this is not a sterile procedure, it is still advised to perform the procedure as cleanly as possible (washed hands and gloves) as the device will be inserted into a patient's upper airway. Clean technique will help to minimize the risk of infection.

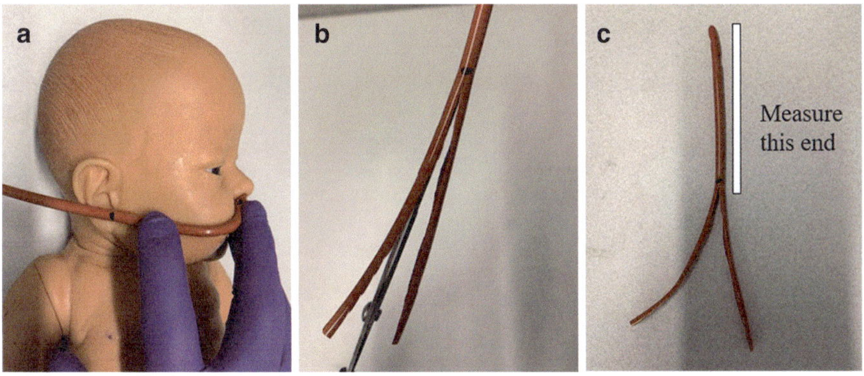

Fig. 6 (**a**) Measuring distance. (**b**) Cutting tube. (**c**) Measuring end that goes into nose

1. Choose an appropriate diameter tube for the creation of the NPA. Choose a size with the diameter a little smaller than the patient's nares. This can often be estimated by looking at the size of the patient's fifth digit.
2. Measure the desired insertion depth of the NPA. This is done by measuring the distance from the lateral rim of the nostril in which the NPA will be inserted to the tragus of the ipsilateral ear [9]. Figure 6a depicts this measurement technique and how the desired depth can be marked on the tubing with a marker.
3. Slice down the length of the tubing, with a clean pair of scissors or a razor blade, starting at the opposite end from the side you measured. Cut all the way up to the NPA depth marking (Fig. 6b). Make a second cut on the other side of the tubing. This should create two tails (Fig. 6c). *If you are using an endotracheal tube, skip this step.* Your NPA is now ready for insertion.

2.2.5 Instructions for Use

It is important to have the patient properly positioned in a sniffing or neutral neck position prior to placement of the NPA. If able, gather resuscitation equipment such as nasotracheal suction, supplemental oxygen, and a bag mask device. Prepare the NPA by liberally covering the insertion end with water-based lubricant jelly. Next, angle the NPA slightly toward the nasal septum and down toward the floor of the nasal cavity (not upwards) as shown in Fig. 7a.

Insert the NPA aiming directly back toward the nasopharynx and allow it to slide along the floor of the nasal cavity to avoid upward displacement. Once the NPA has been inserted to the marked depth, spread the two cut tails over the patient's cheeks (Fig. 7b). Splitting the softer tubes keeps them from migrating in further. Using medical tape, secure the tails using a chevron technique (Fig. 7c). While it can be placed by a single person, a second person may be useful to help apply the tape while the provider inserting the NPA maintains its position.

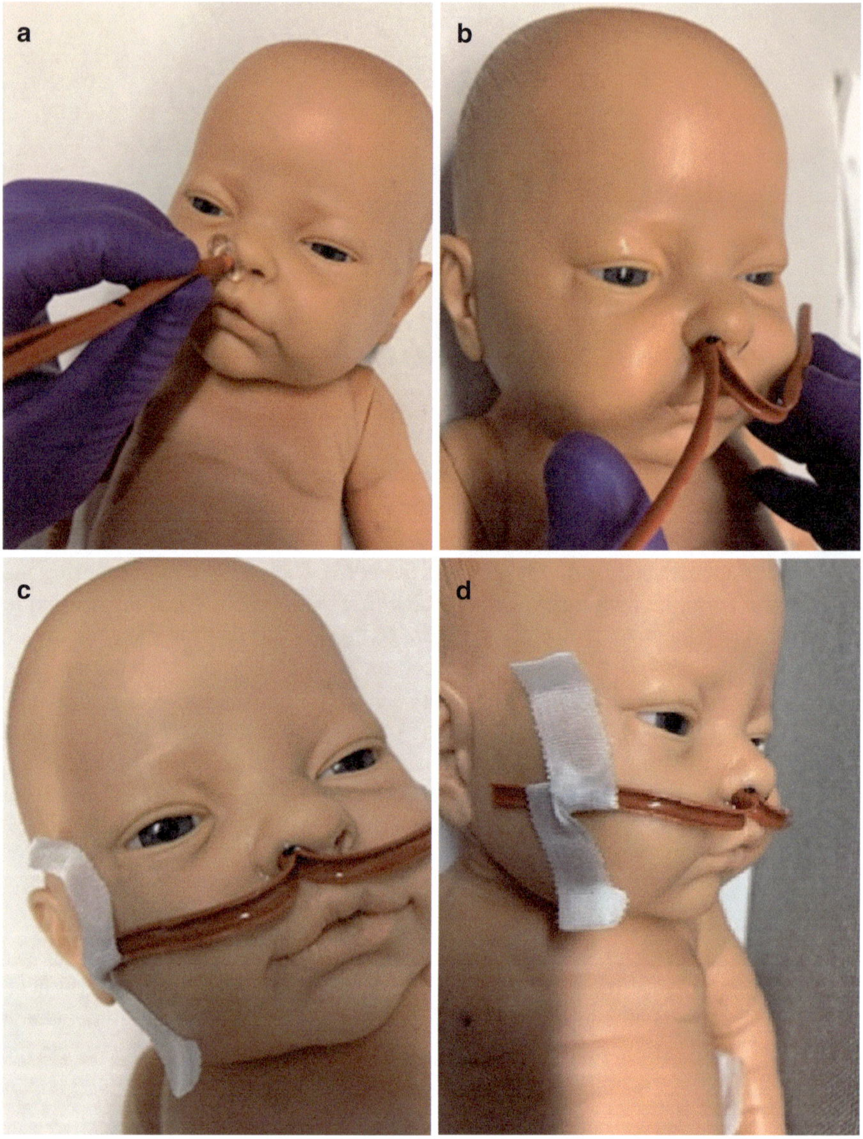

Fig. 7 (**a**) Inserting NPA. (**b**): Showing tails of tube after insertion. (**c**): Securing tails of NPA. (**d**): Securing tails second example

Tubes with greater stiffness, such as endotracheal tubes, do not need to be spliced along their long axis (Figs. 8 and 9). Instead, secure it as you would a nasogastric tube using the chevron tape technique described above.

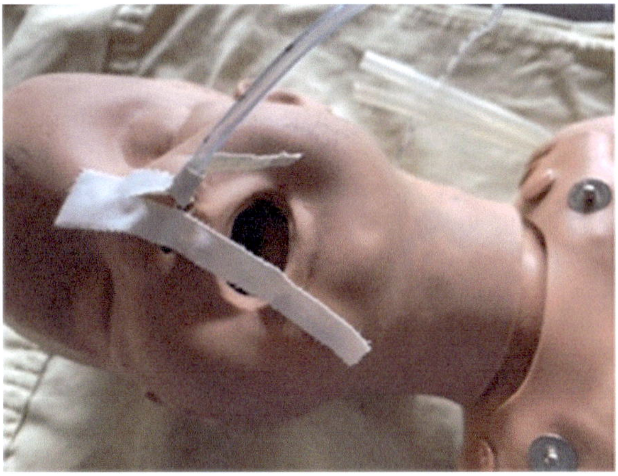

Fig. 8 Securing endotracheal tube used as NPA. (Courtesy of Dr. T. Slusher)

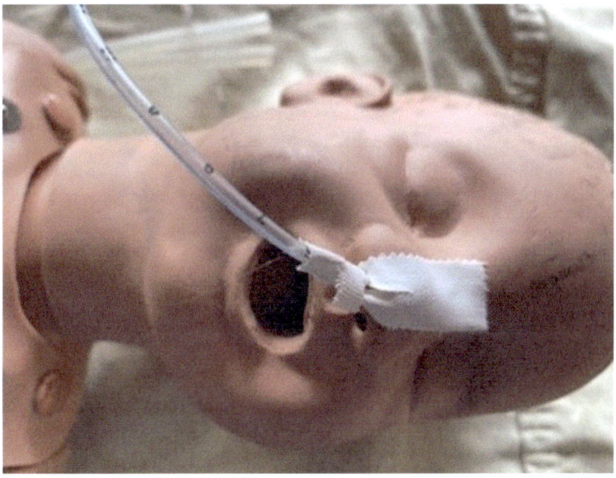

Fig. 9 Securing endotracheal tube used as NPA 2. (Courtesy of Dr. T. Slusher)

2.2.6 Complications

Since the placement of a NPA does not allow direct visualization of the nasal passage with a scope or camera (i.e., blind placement) some complications must be considered.

Nasal Trauma The patient is at risk of nasal skin breakdown and nasal mucosal trauma. To prevent irritation/trauma, insert an NPA whose outer diameter enters the nares easily but stays positioned securely and use lubricating jelly when available. Staff should be advised to monitor the nares for skin breakdown and bloody discharge from the nose or mouth at least once per shift. Additionally, if able, the medical team should consider alternating the nares after 48 hours, or sooner if skin breakdown or mucosal bleeding is seen, to allow for healing.

Positioning Unlike oropharyngeal airways and endotracheal tubes which are placed in sedated patients, NPAs can be placed in conscious or semi-conscious persons. Thus, diligent measurement for insertion depth is critical in order to decrease the risk of triggering a cough or gag reflex, which puts the patient at risk for aspiration. Since the NPA is measured with the neck in a neutral position, staff should first assess to ensure the patient neck has not been hyperextended or flexed as this can result in up to 0.5 cm movement. If the NPA is too short (positioned too high) the patient may continue to have obstruction since the NPA would not be moving the tongue away from the oropharynx to relieve the obstruction. If the patient has significant coughing or gagging, this can be a sign that the NPA is too deep. Coughing/gagging may also signal that the patient is not going to tolerate an NPA. If a patient starts coughing or gagging, first attempt to retract the NPA slightly and re-secure it. If the positioning is still in question, you can obtain a lateral neck radiograph to assess the NPA position.

Brain Injury Finally, while exceedingly rare and only reported in patients with maxillofacial or basilar skull fracture, serious complications such as intracranial mispositioning of an NPA can lead to brain injury [10, 11]. Therefore, **NPA insertion is contraindicated in the setting of maxillofacial or basilar skull fracture.**

2.3 Case Resolution

The infant's airway was cleared with suctioning and a nasopharyngeal airway was fashioned from a flexible red rubber catheter by following the instructions above for measuring, cutting, inserting, and securing the NPA. There was immediate improvement in the stridor and suprasternal retractions. With the NPA in place, the mother was able to breastfeed in a side-lying position.

References

1. Volerman A, et al. Mask use with spacers/Valved holding chambers and metered dose inhalers among children with asthma. Ann Am Thorac Soc. 2021;18(1):17–22.
2. Rodriguez C, Sossa M, Lozano JM. Commercial versus home-made spacers in delivering bronchodilator therapy for acute therapy in children. Cochrane Database Syst Rev. 2008;2:CD005536.
3. Boulet LP, et al. Canadian asthma consensus report, 1999. Canadian Asthma Consensus Group Cmaj. 1999;161(11 Suppl):S1–61.
4. Zar HJ, et al. Home-made spacers for bronchodilator therapy in children with acute asthma: a randomised trial. Lancet. 1999;354(9183):979–82.
5. Butteris SM, et al. Simulation use for global away rotations (SUGAR): preparing residents for emotional challenges abroad--a multicenter study. Acad Pediatr. 2014;14(5):533–41.
6. National Asthma Education, aPP. Expert panel report 3: guidelines for the diagnosis and management of asthma. National Heart, Lung, and Blood Institute; 2007.

7. Stoneham MD. The nasopharyngeal airway. Assessment of position by fibreoptic laryngoscopy. Anaesthesia. 1993;48(7):575–80.
8. Roberts K, Whalley H, Bleetman A. The nasopharyngeal airway: dispelling myths and establishing the facts. Emerg Med J. 2005;22(6):394–6.
9. Shen CM, et al. Nasopharyngeal tract length measurement in infants. Acta Paediatr Taiwan. 2002;43(2):82–5.
10. Muzzi DA, Losasso TJ, Cucchiara RF. Complication from a nasopharyngeal airway in a patient with a basilar skull fracture. Anesthesiology. 1991;74(2):366–8.
11. Schade K, Borzotta A, Michaels A. Intracranial malposition of nasopharyngeal airway. J Trauma. 2000;49(5):967–8.

Bubble CPAP in a Low-Resource Setting

Andrew Wu, Beatrice Odongkara, and Zubin Shah

Abbreviations

BCPAP	Bubble continuous positive airway pressure
CPAP	Continuous positive airway pressure
LFNC	Low-flow nasal cannula
LMIC	Low-and-middle income country
LRTI	Lower respiratory tract infection
PEEP	Positive end-expiratory pressure

1 Case Example

A neonate is delivered at 34 weeks in a hospital in rural Cambodia. The infant is vigorous and crying at the perineum. She is noted to have nasal flaring and intercostal retractions. Given the prematurity, the team is concerned for respiratory distress syndrome of the newborn. The oxygen saturation is 87% on supplemental

A. Wu (✉)
Boston Children's Hospital, Boston, MA, USA
e-mail: andrewwu@umn.edu

B. Odongkara
Department of Paediatrics and Child Health Gulu, Gulu University, Gulu, Uganda

Z. Shah
Division of Neonatology, Nationwide Children's Hospital, Columbus, OH, USA
e-mail: Zubin.Shah@nationwidechildrens.org

T. M. Slusher et al. (eds.), *Pediatric Procedural Adaptations for Low-Resource Settings*, https://doi.org/10.1007/978-3-030-99955-1_18

nasal cannula oxygen. She has increased work of breathing and tachypnea with a respiratory rate in the 80s. A chest radiograph shows ground glass opacities bilaterally. Plans are made to place the neonate on CPAP, however the only commercial CPAP in the nursery is already in use. In order to use CPAP for this neonate, you will need to construct homemade bubble CPAP.

2 Introduction

Forty-five percent of deaths under five years of age worldwide occur in neonates. Respiratory distress is commonly associated with the leading causes of these deaths in neonates – prematurity and birth asphyxia [1, 2]. Respiratory distress develops in more than half of neonates born under 31 weeks of gestation [3]. Additionally, lower respiratory tract infections (LRTIs) are the leading cause of death in children under five years of age around the world, with over 70% of these deaths occurring in low- and middle-income countries (LMICs) [2, 4, 5].

A key component to the management of respiratory illness in neonates and children is the provision of respiratory support. Support may be needed to improve oxygenation, as well as provide positive pressure to decrease work of breathing. Unfortunately, resources for adequate respiratory support options are scarce in LMICs. Low-cost modified bubble CPAP (bCPAP) can be utilized effectively to meet this gap in respiratory support in young children.

Invented in the 1970s, bCPAP is a form of respiratory support that utilizes the pressure created by a column of water to generate positive end-expiratory pressure (PEEP) [6]. This form of respiratory support is significantly less expensive than conventional CPAP; however, commercial BCPAP still costs hundreds of U.S.D [7]. Fortunately, a low-cost version of bCPAP exists that utilizes compressed air and/or oxygen, oxygen tubing, a bottle of water, and a nasal cannula to create the respiratory circuit [8]. This version of bCPAP does not require electricity, can be constructed from readily available materials found at most hospitals in the world, and costs approximately 5 U.S.D. Most importantly, it has been shown to have clinical efficacy when compared to LFNC while also maintaining safety [9].

Bubble CPAP supports respiratory effort through a nasal interface that conducts air pressure to stent open airways and lungs. The expiratory resistance providing alveolar and airway stenting is delivered via a tube whose distal aperture is under water. The height or distance the tube is submerged under water is approximately equal to the pressure generated in the circuit (i.e., a tube aperture under 5 cm of water (H_2O) creates about 5 cm H_2O pressure). The expiratory limb tubing should be as short and large bore as feasible so as to not add additional resistance to the circuit. Additionally, bubble CPAP devices function optimally if there is an adequate seal at the nose and/or mouth interface.

2.1 The Evidence

The population for whom bCPAP has the strongest evidence is neonates (ages 0 to 28 days) from both high- and low-resource settings [6, 7, 10–14]. Most studies conducted in low-resource settings included premature newborns or those with low birthweight; therefore, there is substantially more evidence to support an indication of bCPAP use in this younger, at-risk population compared to that for older age groups. Most studies included neonates with respiratory distress from any cause, though this usually specifically included those with respiratory distress syndrome (RDS), transient tachypnea of the newborn, and meconium aspiration [11]. There is limited data of the use of bCPAP in neonates with respiratory distress in the setting of congenital anomalies and structural pathologies as these children have typically been excluded from bCPAP trials.

A few RCTs have been published that evaluate bCPAP use in children beyond the neonate up to five years of age, but the data is mixed regarding how to best identify the appropriate patient population [9, 15–18]. BCPAP may be helpful in preventing clinical failure or death in children up to 15 months of age when compared to LFNC but may require frequent physician oversight to be of any benefit [9, 15, 17]. These older patients typically have been those with hypoxia and have met WHO criteria for severe pneumonia [19]. A single RCT performed on children up to 13 months of age in Bangladesh demonstrated less treatment failure and fewer deaths with bCPAP compared to LFNC. Of note, bCPAP performed similarly to high-flow nasal cannula (HFNC) [9]. Therefore, it seems the clinical benefits of bCPAP may extend beyond the neonate, but more research is being done on this topic.

In an effort to adapt this low-cost bCPAP to children beyond the neonate, a recently developed, novel modification called SEAL-bCPAP has been made to this design, which will be described and included in this chapter. The modification creates a tighter seal at the level of the nares and can help avoid leak. This modification has been shown to be safe in a clinical trial in Uganda by Dr. Bjorklund, et al. [20] with a trend toward efficacy; however, a clinical trial to more definitively demonstrate the efficacy of this modification is currently being designed.

This chapter reviews how to construct a low-cost bCPAP circuit, the nasal seal adaptation, as well as how to set up and use bCPAP.

3 Indications

bCPAP has the strongest indication in the following population groups:

Neonates:

1. Neonates with respiratory distress syndrome including those with surfactant deficiency
2. Neonates with respiratory distress from any cause, including infectious etiologies

3. Apnea of prematurity

Children <5yo in resource-limited settings

1. Respiratory distress of any cause, most significantly in those with LRTIs
2. Hypoxia not responsive to low flow nasal cannula

4 Contraindications

Conditions that may be worsened by positive airway pressure

- pneumothorax
- certain cyanotic cardiac malformations
- severe asthma exacerbation
- recent abdominal surgery
  - Significant, active epistaxis.
  - Vomiting, with aspiration risk.
  - Malformations that preclude adequate nasal seal may not benefit from bCPAP, such as those with unrepaired cleft lip or palate.

5 Equipment/Supplies

- Nasal cannula (can use infant, pediatric, or adult)
- Sturdy tubing (oxygen tubing or large NG tube)
- Scissors
- Tape (medical or duct tape) and/or Superglue
- Bottle, beaker, or container (a 500 mL plastic water bottle works well)
- Ruler/measuring tape
- Pen/marker
- Oxygen/air source able to provide up to 6 liters per minute (LPM) of flow
- Optional supplies for nasal seal adaption
  1. Soft compressible ear plugs
  2. Small pointed scissors, 18-20G needle, small nail or a pointed toothpick

6 Technique/Instructions for Use

1. **Obtain an appropriately sized nasal cannula prong and circuit**. This should be based on the patient's age:

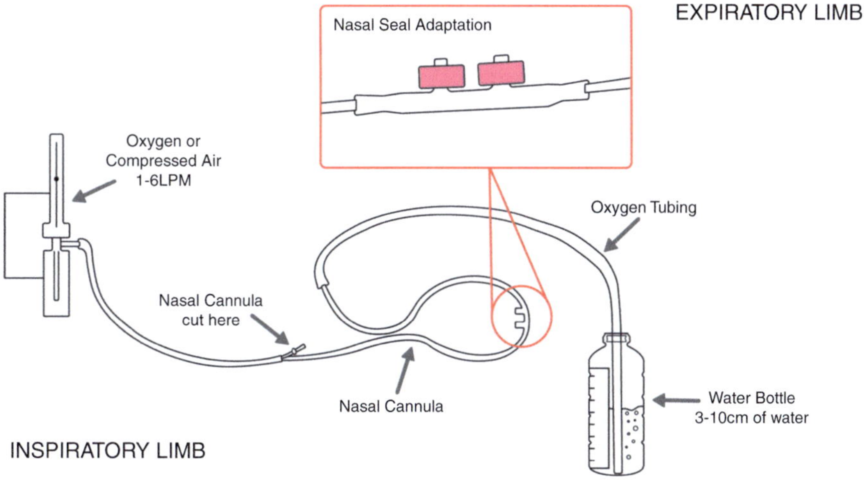

Fig. 1 A completed low-resource bubble CPAP circuit. The SEAL-BCPAP modification is highlighted at the nasal prongs

(a) Neonate – 6 months: use infant nasal cannula if available
(b) 6 months – 12 months: use pediatric nasal cannula if available
(c) >12 months: use pediatric nasal cannula with soft ear plug attachment

It is appropriate to change the size if leak or nasal tissue compression is noted. No pinching of the nasal septum should occur. The ideal prong is the largest that will not pinch the nasal septum.

An adult nasal cannula can be used and modified for most children as well

2. **Using scissors, cut one of the two limbs of the nasal cannula** (Fig. 1). Be sure to leave at least 3-4 cm of length on the short end.
3. **Tie the short end of tubing in a knot.** This will create a one-way passage for air flow.
4. **Insert the longer cut limb into the tubing being used for the expiratory limb (i.e. oxygen tubing or NG tubing)**. This tubing should be long enough to reach the water bottle when the nasal cannula is on the patient and still allow for patient movement. However, it should not be excessively long so as to minimize the resistance of flow in the tubing. **The largest bore tubing available should also be used to minimize resistance to flow**.
5. **Secure the connection of the cut limb and expiratory tubing with tape or super glue.** If using glue, be sure not to occlude the lumen of the tubing with glue.
6. **Label and fill water bottle.** Any container of water is sufficient if it is clean, can stand up on its own, and can contain a water column at least 10 cm high. A 500 mL bottle is sufficient. Using a ruler and a marker or pen, mark measurements along the side of the water bottle to indicate the height of the water column. For readability, these marks can also be made on a strip of tape which is then adhered to the bottle. The 0 cm mark should be at the bottom of the bottle

with the 10 cm mark closer to the aperture/top of the bottle. Generally, the water level is started at 3-5 cm and increased as needed to a max of 10 cm.

7. **Insert the oxygen tubing/expiratory limb into a bottle of water**. The tube should be completely submerged so the tip touches the bottom of the bottle and the CPAP level is then adjusted by adding and removing water without moving the tube. Securing the tubing by taping it in place at the top of the bottle is recommended. An alternative method to this where the expiratory limb is suspended in the water and then moved up and down in the water to adjust CPAP is not recommended. This method introduces the risk of providing too much CPAP as a result of the tube inadvertently falling inside the bottle.
8. **Attach the nasal cannula tubing to the flow meter or oxygen port**. Then turn on the flow.
9. **Test the system by occluding the nasal cannula prongs (i.e., pinch them closed with clean fingers) with the flow on.** You should see bubbles in the water bottle if the circuit is set up correctly without any leaks.

Creating the SEAL-bCPAP modification (Fig. 2). The SEAL-bCPAP modification should be used if the nasal prongs are too small to create a seal in the patient's nares. To construct the modification:

1. Cut a ½ cm- or less wide disc off of the end of the foam ear plug. This is most easily done using scissors to cut a cross section of the plug at the widest end (i.e. the end that remains outside of the ear).
2. Puncture a hole or slit through the center of the disc using one blade of the scissors, a nail, or needle.
3. Fit the nasal cannula prong through this hole so it protrudes through the center of the disc (Fig. 2). The disc will have to be stretched over the prong to make this work.
4. Repeat these steps to create a disc for the other nasal cannula prong.
5. When this is applied to the patient it can either be left outside the nares (commonly in neonates/infants) or compressed and placed in the nares for older children with a larger leak. The ear plug material should be secured to the nasal

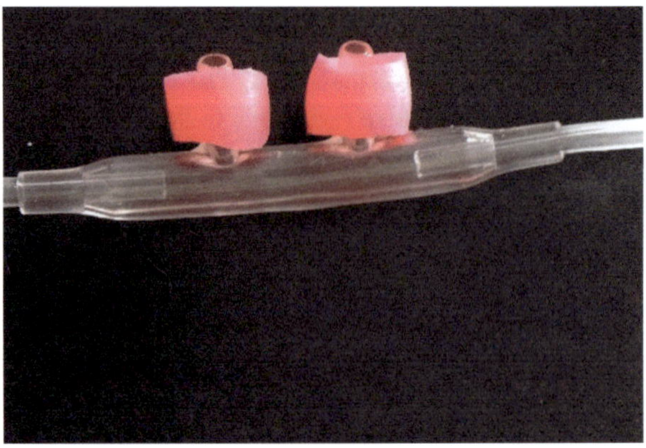

Fig. 2 SEAL-bCPAP modification

prong with a dot of super glue it if is going to be in the nares so as to not create a nasal foreign body.

Adult nasal prong adaptation for infant/child (Fig. 3a–c)

1. If the distance between the two prongs of the cannula is too far apart to fit appropriately in the child's nares, the prongs can move closer together.
2. Cut a small (1/4 cm or less) piece of the tubing between the prongs out. Remove this piece (Fig. 3a).

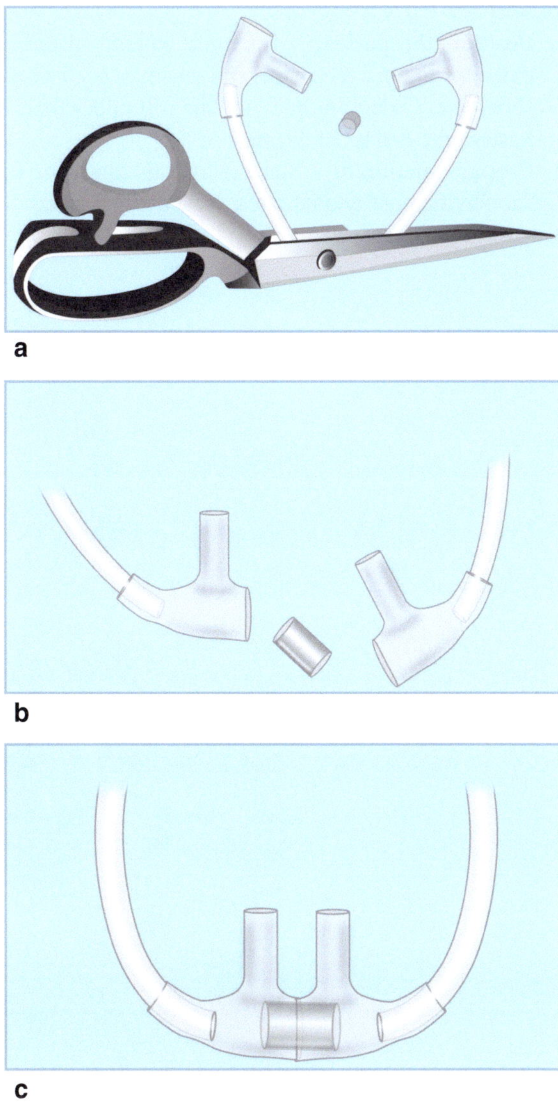

Fig. 3 (**a**) Cut out small piece of tubing between prongs. (**b**) Cut a separate small piece of tube that will hold prongs together. (**c**): Insert small piece without occluding either prong

3. A small piece of tubing that can fit inside the nasal cannula to hold the prongs together can be cut from a different piece of oxygen tubing or a nasogastric tube. This piece of tubing will need to be small enough to fit in the tubing that connects the two prongs and short enough that it does not occlude either prong. It is being used as a bridge to align the 2 prongs (Fig. 3b, c).
4. The tubing bridge described in step 3 should be secured with a dot of super glue. Take care not to occlude either nasal prong. If an appropriate piece of tubing cannot be found, the prongs can be glued together without the bridge, but it is more difficult to get them to align and avoid occluding the prongs when gluing.

Patient Set-Up (Fig. 4)

1. **Position the patient** – Have the patient on their back and the neck slightly extended to open the airway. Infants may need a rolled towel or cloth under their shoulders. Older children may the roll under their neck. If possible, elevate the head of the bed to 30 degrees.
2. **Prepare suctioning** – Since secretions can block CPAP delivery, be prepared to suction the nose and mouth at least every 6 hours.

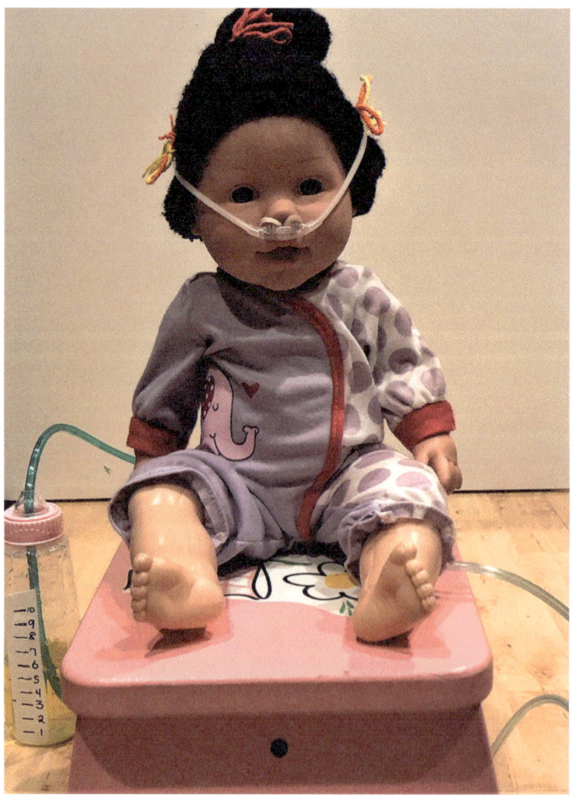

Fig. 4 Doll demonstrating set up including hat to hold tubing showing complete set up except oxygen source

3. **Secure the nasal interface to the patient** – Secure nasal cannula tubing on the child's face using a small piece of tape on each cheek. Instead of tape, a hat and string ties can be used in infants (Fig. 4).
4. **Place a nasogastric tube in selected patients** – Consider placing a small nasogastric tube to vent the stomach, which will decrease discomfort and complications from aerophagia (i.e., air in the stomach). Leave the end open and empty into the inside of a rubber glove.
5. **Set up oxygen monitoring if able –** Ideally continuous oxygen and heart rate monitoring will be utilized, but spot checking can be used if continuous monitoring is not feasible.

7 Instructions for Use

Using bCPAP, while it is on the patient, primarily consists of knowing how to change the CPAP level and how to discontinue bCPAP.

1. **Changing the CPAP level** – If the aperture of the expiratory limb touches the bottom of the bottle (preferred), the CPAP level is approximately equal to the height of the water level in the bottle. Generally, start with 3-5 cm depth of water in the bottle. The CPAP level can be increased by adding water to the desired height. For example, if there is 5 cm of water in the bottle and the desired level is 8 cm, add water until the level reaches 8 cm. To decrease the CPAP level, pour water out to achieve the desired height of water. Water can evaporate, so be sure to add more if the water level is noted to be less than desired.
2. **Weaning/discontinuing bCPAP** – It is recommended to reduce the CPAP level by 1–2 cm H_2O every 4–6 hours as tolerated by the patient once deemed ready to wean. When the CPAP is between 3-5 cm H_2O and the patient's vitals are in normal range for age, bCPAP can usually be discontinued. When discontinuing bCPAP, simply remove the device from the patient. The patient may still need supplemental oxygen via a nasal cannula. Monitor the patient for at least 6 hours after bCPAP is discontinued. If increased work of breathing is noted, place them back on bCPAP.
3. **Assessing for bCPAP effectiveness** – A bCPAP score has been published to quantify the quality of bCPAP delivery. It is recommended to use this score to determine if the bCPAP circuit is delivering appropriate support (Table 1). A score of 0–5 means the circuit is not delivering effective bCPAP. A score of 6–9 means the circuit is delivering inconsistent bCPAP. A score of 10 means the circuit is likely delivering effective bCPAP.

Table 1 The BCPAP score for effectiveness of bubble CPAP delivery

	0	1	2	Score
Bubbles	Not present	Intermittent	Continuous	
Circuit	Contaminated	Clean but small diameter (<1 cm)	Clean and wide diameter (≥1 CM)	
Prongs	Too small	Too large	Occlusive fit	
Airway	Blocked	Partially blocked	Open with bilateral breath sounds	
Pressure	Air leak	Intermittent	Maintained at set level	

Reproduced with permission from Oxford University Press [21]

8 Complications/Monitoring/Troubleshooting

Potential complications of the use of bubble CPAP include nasal erythema, aerophagia, abdominal distension, aspiration and device fragmentation and rarely, pneumothorax, epistaxis, and nasal septum perforation [20]. A recent safety study evaluating SEAL-bCPAP modification found that most of these complications are rare. The most common complications in this study were abdominal distension and nasal tissue irritation.

Therefore, maintenance of the device includes monitoring for signs and symptoms of these complications. This primarily includes regular suctioning to ensure unobstructed flow; monitoring for nasal injury; abdominal decompression; monitoring the integrity of the system; and troubleshooting.

1. **Suctioning** – The nose and mouth should be suctioned at least every 6 hours and more frequently if the patient is noted to have copious secretions. This can be skipped if the medical providers deem this to be unnecessary.
2. **Monitoring for nasal injury** – Septal injury is preventable. Evaluation of the nasal septum should be done at least every 6 hours. Remember to use the correct prong size and secure them in place so they do not move, including twisting of the prongs. If signs of redness or erosion are observed, reposition the prongs. Consider adding the nasal seal adaptation (described above) on the outside of the nares to cushion the nose.
3. **Abdominal decompression** – If abdominal distension is noted, intermittent gastric decompression suctioning can be performed to relieve the pressure in the stomach.
4. **Integrity of the system** – The bedside attendant or parent should be informed to watch to make sure that the bottle continues to bubble. Ideally this would be checked at least every 2 hours for continued bubbling. If there is no bubbling at any point, proceed with troubleshooting.
5. **Troubleshooting** – If no bubbling is present, take the following steps:

    (a) Make sure nasal prongs are in the nose.
    (b) Check the tubing for leaks or obstruction. Start at the flow meter. The most common locations of leak are at the knot tied during construction or the connection between the oxygen tubing and nasal cannula tubing. These connections can be reinforced with tape or glue.

(c) Evaluate the circuit for leaks at the mouth or nasal prongs. A common site of leak is an open mouth, or leak at the nasal prong. Suction the nose, mouth, and adjust the nasal prongs. Consider adding nasal seal adaptation if leak is at the nares.
(d) Increase the flow of oxygen to overcome any leak or resistance that may be present.
(e) If all above fails, replace the system.

9 Case Resolution

Using the equipment available, a bCPAP circuit was used to administer a CPAP level of 6 cm H_2O. Over the course of the first six hours from initiation, the neonates work of breathing improved and vitals stabilized. The bCPAP level was weaned by 1 cm H2O every 4 hours down to 3 cm H2O with no change in O2 saturation, tachypnea, or work of breathing. Bubble CPAP was discontinued after <24 hours.

References

1. Duke T. Neonatal pneumonia in developing countries. Arch Dis Child Fetal Neonatal Ed. 2005;90(3):F211–9.
2. Liu L, et al. Global, regional, and national causes of under-5 mortality in 2000-15: an updated systematic analysis with implications for the sustainable development goals. Lancet. 2016;388(10063):3027–35.
3. St Clair C, et al. The probability of neonatal respiratory distress syndrome as a function of gestational age and lecithin/sphingomyelin ratio. Am J Perinatol. 2008;25(8):473–80.
4. Lozano R, et al. Global and regional mortality from 235 causes of death for 20 age groups in 1990 and 2010: a systematic analysis for the global burden of disease study 2010. Lancet. 2012;380(9859):2095–128.
5. Pneumonia, in Media Centre. 2016, World Health Organization.
6. Lee KS, et al. A comparison of underwater bubble continuous positive airway pressure with ventilator-derived continuous positive airway pressure in premature neonates ready for extubation. Biol Neonate. 1998;73(2):69–75.
7. Boyd J. Clinical study finds 'bubble CPAP' boosts neonatal survival rates. Rice University News and Media [Website] 2014 [cited 2016]; Available from: http://news.rice.edu/2014/01/29/clinical-study-finds-bubble-cpap-boosts-neonatal-survival-rates-2/.
8. Organization, WH. Oxygen therapy for children: a manual for health workers. World Health Organization; 2016.
9. Chisti MJ, et al. Bubble continuous positive airway pressure for children with severe pneumonia and hypoxaemia in Bangladesh: an open, randomised controlled trial. Lancet. 2015;386(9998):1057–65.
10. Chan KM, Chan HB. The use of bubble CPAP in premature infants: local experience. HK J Paediatr. 2007;1(12):86–92.
11. Chen A, et al. Cost-effectiveness analysis of a low-cost bubble CPAP device in providing ventilatory support for neonates in Malawi - a preliminary report. BMC Pediatr. 2014;14:288.
12. Kawaza K, et al. Efficacy of a low-cost bubble CPAP system in treatment of respiratory distress in a neonatal ward in Malawi. PLoS One. 2014;9(1):e86327.

13. Martin S, Duke T, Davis P. Efficacy and safety of bubble CPAP in neonatal care in low and middle income countries: a systematic review. Arch Dis Child Fetal Neonatal Ed. 2014;99(6):F495–504.
14. Yadav S, et al. Bubble vs conventional continuous positive airway pressure for prevention of extubation failure in preterm very low birth weight infants: a pilot study. Indian J Pediatr. 2012;79(9):1163–8.
15. McCollum ED, et al. Bubble continuous positive airway pressure for children with high-risk conditions and severe pneumonia in Malawi: an open label, randomised, controlled trial. Lancet Respir Med. 2019;7(11):964–74.
16. Walk J, et al. Non-invasive ventilation with bubble CPAP is feasible and improves respiratory physiology in hospitalised Malawian children with acute respiratory failure. Paediatr Int Child Health. 2016;36(1):28–33.
17. Wilson PT, et al. Continuous positive airway pressure for children with undifferentiated respiratory distress in Ghana: an open-label, cluster, crossover trial. Lancet Glob Health. 2017;5(6):e615–23.
18. Wilson PT, et al. A randomized clinical trial evaluating nasal continuous positive airway pressure for acute respiratory distress in a developing country. J Pediatr. 2013;162(5):988–92.
19. WHO. Hospital care for children: guidelines for the management of common illnesses with limited resources. 2nd ed. Geneva: World Health Organization; 2013.
20. Bjorklund AR, et al. Use of a modified bubble continuous positive airway pressure (bCPAP) device for children in respiratory distress in low- and middle-income countries: a safety study. Paediatr Int Child Health. 2018:1–8.
21. John SC, Cheng EO, John SP. The BCPAP score: five questions to assess the effectiveness of a bubble CPAP circuit. J Trop Pediatr. 2020;66(5):542–8.

Further Reading

SUGARPREP | Home (https://sugarprep.org)
WHO | Oxygen therapy for children: a manual for health workers, p. 36 (www.who.int/maternal_child_adolescent/documents/child-oxygen-therapy/en/)

Modified Chest Drainage System for Use in a Low-Resource Settings

Rachel Bensman, Agneta Odera, and Biplab Nandi

Abbreviations

CPAP	Continuous positive airway pressure
CT	Computed tomography
CXR	Chest radiograph
IV	Intravenous
LDH	Lactic dehydrogenase
TB	Tuberculosis
USD	United States Dollars

1 Case Presentation

A 4-year-old child presents with a non-productive cough, feeling hot, having night sweats, decreased energy, poor appetite, and weight loss. Parents say her symptoms started last week. Review of systems is otherwise unremarkable. There is no other past medical history, drug history, allergies, or family history. She has no history of any tuberculosis contact. On exam, you note she is febrile to 39.1 °C, tachycardic

R. Bensman (✉)
Cincinnati Children's Hospital, Department of Pediatrics, Division of Emergency Medicine, University of Cincinnati, Cincinnati, OH, USA
e-mail: Rachel.Bensman@cchmc.org

A. Odera
Tenwek Hospital, Bomet, Kenya

B. Nandi
Kamuzu Central Hospital, Lilongwe, Malawi

T. M. Slusher et al. (eds.), *Pediatric Procedural Adaptations for Low-Resource Settings*, https://doi.org/10.1007/978-3-030-99955-1_19

(125 bpm), and tachypneic (24 bpm) with SpO_2 91% on room air, which increases to 96% on low flow O_2 via nasal prongs. She has a normal blood pressure. She appears chronically malnourished and has dry mucous membranes. She is ill appearing with respiratory distress including nasal flaring, intermittent grunting, and mild intercostal retractions. She has good air movement through the right anterior and posterior lung fields without wheezing or crepitations, but she has very decreased breath sounds in the middle and lower left posterior lung fields with distant crepitations and dullness to percussion. Her heart and abdominal exam are unremarkable (no palpable liver or spleen edges).

Chest radiograph (CXR) shows a massive left pleural effusion versus empyema. Ultrasound confirms the presence of a large probable empyema as the fluid is not uniformly echogenic and appears to have possible septations. Under ultrasound guidance, the clinician aspirates pus and appropriately determines that the child needs a chest tube and drainage of the empyema. The medical student visiting from the USA wants to place the chest tube; however, the Malawian doctor reminds him that only clinicians already skilled in placing chest tubes should do so. They place her on intravenous (IV) antibiotics and consult the surgeon who is skilled in placing chest tubes. He is unaware of the options for the chest tubes and discovers that there are no commercial chest tubes available in this rural hospital.

2 Introduction

Accumulated air, blood, or other fluids within the pleural cavity may cause compression of the lung(s), resulting in difficulty breathing, hypoxia, and/or inadequate ventilation. A chest drain/chest tube may be needed to decompress the air or fluid and improve pulmonary function/respiratory stability. In all settings, the risk of the procedure versus the benefit should be considered and in low-resource settings, additional precaution should be taken to carefully consider the complications of such an invasive procedure, including pain, infection, immobility, fistula formation, and human resource needs prior to placement. Safe insertion and management must be ensured.

While often necessary for patient treatment, the decision to place a chest drain should not be undertaken lightly. This is especially important in low-resource settings where monitoring may be lacking, complications more common, and the ability to manage the chest tube may be more challenging. Where provider/nurse-to-patient ratios are low, there is also opportunity cost in inserting and managing a chest drain when the disease may have improved without one. Most non-infective causes of effusions will resolve if the cause is treated without the need of a chest drain and its associated morbidity. Chest drains more quickly improve dyspnea but consider if a pleural tap to dryness may provide adequate relief while reducing exposure to pain and complications.

Insertion of a chest drain includes considerations for both the tube thoracostomy procedure as well as the drainage system to be attached. Guidance is provided here with the assumption that proceduralists are competent in the tube thoracostomy procedure. The purpose of this chapter is to describe the creation of a chest drainage system when a commercial unit (such as a Pleuravac©) is not available, as well as to highlight equipment alternatives and procedural pearls for operating in a limited resource environment.

3 Indications

3.1 Pleural Effusion

Pleural effusions may be transudative, exudative, or gross pus (Table 1). The decision to insert a chest drain for effusions requires careful considerations around severity of symptoms, likelihood of resolution of effusion without intervention, and

Table 1 Evaluation of fluid in the chest [1]

Type of effusion	Transudative effusion	Exudative effusion	Empyema
Causes	Heart failure Hepatic failure Renal failure	Malignancy Tuberculosis (TB) Infection (parapneumonic)	Infection
Pathophysiology	Oncotic pressure leading to plasma leak and decreased lymphatic return	Inflammation leading to vascular permeability	Local bacterial invasion
Exam findings	Typically symmetric lower chest dullness and dyspnea	Greater pleuritic pain and splinting; unilateral decreased chest expansion and dullness	Greater pleuritic pain and splinting; fever, signs of sepsis
Chest X-ray	Gravity-dependent fluid or white-out without air-fluid levels; more often bilateral	May have air-fluid levels or loculation which prevents free flowing between upright and decubitus films; more often unilateral	May have air-fluid levels or loculation which prevents free flowing between upright and decubitus films' more often unilateral
Ultrasound	Free flowing, gravity-dependent fluid	May have loculations or pleural thickening and/or nodules	May have loculations
Fluid appearance	Clear to straw colored	May be straw colored, purulent, bloody	Cloudy or purulent
Fluid analysis	Lactic dehydrogenase (LDH) is not raised Protein is not raised Glucose is not low	Leukocytes on gram stain or cytology (neutrophils in parapneumonic, lymphocytes in TB, abnormal in malignancy) Positive acid-fast bacilli stain (TB)	Bacteria on gram stain and culture Leukocytes with neutrophil predominance on gram stain or cytology

Adapted from Balfour-Lynn, 2005

risk of complications for unevacuated effusions. Patients who are significantly symptomatic from effusion will certainly benefit from drainage of fluid, but large transudative and even simple exudative effusions can often be drained by one-time or intermittent thoracentesis with small bore catheter, thus eliminating the need for tube thoracostomy and maintenance of a chest drain.

A reasonable approach to decision-making around the need for placement of a chest drain in a patient without severe symptoms is to first evaluate the characteristics of the effusion by sampling the fluid by needle thoracentesis and/or draining with a small bore catheter. In the absence of laboratory capabilities, overtly purulent fluid indicates the need for evacuation by tube thoracostomy with chest drain. If laboratory analysis is available, transudative effusions are better managed medically in the absence of severe symptoms. Exudative effusions, especially parapneumonic effusions, may require chest tubes for resolution. Malignant effusions may appear yellow, bloody, or milky. To this point, a chylothorax may be traumatic, iatrogenic, or, most commonly in the authors' experiences in sub-Saharan Africa, secondary to pleural Kaposi's sarcoma [2]. This will resolve with chemotherapy and in our experience does not require drainage.

Inserting a chest drain when the pleural fluid is not purulent, or not due to a parapneumonic effusion, may lead to complications such as ongoing fluid losses, infection, or fistula formation, without expediting cure of the underlying condition. While a chest drain is curative for an empyema, in most simple effusions it only provides symptomatic relief of dyspnea. If in doubt of whether a chest drain is indicated, one can try a therapeutic pleural tap to dryness. A three-way tap or large (50-60 ml) syringes (at least 2) are helpful to facilitate drainage. If "tap to dryness" produces significant relief from dyspnea, the potential complications, pain, and decreased mobility associated with placement of a chest tube may be warranted. However, in the authors' experience, this is rarely the case.

3.2 Hemothorax

Traditional teaching and guidelines recommend that traumatic hemothorax or hemopneumothorax generally requires placement of a chest tube [3]. However, there is some evidence that smaller hemothoraces, in hemodynamically stable patients, may be treated conservatively with better outcomes [4].

3.3 Pneumothorax

A pneumothorax may be spontaneous, traumatic, post-operative, or related to infection. Traumatic hemopneumothorax and pyopneumothorax, including bronchopleural fistula, are common combination collections. The decision to place a chest drain/tube for pneumothorax in a low-resource setting should primarily be driven by patient stability and degree of symptoms. The patient who is dyspneic and hypoxic from a moderate pneumothorax will benefit from placement of a chest drain, while patients with even large pneumothoraces can be managed expectantly if they are stable. In addition, it is reasonable to attempt only needle aspiration first with any size pneumothorax, potentially avoiding the need for tube thoracostomy [5]. However, tension pneumothoraces with evidence of cardiovascular compromise, such as hypotension, due to compression of the heart and great vessels, require immediate decompression with needle thoracostomy followed by tube thoracostomy.

It is also incredibly important to ensure that you have not mistaken another pathology for a pneumothorax. Specifically, radiography should be performed to evaluate for bullae, pneumatocele, or a diaphragmatic hernia in which case a chest drain is contraindicated (Fig. 1). If in doubt, a computed tomography (CT) scan may also be helpful. These pathologies are more likely to present in low-resource settings, either due to underlying disease or delayed diagnosis of congenital disorders. Another relevant differential diagnosis in Sub-Saharan Africa is hydropneumothorax from thoracic hydatid disease. With hydatid cysts, in asymptomatic patients, chest tube insertion should be avoided. Emergent chest tubes in this condition are only recommended if there is rupture of the cyst and the patient presents with symptomatic tension pneumothorax.

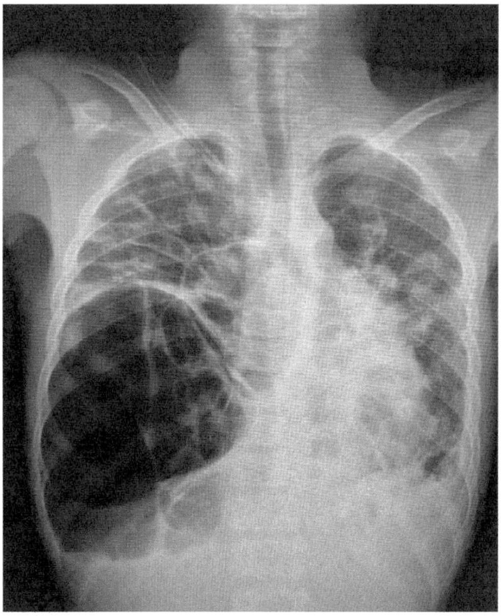

Fig. 1 Large bullae can be mistaken for pneumothorax. A chest drain is contraindicated. (Figure used with permission from Dr. Nandi)

4 Contraindications

There are no true absolute contraindications to tube thoracostomy for confirmed pneumothorax, hemothorax, or effusion, although entry to the chest through localized skin or soft tissue infection should be avoided. Relative contraindications include coagulopathy, thrombocytopenia, and anticoagulation therapy; risks of bleeding should be weighed against the benefit and urgency of need for chest drainage. Caution should be used in patients known to have pulmonary bullae or pleural or diaphragmatic adhesions.

5 Equipment

A. Supplies needed for tube thoracostomy

1. Skin cleansing agent/applicator (chlorhexidine, alcohol, betadine, with sterile gauze, cotton wool, or applicator wands)
2. Local anesthetic, needle, and syringe for injection of local anesthetic (if available)
3. Sedation medications and personnel depending on available expertise and patient stability [6]
4. Scalpel
5. Kelly clamp or similar device for blunt dissection
6. Sutures – ideally silk/nylon/other non-absorbable suture. The size will depend on the size of child/tube but usually between 4–0 and 2–0
7. Needle driver
8. Monitoring equipment (if available; a pulse oximeter provides at least heart rate and oxygen) and a second person to monitor the patient and vital signs while the procedure is being performed
9. Chest tube:
   (a) When an appropriately sized pediatric chest tube is available, use the following size guide [7] (Table 2)
   (b) If the appropriate size tube is unavailable, a chest tube may be improvised as discussed below

Chest tubes tend to have one hole at the end and multiple side holes for a short distance, so that the holes remain inside the chest. They may have a radiopaque marker line. More recently pigtail and Seldinger catheters are also available.

In resource-constrained settings, you may not be able to find an appropriately sized chest tube. When improvising a tube one should consider its stiffness, presence of end hole/side holes and how far they extend, length, and distal structure for attachment to the drainage system (Table 2). A tube that is too floppy may occlude or be difficult to insert through the chest wall. For air and thin pus, the size and quantity of the holes is likely less important. When pus is thick one can consider

Table 2 Chest tube sizes by patient weight

Chest tube sizes by patient weight		
Age	Weight	Chest tube size
Newborn to 1 year	3–5 kg	10–12 Fr
1–2 years	6–9 kg	12–16 Fr
2–4 years	10–11 kg	16–20 Fr
	12–14 kg	20–22 Fr
5–7 years	15–18 kg	22–24 Fr
	19–22 kg	24–28 Fr
8–11 years	23–30 kg	28–32 Fr
Greater than 11 years	>30 kg	32–42 Fr

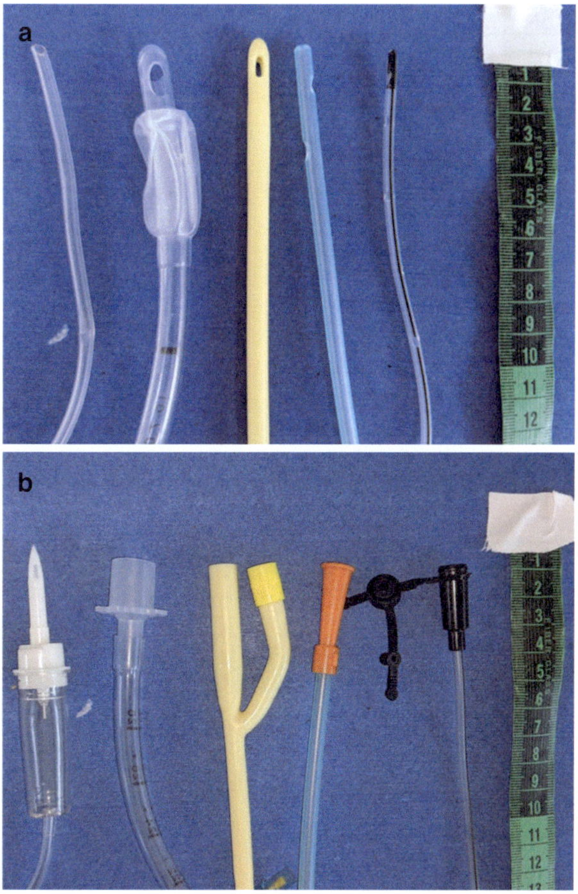

Fig. 2 (**a**) Improvised chest tubes proximal ends (Figure used with permission from Dr. Nandi). From left to right: cut giving set, endotracheal tube, foley catheter, suction catheter, nasogastric tube. (**b**) Improvised chest tubes distal ends. From left to right: cut giving set, endotracheal tube, foley catheter, suction catheter, nasogastric tube. (Photos courtesy of Dr. Nandi)

bending the tube and cutting side holes (Fig. 2a and b) but beware this is likely to weaken the tube and may cause a fragment to be retained on removal. For pus, any tube is probably better than no tube. Figure 2a and b and Table 3 illustrate and describe tubes that can be considered.

Table 3 Considerations for the choice of an improvised chest tube

Tube	Advantages	Disadvantages	Considerations
IV giving set with distal end cut off	Readily available, small size good for infants, stiff enough	Single-end hole, no side holes	Long length so can be inserted directly into drainage bottle without additional connections needed. Good option in newborns with thin pus, or when nothing else is available
Endotracheal tube	Good stiffness, large end hole, often a side hole	Short – Will need connection to a longer tube	A good option if available in correct size but consider how to connect to drainage system securely. Cuffed tubes may be difficult to insert but the cuff can be cut off
Urinary "Foley" catheter	Readily available in a variety of sizes, side holes only	Floppy, especially small sizes, takes creativity to connect	Smaller Foley may not be stiff enough, using a "red rubber catheter" an option
Suction catheter	End hole and side holes, stiffer than Foley	May be small for some patients but comes in many sizes	Generally a good option
Nasogastric tube	May be long enough not to need connectors	No end hole, side holes extend some distance and risk sitting outside chest	Consider cutting the end off to create an end hole and reduce number of side holes

B. Supplies needed for drainage system

1. If a reliable suction source is available, this should be prepared
2. 1 to 3 large collection containers with tight-fitting wide plastic lids

   (a) Number of containers depends on type of system (Fig. 3a–d)
   (b) Size depends on child: 50 ml for neonates to 1 liter for older children
   (c) Examples: dextrose bottles, IV fluid bottles, large plastic jars

3. Ruler and marker
4. Flexible tubing to connect containers to each other and to chest tube

   (a) Length: 1 to 2 meters total
   (b) Examples: pieces of Foley catheter, suction tubing, or bubble continuous positive airway pressure (BCPAP) tubing

5. Rigid tubing or straws

   (a) Length:

      1. 1 to 2 pieces – depending on type of container system – deep enough to reach the bottom of the containers
      2. 1 to 5 shorter pieces (at least 5 cm)

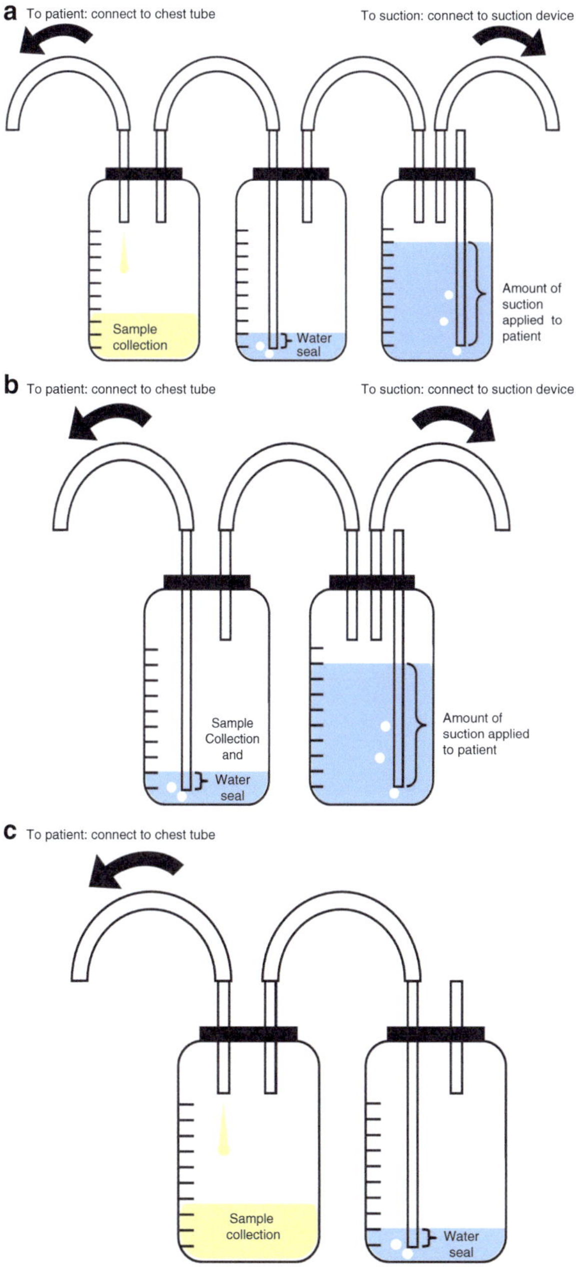

Fig. 3 (**a**) 3-container drainage systems [9]. (**b**) 2-container drainage systems with suction [9]. (**c**) 2-container drainage systems without suction [9]. (**d**) 1-container drainage systems [9]. (Chest drainage design credit - Dr. Ainhoa Costas-Chavarri)

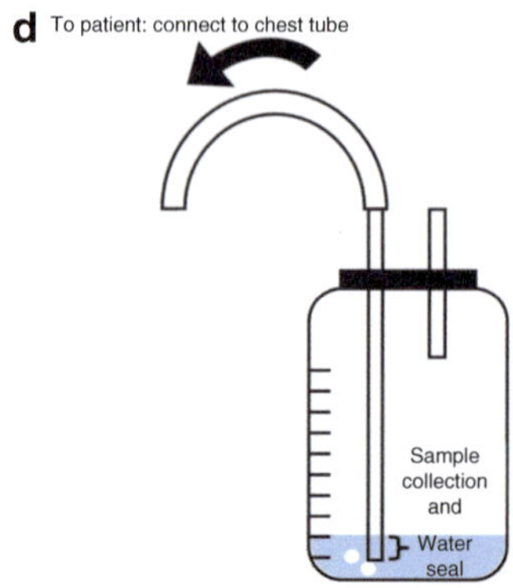

Fig. 3 (continued)

(b) Example: manometers, 1 to 5 ml syringes
(c) These are optional. System can be created from flexible tubing alone if needed.

6. Tape, super glue/epoxy, and/or adaptors for connecting tubing
7. Drill with drill bit or a punch device to create hole in the lid of the containers
8. Water (sterile if possible but can function with non-sterile)

6 Technique

An understanding of the mechanics of a chest drainage system is necessary to build and troubleshoot one. A chest drainage system is composed of one to three connected airtight chambers sealed at one end to the patient and the other end to a column of water, known as a water seal, with or without additional extrinsic suction applied. The purpose of the drainage system is to allow evacuation of air and fluid from the pleural space while minimizing the risk of introducing air into the space and while controlling suction pressure (if available). It uses pressure created by columns of water to do so. If using suction, for example, a column of 20 cm water is applied to a pop-off valve to limit the suction applied to the pleural space to -20 cm water. A water seal is generally created by placing the distal-most end of the tube contiguously connected to the patient under 2 cm water. Thus, air escapes the system when evacuated air or fluid pressure exceeds 2 cm water pressure.

Commercial chest drainage systems such as Pleuravac© are typically integrated 3-chamber systems designed to allow measurement of fluid output under titratable suction with an intervening water seal [8]. A 3-container system is the ideal set-up when possible because of these added benefits but requires continuous suction which is not often available in low resource settings (Fig. 3a) [9]. Furthermore, manual creation of a 3-container system requires additional time and materials that are unlikely to convey added benefit in most patients. A 2-container system

(Fig. 3b and c) [9] provides the benefit of separating sample collection from water seal and can be used with or without suction. However a sample can be readily obtained with a pleural tap, so unless suction is required, a 1-container system (Fig. 3d) [9] is likely adequate for most patients. A 1 container system is simplest to set up. The primary downside of a 1 container system is that fluid drained from the chest mixes with the water seal, introducing variability in the depth of the water seal [9].

Creation of a 3-Chamber System (Requires Suction)

A. Preparing the containers

1. Label containers 1, 2, 3.
2. Mark the sides of each of the 3 containers at 1 cm intervals up to at least 20 cm.
3. Create holes in the lids of each container. We suggest using a drill or a punch device to create a hole about the diameter of the tubing you have available. These should be opposite one another on the top surface location on the lid.
   (i) Containers 1 and 2: Create two holes in each lid
   (ii) Container 3: Create three holes in the lid.
4. If rigid tubing is available, you will need to prepare the following: (*If unavailable, skip this step and use the flexible tubing as described below.*)
   (i) 2 long pieces of tubing (long enough to extend into the container until it is about 1 cm from the bottom with 2-3 cm extending out of the lid)
   (ii) 5 pieces of short tubing 3-6 cm (extend a few cm into the container with a few cm extending out of the lid).
5. Insert the long rigid tubing into one hole in each of the lids of containers 1 and 3. This tube should end near the bottom of the container (ideally at the 1 cm mark). Seal the connection with glue/epoxy or adhesive tape.
6. Insert the short rigid tubing into the holes in the rest of the containers. These tubes should extend a few cm into the container. Seal the connection with glue/epoxy or adhesive tape.
7. Add water to container 2 to create the water seal. The long tube should be submerged 2-3 cm.
8. Add water to container 3 to create the pressure pop-off valve. The long tube should be submerged 20 cm or whatever degree of suction is desired.

B. Connecting the containers

1. Tape the 3 containers together in a straight line.
2. Prepare 4 pieces of flexible tubing that are long enough to easily connect the protruding rigid tubing from one bottle to the next and extend to both the chest tube and the suction source (Fig. 3a).
3. Connect flexible tubing to the rigid tubing as shown in the figure below. If rigid tubing is unavailable, insert flexible tubing through the holes in container lids and down into the water to the depths described above.

4. Secure each connection with tape or glue.
5. Once the chest tube is inserted into the chest (as discussed above), connect it to container 1.
6. Connect container 3 to suction.

Creation of a 2-Chamber System

A. With suction: Use containers 2 and 3 from the 3-container system.
B. Without suction: Use containers 1 and 2 from the 3-container system.

Creation of a 1-Chamber System

A. Only for use without suction.
B. Use container 2 from the 3-container system.
C. If fluid is draining from the patient, be sure to empty it and refill water seal to a level above the end of the long tubing. Of note: as the container fills additional water seal pressure is being applied, making it more difficult to continue to drain or evacuate air.

6.1 Heimlich Valve

The Heimlich valve is a small one-way valve used for chest drainage that empties into a flexible collection device and prevents return of gases or fluids into the pleural space (Fig. 4). It was developed so that the process of draining the pleural cavity could be accomplished in a safe, relatively simple, and efficient manner. This valve system has replaced the cumbersome underwater drainage bottle system in some situations. The system connects to chest tubing and allows fluid and air to pass in

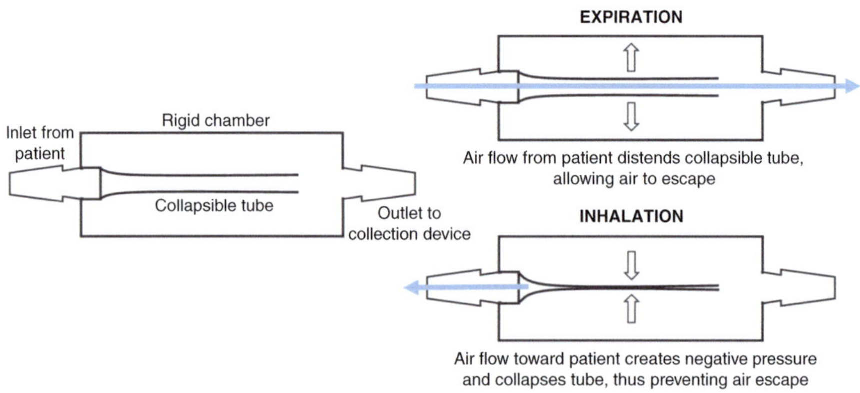

Fig. 4 Heimlich valve physiology. (Figure used with permission from Dr. Rachel Bensen)

one direction only. This system functions in any position, and it does not ever need to be clamped. A regulated suction can be attached to it if necessary.

A. *Advantages:*

(a) The valve drains into a plastic bag that can be held at any level, allowing the patient undergoing chest drainage to be ambulatory simply by carrying the bag.
(b) It does not need to be kept upright like the underwater seal drainage system.
(c) It can be used for both in-patient and out-patient setting.
(d) It is suitable for aeromedical transport.

B. *Disadvantages:*

(a) For pneumothorax, the distal end must be kept open to the atmosphere.
(b) Very thick fluid discharges may block the valve resulting in tension pneumothorax or hydrothorax.
(c) It is not suitable for very large volumes of fluid requiring frequent emptying of the drainage bag.

C. *Commercial options:*

(a) Currently, there are several systems in the market.
(b) A Pneumostat Chest Drain valve device has also been modified for use in the place of a Heimlich valve [10].
(c) The cost of each Heimlich valve is about three (3) United States Dollars (USD) compared to 35 USD for the standard underwater seal drainage system and 87 USD for the Pneumostat device.

D. *Modification of the Heimlich valve for low resource setting*

(a) See detailed illustrations in Fig. 5a and b.
(b) Assembly should be performed in sterile fashion.
(c) Note that the tubing should be cut as short as possible to avoid unnecessary length (a risk for accidentally dislodging or damaging the chest tube).
(d) The infusion set white clamp may be removed or used to regulate the rate of drainage as needed. It should be noted, however, that a chest drainage system should never be left clamped for no specified reason and without health providers' attention.

6.2 Procedure Preparation

If the patient is stable, it is preferable to create the drainage system prior to tube insertion. Alternatively, the tube can be inserted first, allowed to partially drain under careful observation, and then clamped while the drainage system is set up.

While the review of the tube thoracostomy procedure is beyond the scope of this chapter, we do want to emphasize certain aspects in a low-resource environment. As discussed in the intro of this book, the overall principle with all of these procedures is to first, do no harm. The introduction sections of this chapter were chosen to emphasize being very critical in selecting patients which are appropriate for

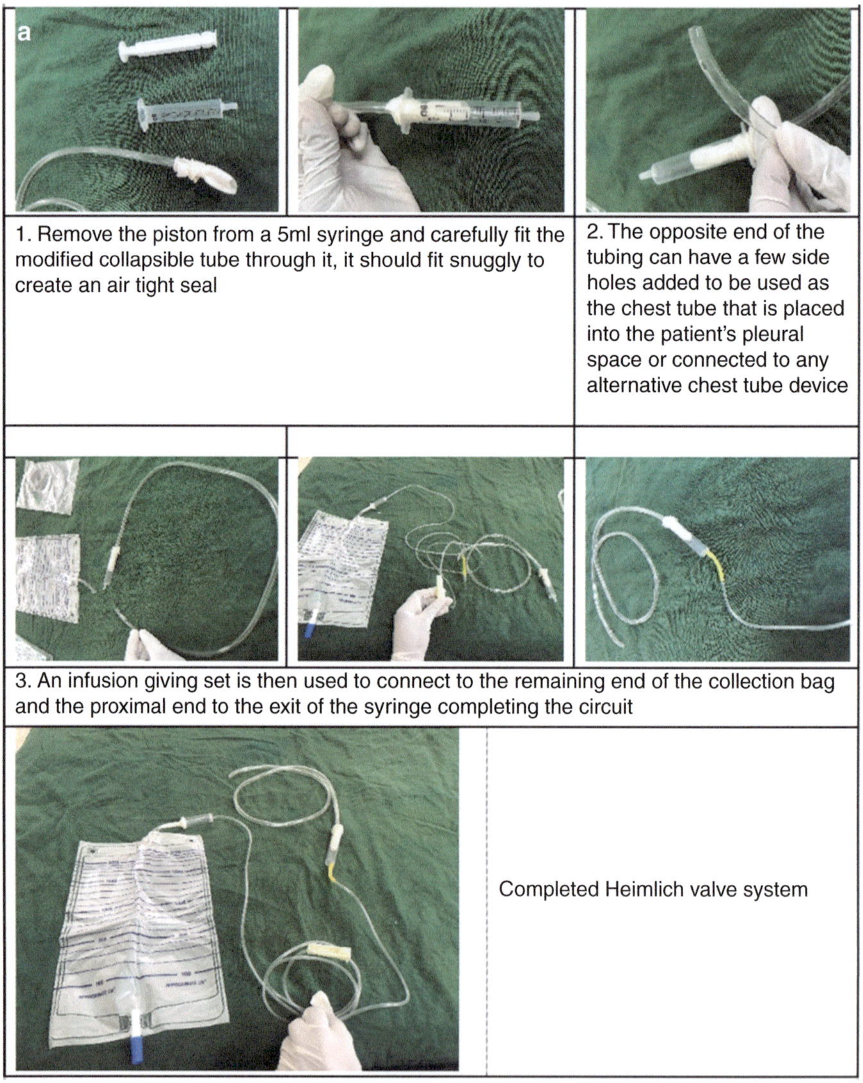

Fig. 5 (**a**) Stepwise assembly of modified Heimlich valve system (Firgure used with permission from Dr. Odera). (**b**) Stepwise assembly of modified Heimlich valve system. (Firgure used with permission from Dr. Odera)

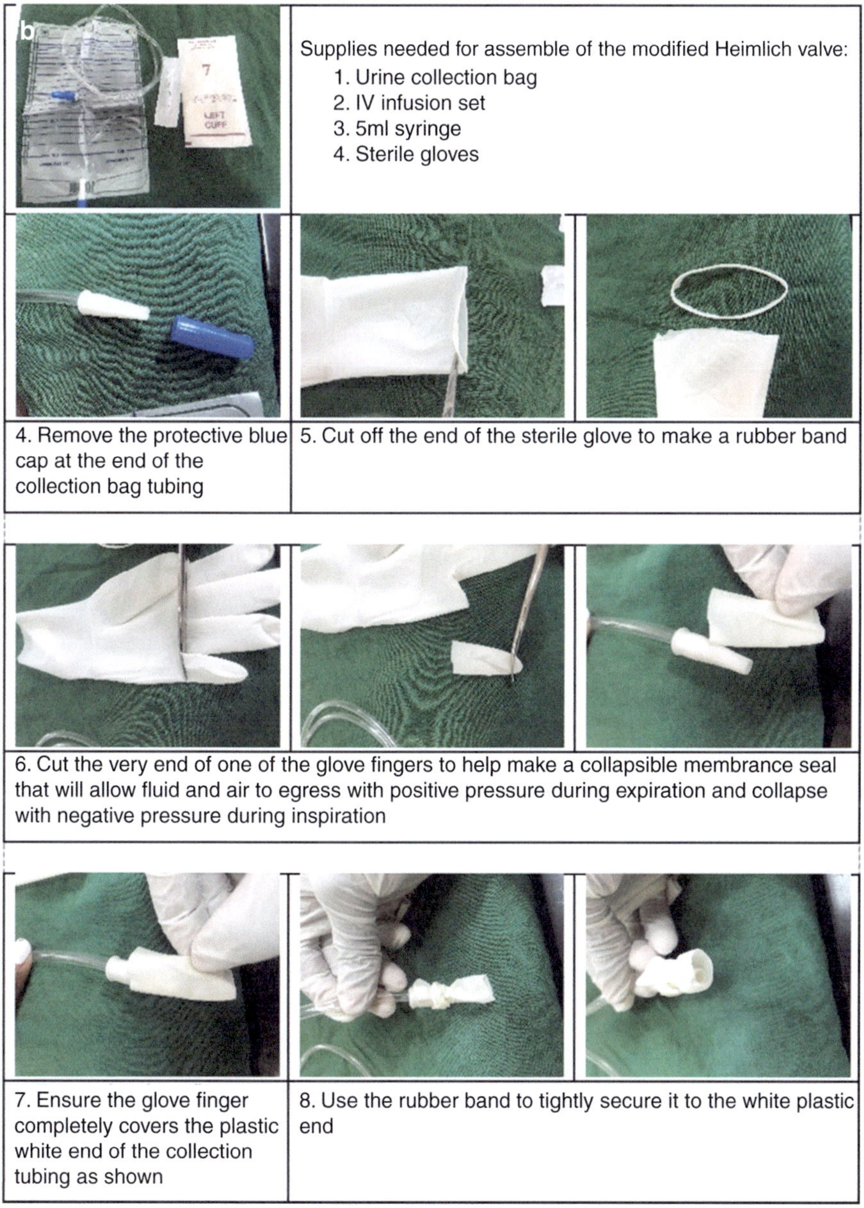

Fig. 5 (continued)

placement of a chest tube. There are going to be situations where it is indicated, and therefore this procedure and set up is essential to know for those situations. Using sterile procedure (reduce iatrogenic infection) is essential.

6.3 Monitoring

In an ideal scenario, continuous heart rate and oxygen saturation with frequent intermittent blood pressure readings will be monitored during chest drain insertion. Especially in small, critically dyspneic children, chest drain insertion can precipitate apnea and expedite death if appropriate resuscitative measures are not available. Careful counseling is required. A fingertip pulse oximeter can provide reasonable monitoring. Sudden changes in heart rate or decreasing oxygen levels may indicate procedural complication such as pneumothorax or hemorrhage. It is helpful but not always necessary to measure the volume of fluid or blood removed.

Second, a plan for monitoring and nursing care must be established prior to insertion of the tube. Maintenance of a chest drain requires ongoing patient monitoring and interval checks of the system.

6.4 Procedural Sedation and Pain Management

Patient discomfort is a major concern in the consideration tube thoracostomy and chest drain maintenance. The intercostal space is quite sensitive and care must be taken to reduce pain as much as safely possible. If local anesthetic is available, it should be utilized.

If procedural sedation is possible, it should be utilized during tube thoracostomy as patient stability allows. The Every Second Matters – Ketamine Package provides checklists and guidance for safely administering ketamine sedation in emergent situations [6].

Continued presence of a tube in the chest wall ranges from uncomfortable to quite painful, therefore care should be taken to continue to assess and treat pain after placement. Intermittent dosing of analgesics per local formulary and guidelines should be used as needed during the maintenance of the chest drain.

7 Troubleshooting

The output and fluid column in the tubing should be checked regularly to determine timing of removal or further interventions. After drainage of any fluid, the fluid column may bubble, swing, or be stationary.

Stationary Column Suggests that the tube is blocked, kinked, disconnected, or displaced such that some of the drainage holes are open to air or the lung has sealed around the tube.

- There is no purpose in maintaining a chest drain with a stationary water column.

Troubleshooting (Proceed Stepwise)

1. If possible, ask the child to cough.
2. Evaluate for displacement, disconnection, or kinking.
3. Attempt to clear blockage by flushing the tube with sterile water or saline.
4. If none of the above induces swinging, draining, or bubbling, consider removing the tube.
5. If a chest drain is still needed, consider whether the previously chosen tube lacked adequate rigidity to prevent kinking or caliber (such as in cases of thick empyema).

Swinging Column Swinging movement according to changing intrathoracic pressure of respiration implies the tube is still well connected to the pleural space but the pathology may have resolved. Consider removal.

Management/Troubleshooting

1. Clamp the tube for at least several hours and observe for deterioration
2. If deteriorates, unclamp, reposition, and flush as necessary.
3. If remains well, remove the tube and apply a bandage to the site.
4. A chest X-ray is not necessary prior to removal but may help evaluate the status of the collection or serve as a new baseline in case of clinical worsening after removal [11].

Bubbling Chest Drain Sign of an ongoing air leak. If bubbling continues for several days post-insertion, it may indicate alveolar-pleural or broncho-pleural fistula.

- Never clamp a bubbling chest drain as this can cause a tension pneumothorax.

Management/Troubleshooting

1. Fistula generally requires specialist care and the method will depend on locally available expertise, equipment, and type and cause of fistula [12].
2. Options include Heimlich valve, pleurodesis with chemical agents/autologous blood products, bronchoscopic/thoracoscopic/open procedures.

8 Complications

- **Fistula formation/**non-healing chest tube site.
- **Infection:** Entry into the chest cavity poses a risk of introducing infection. Sterile instruments and tubes must be used to minimize this risk. Care must be taken to cleanse the entry site and to avoid entry through infected skin or soft tissue.
- **Chronic drainage**: results in fluid, protein, and nutrient loss.
- **Tension Pneumothorax:** A continuously bubbling chest drain suggests an air leak and should never be clamped as there is risk for development of tension pneumothorax. If a patient with a clamped tube complains of increasing shortness of breath, the tube should be immediately unclamped due to concern for developing tension pneumothorax [1].
- **Re-accumulation of pneumothorax or pleural effusion loss of suction or water seal.** Consider the rigidity of the devices and tubing you have chosen to create the device and perform a thorough evaluation of the drainage system from patient to suction source or last container. Tube kinking, compression, or obstruction can result in re-accumulation of pneumothorax or pleural effusion.

8.1 Procedural Complications

- **Injury** to various critical structures, such as lungs, heart, liver, spleen, nerves, and soft tissue during placement.
- **Bleeding:** Damage to intercostal vessels are the primary source of clinically significant bleeding

9 Pearls

1. Carefully consider your local context and whether the tube can be inserted safely, connected securely, and cared for appropriately on the ward. Many non-purulent effusions will resolve if the underlying cause is treated without need for a chest drain.
2. Chest tube insertion in small critically dyspneic children can precipitate demise. Have the best team available ready for resuscitation and counsel the guardians well.
3. Good preparation in settings where specialized chest drains or procedure packs are not available is crucial. Have a checklist of equipment.
4. A one-chamber under-water seal device is easier to construct and manage, and will suffice for most applications.

5. The best air-tight seals are made by connecting rubber to plastic, and not rubber to rubber or plastic to plastic. This is important to avoid iatrogenic pneumothorax, no matter which system is used.
6. To avoid bottles in the drainage system being knocked over, consider taping to the leg or base of the bed.
7. Prompt removal will improve discomfort, reduce complications, and hasten discharge. A stationary water column means you need to troubleshoot or remove the drain.
8. If chest tube will not drain fluid despite all troubleshooting, consider whether an organizational effusion with pleural thickening and peel is preventing lung re-expansion. Surgical consultation is needed in these cases.

10 Case Resolution

Five days after the chest tube is placed, the drainage stops, the chest tube is maintained with water seal for 1 more day and then removed. A follow-up CXR reveals almost complete resolution of the pneumonia and no pneumothorax. The child is discharged on oral antibiotics to return to see the clinician in one week.

References

1. Balfour-Lynn IM, et al. BTS guidelines for the management of pleural infection in children. Thorax. 2005;60(Suppl 1):i1–21.
2. Shah K, Gulati S. Disseminated kaposi sarcoma presenting as chylothorax. American Thoracic Society Conference; 2020. p. 2.
3. Mowery NT, et al. Practice management guidelines for management of hemothorax and occult pneumothorax. J Trauma. 2011;70(2):510–8.
4. Stafford RE, Linn J, Washington L. Incidence and management of occult hemothoraces. Am J Surg. 2006;192(6):722–6.
5. Kirmani B, Zacharias J. Insertion of a chest drain for pneumothorax. Anaesthesia Intens Care Med. 2016;17(4):196–8.
6. Schwartz KR, et al. An innovative safe anesthesia and analgesia package for emergency pediatric procedures and surgeries when no anesthetist is available. Int J Emerg Med. 2016;9(1):16.
7. Lopushinsky, S.M.D.M., Tube Thoracostomy for trauma. 2019.
8. George RS, Papagiannopoulos K. Advances in chest drain management in thoracic disease. J Thorac Dis. 2016;8(Suppl 1):S55–64.
9. Butteris S, M.P.a.t.M.C.o.G.C.H.E. Sugarprep. [cited 2021 9/9/2021]; Available from: https://sugarprep.org/.
10. Narasimhan A, Ayyanathan S, Krishnamoorthy LR. Re-discovering the Heimlich valve: old wine in a new bottle. Lung India. 2017;34(1):70–2.
11. McGrath E, et al. Is a chest radiograph required after removal of chest tubes in children? J Pediatr Health Care. 2017;31(5):588–93.
12. Kurman JS, Hogarth DKJAMJ. Minimally invasive persistent air leak management. 2018, 2018.

Further Reading

Bliss D, Silen M. Pediatric thoracic trauma. Crit Care Med. 2002;30(11 Suppl):S409–15. https://doi.org/10.1097/00003246-200,211,001-00005.

Gogakos A, Barbetakis N, Lazaridis G, et al. Heimlich valve and pneumothorax. Ann Transl Med. 2015;3(4):4–8. https://doi.org/10.3978/j.issn.2305-5839.2015.03.25.

Kwiatt M, Tarbox A, Seamon MJ, Swaroop M, Cipolla J, Allen C, Hallenbeck S, Davido HT, Lindsey DE, Doraiswamy VA, Galwankar S, Tulman D, Latchana N, Papadimos TJ, Cook CH, Stawicki SP. Thoracostomy tubes: a comprehensive review of complications and related topics. Int J Crit Illn Inj Sci. 2014;4(2):143–55. https://doi.org/10.4103/2229-5151.134182. PMID: 25024942; PMCID: PMC4093965

Menegozzo CAM, Utiyama EM. Steering the wheel towards the standard of care: Proposal of a step-by-step ultrasound-guided emergency chest tube drainage and literature review. Int J Surg. 2018;56(April):315–9. https://doi.org/10.1016/j.ijsu.2018.07.002.

Millar FR, Hillman T. Managing chest drains on medical wards. BMJ. 2018;363:1–7. https://doi.org/10.1136/bmj.k4639.

Redden MD, Chin TY, van Driel ML. Surgical versus non-surgical management for pleural empyema. Cochrane Database Syst Rev. 2017;2017(3) https://doi.org/10.1002/14651858.CD010651.pub2.

Sundaralingam A, Banka R, Rahman NM. Management of pleural infection. Pulm Ther. 2020; https://doi.org/10.1007/s41030-020-00140-7.

Toth JW, Reed MF, Ventola LK. Chest tube drainage devices. Semin Respir Crit Care Med. 2019;40(3):386–93. https://doi.org/10.1055/s-0039-1,694,769.

Tovar JA, Vazquez JJ. Management of chest trauma in children. Paediatr Respir Rev. 2013;14(2):86–91. https://doi.org/10.1016/j.prrv.2013.02.011.

For video review of the major points described here, we recommend using the resources available at www.sugarprep.org/PEARLS.

Performing Lumbar Puncture in a Low-Resource Setting

Olumide T. Adeleke

Abbreviations

CNS	Central nervous system
CSF	Cerebrospinal fluid
LMICs	Low-middle income countries
LP	Lumbar puncture

1 Case Example

A previously healthy 6-year-old girl is brought to the emergency room in Nigeria with a one-week history of fever, headache, and new onset of convulsions and lethargy. She has just completed antimalarial drugs. On examination, she is noted to be febrile, tachypneic, and tachycardic with normal blood pressure and oxygen saturation. She is lethargic with positive Kernign's and Brudzinski's signs and no focal neurologic findings. Abdominal, respiratory, and cardiovascular examinations are normal except for tachypnea and tachycardia. She has warm extremities with a brisk capillary refill and no noted rashes.

Her laboratory results show a negative malaria test, normal random glucose test, and elevated white cell count. Based on her presentation a lumbar puncture for cerebrospinal fluid analysis is indicated, but a commercial lumbar puncture set is unavailable.

O. T. Adeleke (✉)
Department of Family Medicine, Bowen University Teaching Hospital, Ogbomoso, Nigeria

T. M. Slusher et al. (eds.), *Pediatric Procedural Adaptations for Low-Resource Settings*, https://doi.org/10.1007/978-3-030-99955-1_20

2 Introduction

A lumbar puncture (LP) is indicated for many diagnostic and therapeutic purposes. The most common indication for lumbar puncture in the pediatric age group is for the diagnosis of meningitis [1]. The cerebrospinal fluid (CSF) may be examined for signs of infection by studying it for microbes, cells, glucose, protein, and culturing the CSF for organisms. Other common indications for a LP include the injection of central nervous system (CNS) chemotherapeutic agents and spinal anesthesia especially in older children.

Lumbar puncture is a relatively simple procedure [2, 3]. The procedure is by no means innocuous as poor knowledge of the contraindications, regional anatomy and rationale of the technique as well as inadequate prior skills practice may result in failure or complications. These complications can be mitigated by the appropriate understanding of the indications, contraindications, and procedural techniques. This chapter explains modifications to performing a lumbar puncture (LP) in a low-resource setting. LPs should only be performed by experienced providers trained to do them or by learners under the guidance of experienced providers.

3 Indications

- Evaluation of CSF to assist with CNS disease diagnoses:
  - Infections (meningitis, encephalitis, myelitis)
  - Inflammatory or demyelinating disease (multiple sclerosis, Guillain-Barre disease)
  - Subarachnoid hemorrhage
  - Oncologic disease (ex: leukemia staging)
- *Therapeutic Indications*
  - Intrathecal administration of medications (chemotherapeutic agents, antibiotics, analgesics)
  - Therapeutic relief of pseudotumor cerebri through CSF drainage (idiopathic intracranial hypertension) [4]

4 Contraindications

- LP is *relatively* contraindicated with
  - Cardiorespiratory instability
  - Spinal deformities that make the procedure difficult

- LP is *absolutely* contraindicated with
  - New focal neurologic deficits (except in the neonate who does NOT have evidence of increased ICP; generally focal neurological in the neonate are not a contraindication)
  - Concern for increased ICP in any age (unless head imaging has ruled out mass effect). Removal of CSF in a patient with mass effect/increased ICP has a risk of herniation
  - Infection at the site of needle insertion
  - Coagulopathy or other bleeding diatheses

5 Equipment/Supplies

Most hospitals in high-income countries have commercially available LP kits/trays (Fig. 1a, Table 1), which contain all the necessary supplies. These kits include sterile drapes (2), cleaning sponges (3) and cleaning solution, 22- or 20-gauge spinal

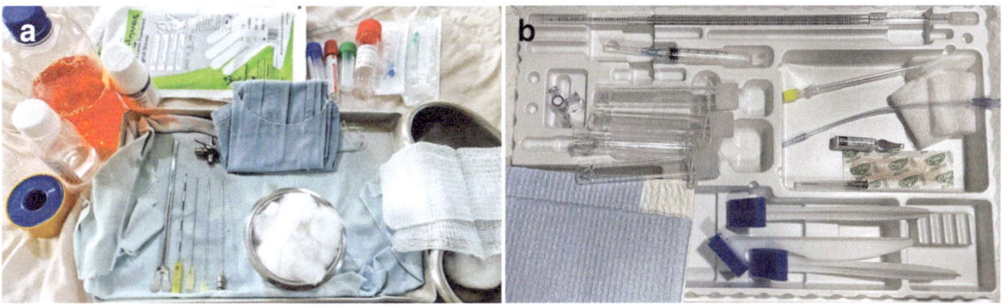

Fig. 1 (**a**) Commercial LP kit. (Figure used with permission from Dr. T.O Adeleke). (**b**) Locally adapted LP equipment. (Figure used with permission from Dr. T.O Adeleke)

Table 1 Commercial LP kit and local adaptations

Commercial LP kit	Local adaptations
Spinal needles	Hypodermic needles (size 22–18 G)
Sponge sticks	Sterile gauze
Povidone cleaning solution	Methylated spirit solution
Commercial dressing	Plaster/tape and gauze
Manometer	Qualitative observation of the CSF flow rate IV giving set tubing as an alternative manometer
Sterile drapes	Inside of the sterile glove paper wrapping
Collection vials	Any small container with a sterile inside and cap/securable cover (i.e., lab tubes, urine cups, sterile syringes – Care must be used not to lose the CSF when replacing the plungers)

needle (1), a 25-gauge and a 20-gauge needle for anesthetic infiltration, 3 ml syringe (1), vial of 1% lidocaine for anesthesia (1), pressure manometer with tubing (1), collection vials (4), a dressing (1), and stopcock (1). Additional equipment required for the procedure includes sterile gloves, a facemask, and a povidone cleaning solution. Some providers wear a full sterile gown as well.

However, in low- and middle-income countries (LMICs), commercial LP kits are often very costly, and unavailable. Clinicians practicing in such resource-limited settings, therefore, need to modify and adapt available supplies for use (Table 1).

5.1 Technique/Instructions for Use

5.1.1 Procedure with Adaptations

1. Obtain informed consent – per the standards of the institution
2. Personnel, Positioning, and Holding the Infant/Child

At least two personnel are usually required to perform the procedure in pediatrics (a trained proceduralist (physician, provider) and at least one assistant trained to hold the child) (Figs. 2 and 3).

Since moderate or deep sedation for LPs can rarely be done in LMICs, it is extremely important that the child be held securely to perform the procedure quickly without performing a traumatic tap and decreasing the trauma to the infant/child if multiple sticks are done to secure the spinal fluid [5].

Neonatal/Infant Hold: In the neonate and small infant, the holder can use one hand to hold the infants' knees and elbows/hands and the other to bend the neonates' shoulders when the clinician is ready to perform the tap (Fig. 2a, b). Pay attention to which extremity the intravenous catheter is in and make sure to protect the intravenous site. Do not bend the neck down until the clinician is ready to insert the needle to decrease the chances of respiratory compromise of the infant in this position. Allow the neck/shoulders to extend again once the needle is in place and observe the infant closely for respiratory distress. If possible, place the child on a pulse oximeter during the procedure [6].

Child Hold: In the older child have the holder put one elbow behind the patient's neck and the other behind the patient's knees (Fig. 3). The patient's hands are then held by the holder. This allows a secure hold again helping assure a fast and atraumatic LP (Fig. 3).

Sitting Hold: Alternatively, the patient may be in a sitting position. For this procedure, the patient leaning forward and resting their arms on a tray stand with the neck and back fully flexed. Flexion facilitates the course of the needle by widening the gap between adjacent lumbar spinous processes. Good positioning and landmark identification are very important steps in performing the procedure successfully [7].

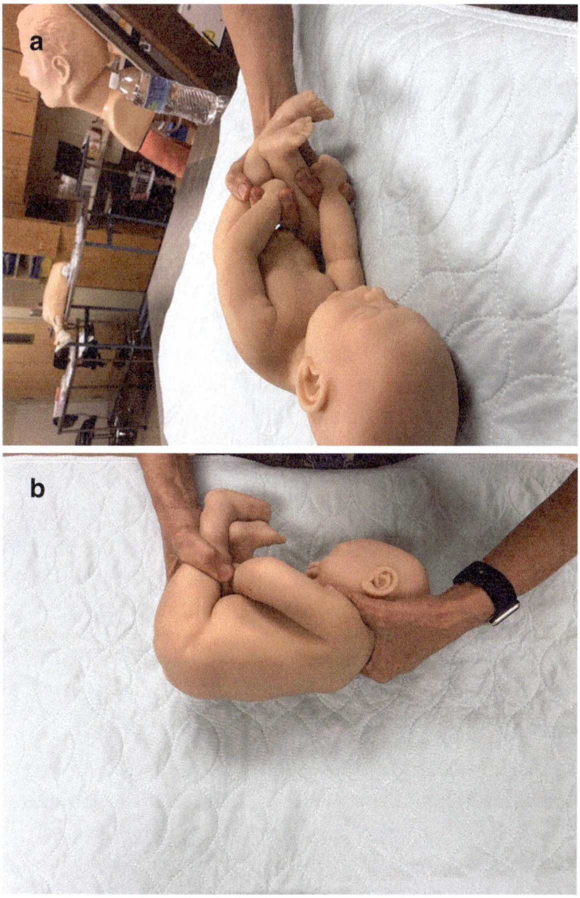

Fig. 2 (**a**) Holding knees and hands with one hand. (Figure used with permission from Dr. Tina Slusher). (**b**) Holding hands (or elbows) and knees in one hand and bending neck down with other. (Figure used with permission from Dr. Tina Slusher)

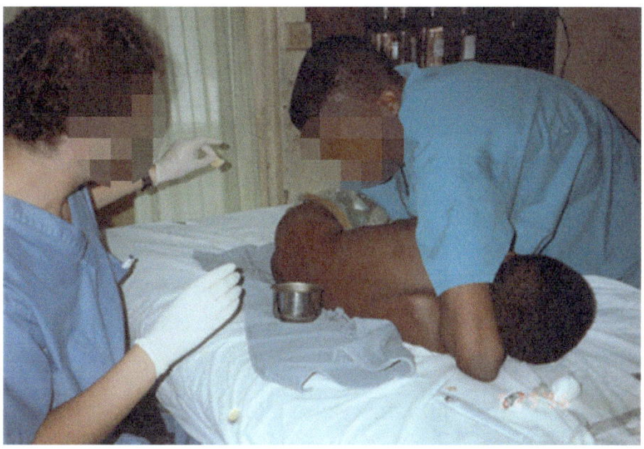

Fig. 3 Holding an older child for an LP. (Figure used with permission from Dr. Tina Slusher)

In sick neonates, studies have shown that hypoxemia is higher in the conventional lateral knee-chest position. Therefore, consider the sitting position for neonates as well. The neonate may be rolled over a blanket [6].

3. *Prepare and drape the patient*. Clean using the solution available at your hospital or clinic. If sterile drapes are in short supply *the sterile inside of the glove paper can be used as a sterile drape*. If not able to fully drape the area because of limited drapes clean broadly including the iliac crest.
4. *Select your needle*. Whenever possible use commercially available one-time use 22-gauge spinal needles in 1.5 inches for infants and young children and 2.5 inches for older children and 3.5 inches for adolescents. When spinal needles are not available a *plain 22- or 23-gauge hypodermic needle* can be substituted, acknowledging the extremely small risk of introducing epidermoid tissues into the spinal canal causing an epidermoid cyst. This is extremely rare but can be prevented by using a stylet which should be done whenever possible.
5. *Use local anesthesia and acute pain management modalities*. Many physicians consider local anesthesia with lidocaine infiltration before LP optional; however, it is extremely helpful in assuring atraumatic tap and allowing for more than one puncture without further traumatizing the child if necessary. Lidocaine 1% with a small (25-gauge) needle is recommended.

Other modalities of acute pain management in LP include topical anesthetic cream, oral sucrose for infants <3 months, analgesics, nitrous oxide, and other sedation but these are often not feasible in LMICs.

6. *Perform the procedure*. Perform the procedure as you have been trained to do, with the noted supply/set up modifications discussed above as indicated.
7. *Measure opening pressure and collect samples for CSF analysis***.** If you are measuring opening pressure, the manometer is attached to the spinal needle and the stopcock is opened to allow for CSF to fill the manometer. The standard method of measuring CSF opening pressure is with a spinal manometer, but in many resource-limited centers, manometers are not readily available. *Alternative ways to measure CSF opening pressure without a manometer* include a qualitative assessment of CSF flow rate, i.e., whether the flow is like a jet (under pressure or not) and the use of intravenous giving set as an alternative to the spinal manometer for quantitative measurement of CSF opening pressure [8].

Collect CSF into the sample bottles/tubes for appropriate testing as noted in the chart above. The amount of CSF collected for diagnostic purposes should be restricted to the smallest volume necessary. For children, this is typically 0.5 ml/tube and not more than 3 ml in total.

8. *Post lumbar puncture care***.** Clean and cover the LP site with the semi-occlusive dressing. Ensure that all the cleaning solution is washed off the skin [9].

5.2 *Complications*

- Procedural complications include
  - Bleeding
  - Infection
  - Spinal cord injury
  - Herniation
  - Headache
  - CSF leak
- Positioning complications include
  - Respiratory compromise
  - Aspiration

6 Case Resolution

The patient's LP was performed safely and successfully. The CSF was noted to be purulent. She was admitted to the pediatric ward and treated with a meningitic dose of empiric antibiotic therapy and adjunctive therapies/monitoring pending CSF culture results. The result of CSF analysis was consistent with features of acute bacterial meningitis. Her cultures revealed that her micro-organism was sensitive to the antibiotic she had been placed on. Her antibiotic therapy was completed, and she was discharged home to return to the clinic in one week.

References

1. Bonadio W. Pediatric lumbar puncture and cerebrospinal fluid analysis. J Emerg Med. 2014;46(1):141–50.
2. Farah A. Lumbar puncture. Dia Med. 1962;34:837–40.
3. Ellenby MS, et al. Videos in clinical medicine. *Lumbar puncture*. N Engl J Med. 2006;355(13):e12.
4. Sherman SC, Cico SJ, Nordquist E, Ross C, Wang E. Atlas of clinical emergency medicine. 1st ed. Sherman SC, editor. Lippincott Williams & Wilkins; 2015.
5. Srinivasan L, et al. Traumatic lumbar punctures in infants hospitalized in the neonatal intensive care unit. Pediatr Infect Dis J. 2013;32(10):1150–2.
6. Abo A, et al. Positioning for lumbar puncture in children evaluated by bedside ultrasound. Pediatrics. 2010;125(5):e1149–53.
7. Boon JM, et al. Lumbar puncture: anatomical review of a clinical skill. Clin Anat. 2004;17(7):544–53.
8. Mogambery TA, Moodley A, Connolly C. Is the intravenous giving set a reliable alternative to the spinal manometer in measuring cerebrospinal fluid opening pressure? S Afr Med J. 2018;108(10):865–9.
9. Doherty CM, Forbes RB. Diagnostic Lumbar Puncture. Ulster Med J. 2014;83(2):93–102.

Peritoneal Dialysis in a Low-Resource Setting

Michael A. Alao, Dennis Palmer, Norah Ndi Nyah Njini, and Olayinka R. Ibrahim

Abbreviations

AKI	Acute kidney injury
HD	Hemodialysis
KRT	Kidney replacement therapy
LMICs	Low-middle-income countries
PD	Peritoneal dialysis

1 Case Example

A five-year-old female presents to your hospital in Cameron after a four-day history of fever, malaise, and passage of dark brown urine. The patient had presented at two other health facilities before arriving. She has been diagnosed with malaria and prescribed appropriate treatment. On arrival, she is acutely ill-appearing with generalized edema. She is noted to have decreased urine output and has been passing "Cola" colored urine. She is afebrile. Her initial laboratory results show a

M. A. Alao (✉)
Department of Paediatrics, University College Hospital, Ibadan, Nigeria
e-mail: michael.alao@uch-ibadan.org.ng

D. Palmer
Baptist Institute of Health Sciences, Mbingo Baptist Hospital, Bamenda, Cameroon

N. N. N. Njini
Baptist Institute of Health Sciences, Mbingo Baptist Hospital, Bamenda, Cameroon

Loma Linda University, Loma Linda, CA, USA

O. R. Ibrahim
Department of Paediatrics, Federal Medical Centre, Katsina, Nigeria

T. M. Slusher et al. (eds.), *Pediatric Procedural Adaptations for Low-Resource Settings*, https://doi.org/10.1007/978-3-030-99955-1_21

hemoglobin of 7 gm/dl, a serum creatinine of 9.9 mg/dl, a blood urea nitrogen of 312 mg/dl, and a serum potassium of 4.8 mmol/l. You diagnose acute kidney injury secondary to malaria and recognize that peritoneal dialysis is necessary, but your surgeon does not have a commercial peritoneal dialysis catheter available and hemodialysis is not feasible given the intensive care needs and equipment. Commercial peritoneal dialysis fluid is not available.

2 Introduction

Acute kidney injury (AKI) is a relatively common clinical condition in the critically ill child [1, 2]. It is often associated with poorer outcomes in low-resource settings compared to high-income settings [3]. Factors that contribute to poor outcomes include lack of access to dialysis due to prohibitively expensive cost of consumables, non-availability of consumables, and technical requirement for some kidney replacement therapy such as hemodialysis [3].

Although there are different kidney replacement modalities, peritoneal dialysis (PD) appears to be one of the most feasible and accessible forms of kidney replacement therapy in low-middle-income countries (LMICs) [4]. PD requires the least technical requirements among the various modalities of treatment, which makes it possible (even for patients) to administer the physician prescriptions at home [5]. Additionally, PD is the preferred modality in neonates and infants, in hemodynamically unstable patients, and patients who cannot tolerate anticoagulation. PD provides a slower clearance rate, which limits the risk for dialysis disequilibrium syndrome, a syndrome that is often associated with hemodialysis. All of these advantages make PD a modality of choice for renal replacement therapy in LMICs.

The attainment of zero preventable death from AKI by 2025 (0 by 2025), proposed by the International Society of Nephrology, can only be achieved through scale-up of access to dialysis in LMICs [6, 7]. Access to dialysis can be improved through the use of adaptable methods in low-resource settings [5, 8]. This chapter describes indication for dialysis and options for a modified peritoneal catheter. This section also describes the PD procedure, including options for dialysates and complications for low-resource settings.

3 Indications

The indications for kidney replacement therapy (KRT) can be categorized into clinical and laboratory indications (Table 1).

4 Contraindications

The contraindications include known allergy to any of the PD fluid constituent, previous major recent abdominal surgery, acute abdomen, intraabdominal abscess, and peritoneal membrane failure.

Table 1 Indications for PD

Clinical	Laboratory
Uremic syndrome Stage 3 AKI Fluid overload not responding to medical treatment Persistent oliguria/anuria	Rapidly rising azotemia Severe hyperkalemia (K + $\geq$ 6.5 mmol/l) with failed medical treatment Severe metabolic acidosis (HCO_3+ $\leq$15 mmol/l) Severe hypernatremia >180 mmol/l Severe/intractable hypercalcemia Severe/intractable hypocalcemia
PD > HD	
Un-affordability of HD in patient requiring RRT hemodynamic instability Preference for PD Weight <10 kg Anticoagulant intolerance Bleeding diathesis Poor cardiac function HD vascular access failure Congestive heart failure	

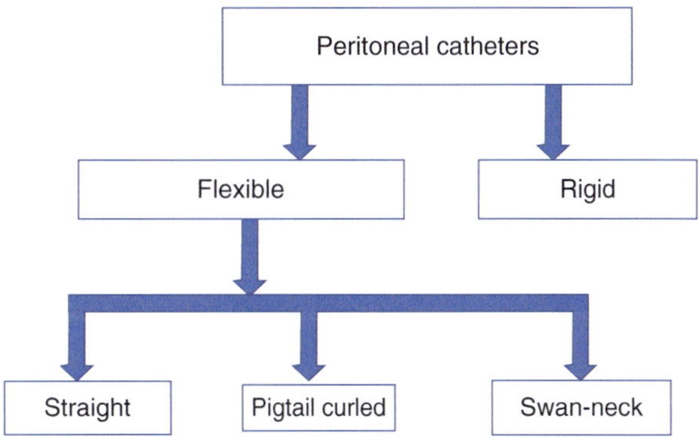

Fig. 1 Types of PD catheters

5 Supplies/Equipment

5.1 PD Catheter Options

Peritoneal dialysis catheters are tubes or rods with an open-end port and side fenestrations. They come in various shapes and tensile strengths. They may either be flexible or rigid. Over the years, the flexible catheters have become the most preferred, but the reusable rigid catheters may be useful where the former is not available. In terms of shapes; catheters may be straight (typical of the adaptable/improvised catheters), pigtail curled, and swan-neck (Fig. 1).

They may be of various lengths and may have cuffs for retention in the anterior abdominal wall. A typical example includes Tenckhoff™ and Dacron™ catheters. In resource-limited settings, the commercial catheters are often not available and where they are available, they are not affordable ($40). In place of the commercial catheter, other tubes/catheters can be adapted and modified for use as a PD catheter. Commonly adapted equipment includes use of feeding tubes of various sizes depending on the patients' age and weight (Table 2). Similar sized urethral catheters could also be improvised in place of feeding tubes with similar efficacy.

5.1.1 Supplies Required for PD Catheter Placement (Fig. 2)

- Bedside table
- Surgical masks (2)
- Sterile towels* (2)
- Small sterile bowl*
- Sterile forceps*
- Sterilizable stylet or bicycle spoke
- Scissors
- Artery forceps
- Sterile cotton swabs* (2)
- Squares sterile gauze* (4)
- Sterile 4×4 gauze*
- Lactated Ringer (LR) – ordered amount*
- D50W – ordered amount*

Table 2 Recommended feeding tubes size for PD catheter based on weight

Weight	Recommended feeding tube sizes (FG)
Less than 10 kg	Size 8
10–20 kg	Size 10
21–30 kg	Size 12
Greater than 30 kg	Size 14–18

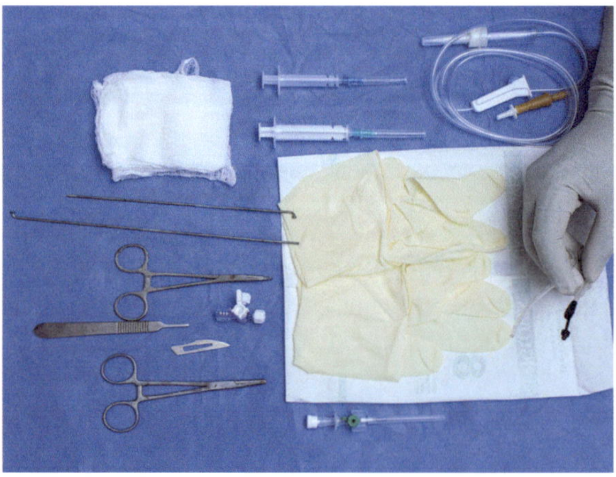

Fig. 2 Basic consumables for peritoneal dialysis

- Large syringe with needle
- Infusion Set – may be reused for 24 h if sterility is maintained
- Urinary catheter bag*
- Container with a lid containing 90% alcohol (change weekly)
- 3-way stopcock (in open-all-ways position in 90% alcohol)
- 4–5 cm section of suction tubing (in 90% alcohol)
- Sterile gloves* (2 pairs)
- Non-sterile kidney basin or bowl for discarded fluid
- Bucket for drained dialysate

*indicates items that are NOT reused, they are NEW with every exchange

5.2 *Technique*

5.2.1 How to Make or Obtain PD Fluid and PD Fluid Sustainability

PD fluid is referred to as dialysate. This fluid is composed of water, physiologic concentrations of electrolytes, and an osmotic agent. Commonly glucose is the osmotic agent, which pulls toxins including waste products, excess body water, and electrolytes from the body. The PD fluid composition is shown in Table 3. PD fluid can either be commercially prepared or locally constituted by the healthcare provider. Usually, glucose is added to intravenous fluid such as ringer lactate or saline at various concentrations. Higher dextrose concentration would generate more osmotic pressure and drag to pull in excess body water in a hypervolemic state. The efficacy and safety of the locally prepared fluid are well documented in the literature [9].

Table 3 Composition of PD fluids

	Commercial produced	Locally prepared fluid using Ringer's lactate
Composition[a]	Per liter	Per liter
Sodium	134	130
Potassium	0–2	0–4
Calcium	1.75	2.7
Magnesium	0.5	–
Chloride	103.5	109
Lactate	35–40	28
Glucose[b]	1.5–4.25%	1.5–4.25% (Table 4)
pH	5.5	6.5

[a]May add heparin and antibiotics (100 IU/L of heparin and 4 mg/L of gentamycin)
[b]15ml, 23 ml, or 42.5 ml of 50% dextrose is added to 500 ml of the primary fluid to make a 1.5%, and 2.3% or 4.25% dextrose concentration strength PD fluid 4.25%

Table 4 Mixing PD dextrose compositions

PD dextrose concentration	Primary fluid (ml)	D50 (ml)
1.5%	500	15
2.3%	500	23
4.25%	500	42.5

(a) *Commercial PD Fluid*

The various available commercial PD fluids include a 1.5% or 2.3% glucose strength. The choice of the glucose concentration is determined by the patient's fluid status. For instance, where there is significant fluid overload/retention, a higher (2.3%) glucose concentration should be selected as the fluid of choice (Table 3).

(b) *Locally Prepared PD Fluid*

When commercial PD fluids are not available, intravenous fluids with a physiologic constituent of electrolyte should be prepared by the team. *Strict aseptic technique* is important during the entire process of the fluid constitution in order to minimize the risk of bacterial contamination and subsequent peritonitis; a common complication of PD.

The fluid composition that is prepared should be as close as possible to the electrolyte composition of commercial PD fluid. Using locally prepared solutions is advantageous as the needed solutions can be readily made available in the concentration needed. Typically, Ringer's lactate or Hartman's solution is used but normal saline may be used if necessary (Table 3). Dextrose 50% is added to the primary solution to produce the desired concentration of PD solution. Antibiotics may be added to the PD solution to reduce the incidence of peritonitis or for treatment depending on the risk factors and concern level for infection. Heparin may also be added to the PD fluid to prevent fibrin clots from blocking the PD catheter. If the patient is hypokalemic, potassium chloride may be added to the constituted fluid as well.

(c) *Adaptation for Sustainability – PD Fluid Revolving Fund Model*

A major barrier to PD is the availability of PD fluid. Where commercial PD fluid is available, a model that has been proven to be efficient in making commercial PD fluid use possible is the use of a "PD revolving fund'. This model followed a key strategy for health care financing "the drug revolving fund model". A revolving fund is a fund that is always available to finance an organizations continuing operations – it is replenished by the organization anytime funds are used and does not have fiscal year limitations. This model, when applied to PD fluid, ensures PD fluid is stocked and made available and accessible when needed. The seed funding for this model may be obtained from a donor for the acquisition of the initial stock of PD fluids. Fluids are then replenished at restocking cost to always have a constant available level. A marginal profit may be added to the cost to ensure sustainability and to account for the care of indigent patients who may not be able to pay for cost recovery. Adoption of this model has been shown to improve commercial dialysis access rate to well above 90% and demonstrated a low infection rate of 0.5% in a single-center experience in Nigeria. This model is recommended where infection control and prevention are of major concern since the risk of contamination, a key challenge with manually constituted fluids, is avoided.

(d) *PD Catheter Insertion Procedure*

PD catheter insertion should be performed by an experienced member of the team who has previously been trained to perform this procedure. Trainees must always be supervised by experienced trained providers. It is beyond the scope of this book to teach the entire PD catheter placement procedure, what is described here is to show modifications of what can be used for an experienced provider to place the PD catheter.

The procedure should follow a strict aseptic pre-condition in line with global standard practice for infection prevention and control policy. Sterile materials from the central sterilizing unit should be available for the procedure. All eligible patients are catheterized to ensure the bladder is empty and for monitoring of urine output.

The catheter insertion can be done in a dedicated room or at the patient's bedside. About 30 min before PD catheter insertion an intravenous 2 mg/kg of intravenous ethamsylate should be administered to the patient for maintenance of good homeostasis. The peritoneal cavity should be filled with 10 ml/kg of normal saline through a sterile needle inserted into the left iliac fossa so the abdominal organs could be freely displaced during catheter insertion. A video of the procedure is accessible through this link below:

- https://www.youtube.com/watch?v=-pB7kPT4gfc&t=22s&ab_channel=DennisPalmer: PD Catheter Placement Video used with permission from Dr. Dennis Palmer

In brief, the anterior abdomen should be cleaned with an antiseptic (povidone-iodine), and the surgical site infiltrated with 0.5% lidocaine at 4 mg/kg (Fig. 3). Thereafter, a 0.5 cm incision should be made about 2.5 cm below the umbilicus with a size 15 surgical blade deep through to the fascia.

If a sterile, reusable stylet is not available, an adapted, sterile bicycle spoke can be inserted into a fenestrated size 10 feeding tube for resilience through the skin nick with sustained pressure until a feel of some "give" is experienced. The adapted stylet should be removed, and the tube should be gently advanced into the peritoneal cavity (Fig. 3). A deep subcutaneous purse-string suture should be applied if the catheter moves loosely through the incision as shown in Fig. 3. The improvised PD catheter can be connected to a 3-way tap (Fig. 2), with the second end connected to the PD fluid tubing, while the third limb is connected to a urinary bag (waste bag) to drain the effluent. The PD fluid may have 100 IU/L of heparin and 4 mg/L of gentamycin added as indicated.

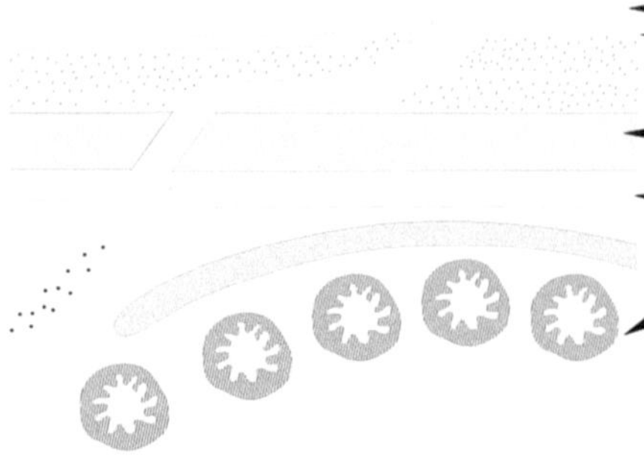

Fig. 3 Peritoneal catheter insertion site

6 Instructions for Use

6.1 Basics on How to Do PD

The PD should be carried out in a dedicated room in the ward where the patients requiring dialysis are located. However, where this is not available, a dedicated part of the ward may be screened for this purpose.

6.2 PD Cycling

There are three phases in one cycle of peritoneal dialysis (PD), they are: Fill, Dwell, Drain. During each exchange, the first phase is draining from the previous cycle and then filling to begin the next cycle.

To start with, a 5–10 mL/kg PD fluid is instilled to the peritoneal cavity for the first three cycles without a dwell time to ensure smooth ruining of the circuit. The PD cycling volume may be increased to 20 and up to 40 mL/kg depending on patients' tolerability and absence of respiratory distress. Cycles of PD should be performed until patients regained full consciousness, urinary output improves ≥1.5 mL/kg/h and patients become ambulant. However, in the event of recurrence of oliguric, anuric, or rising azotemia or worsening encephalopathy, dialysis should be re-commenced. If the patient's serum potassium falls below 4 mmol/l, a potassium supplement of 4 mmol/l should be added to 1 l of the PD fluid. Patients' vital signs are to be closely monitored throughout the procedures. The presence of abdominal pain, tenderness, guarding, and cloud effluent of PD fluid should be suggestive of peritonitis.

Further details are shown in Appendix I (Peritoneal Dialysis Procedure – Mbingo Baptist Hospital).

7 Complications/Troubleshooting

1. Peritonitis: The most common complication of PD is peritonitis, the tell-tale signs which include cloudy effluent, abdominal pain, and tenderness. Detailed attention should be paid to the color of effluent which should be normally clear. Where peritonitis is suspected, PD fluid sample and or PD catheter tip should be sent for culture and sensitivity test. The patient should be commenced on broad-spectrum antibiotics and revised with the culture result.
2. Catheter malfunction: Partial or complete catheter malfunction can occur. This may be due to kinking or intraluminal obstruction by clots or tissues. In such an instance, the patient should be repositioned and the catheter can be re-adjusted. If no improvement with such manipulations a new catheter may be re-inserted.
3. Other complications:

    (a) Hemorrhage from the surgical insertion site.
    (b) Hypokalemia. Close monitoring of electrolytes is essential and where hypokalemia ensure, potassium should be added to the dialysate.
    (c) Hypocalcemia. Hypocalcemia should be corrected with calcium gluconate.
    (d) Scrotal or abdominal wall edema. The scrotum should be elevated.
    (e) Hyperglycemia.

8 Case Resolution

A modified peritoneal dialysis catheter was inserted by the surgical team and PD was initiated. The child is commenced on PD using locally prepared fluid. Fifteen ml of 50% dextrose water was added to each 500 ml of ringer lactate solution to prepare an isotonic PD fluid of 1.5% strength. The PD was dosed at 10–30 m/kg per session of the dialysis with a dwell time of 45 min and let in and let out time of 15 min each. She received 36 sessions of peritoneal dialysis and was discharged home with improved renal function. At discharge, her serum creatinine was 7.0 mg/dl and the blood urea was 109 mg/dl.

At her one-month follow-up visit, her serum creatinine was 1.8 mg/dl and the blood urea was 41 mg/dl.

References

1. Kellum JA, et al. Kidney disease: improving global outcomes (KDIGO) acute kidney injury work group. KDIGO clinical practice guideline for acute kidney injury. Kidney Int Suppl. 2012;2(1):1–138.
2. Hessey E, et al. Acute kidney injury in critically ill children and subsequent chronic kidney disease. Can J Kidney Health Dis. 2019;6:2054358119880188.

3. Olowu WA, et al. Outcomes of acute kidney injury in children and adults in sub-Saharan Africa: a systematic review. Lancet Glob Health. 2016;4(4):e242–50.
4. Li PKT, Burdmann EA, Mehta RL. Acute kidney injury: global health alert. Arab J Nephrol Transplant. 2013;6(2):75–81.
5. Alao MA, et al. Acute pediatric peritoneal dialysis: impact of an opt-out model and adaptable methods in a hospital in Nigeria. Med J Indonesia. 2020;29(4):386–91.
6. Mehta RL, et al. International Society of Nephrology's 0by25 initiative for acute kidney injury (zero preventable deaths by 2025): a human rights case for nephrology. Lancet. 2015;385(9987):2616–43.
7. Raimann JG, Riella MC, Levin NW. International Society of Nephrology's 0by25 initiative (zero preventable deaths from acute kidney injury by 2025): focus on diagnosis of acute kidney injury in low-income countries. Clin Kidney J. 2018;11(1):12–9.
8. Alao MA, et al. Long-term survival of children following acute peritoneal dialysis in a resource-limited setting. Kidney Res Clin Pract. 2020;39(4):469.
9. Palmer D, et al. Peritoneal dialysis for AKI in Cameroon: commercial vs locally-made solutions. Perit Dial Int. 2018;38(4):246–50.

Wound Vacuum-Assisted Closure Therapy in a Low-Resource Setting

Justin Y. Lim, Shady Fayik, and Paul K. Lim

Abbreviations

NGFT	Nasogastric feeding tube
NPWT	Negative pressure wound therapy
OR	Operating room
VAC	Vacuum-assisted closure

1 Case Example

An 8-year-old girl presents to your emergency room in Egypt with a large wound to most of the dorsum of her left foot from a motorcycle accident. There are some small areas of exposed tendons making the wound not appear amenable to closure with a skin graft. Dressing changes are very painful to her such that she needs to be anesthetized for them. She is brought to the operating room (OR) and undergoes debridement of the wound. Plans are made to apply negative pressure wound therapy (NPWT); however, no commercially manufactured units are available.

J. Y. Lim · S. Fayik
Harpur Memorial Hospital, Menoufia, Egypt

P. K. Lim (✉)
Harpur Memorial Hospital, Menoufia, Egypt

Department of Surgery, University of Minnesota, Minneapolis, MN, USA
e-mail: Limxx038@umn.edu

T. M. Slusher et al. (eds.), *Pediatric Procedural Adaptations for Low-Resource Settings*, https://doi.org/10.1007/978-3-030-99955-1_22

2 Introduction

The first commercially available negative pressure wound therapy (NPWT) device was invented by Argenta and Morykwas in 1990, patented in 1991, and approved for use by the United States (US) Food and Drug Administration in 1995 as the V.A.C.®, or vacuum-assisted closure (VAC), device [1]. The VAC system includes multiple components: a wound-dressing interface (different types of foam sponges), dressing sealant, multi-channel suction tubing, and a sophisticated electric-powered suction device (seal monitor, adjustable pressure and time cycles, alarms, etc.) [2]. Over the years, clinical research articles have documented the effectiveness of VAC therapy as an adjunct to wound closure. Prior to its development, the mainstay of treating wounds, either primarily or in preparation for surgical closure, was simple dressing changes, a therapy which has been effectively unchanged for decades if not centuries. In many ways, the VAC has been nothing short of revolutionary in the treatment of wounds. However, due to its prohibitively high cost, estimated to be $120 per therapy day, it remains unaffordable to most patients in low- and middle-income countries (LMICs) [3]. In this chapter, we describe the use of NPWT as well as a way to use materials locally available to make a "home-made" VAC in many such contexts.

NPWT assists in wound closure by multiple mechanisms: the sealed wound-dressing interface keeps the wound moist (wound surface desiccation impairs healing); the active suction effect reduces surface bacterial load, reduces edema, and stimulates blood flow; and, when used on skin graft recipient sites, NPWT securely immobilizes the graft to improve take by reducing shearing and, thus, improving vascularization.

3 Indications

NPWT is indicated for use on open wounds to promote healing by secondary or tertiary intention. Tertiary, also known as delayed-primary, closure is the process by which a wound is first allowed to heal to a degree by secondary intention. Then, when amenable, the wound is surgically closed, for instance, by direct suture closure or skin graft closure.

3.1 Open Wound Categories

- Acute, subacute, chronic
- Dehisced
- Burns
- Ulcers (such as pressure, neuropathic, and venous stasis)
- Skin grafts (at time of grafting, on the recipient site as a bolster, and on the donor site for patients with significant edema such as with capillary leak from SIRS)

It may also be used on wounds closed by staples or sutures which have continuous drainage. In this situation, NPWT acts as an "external drain" by removing exudate while protecting the surrounding skin.

3.2 Contraindications

The dressing-wound interface should not be placed directly on exposed

- Blood vessels
- Anastomotic sites
- Organs
- Nerves

NPWT should not be used on wounds from

- Malignancy
- Untreated osteomyelitis
- Non-enteric and unexplored fistulas
- Necrotic tissue with eschar

3.3 Relative Contraindication: Elevated Bleeding Risk

Weakened or friable vessels in the wound from

- Suturing of blood vessels
- Infection
- Trauma
- Radiation
- Inadequate hemostasis
- Hypo-coagulable state and/or reduced thrombosis function condition
- Inadequate tissue coverage over blood vessels
- Sharp edges from bone fragments which may shift and lacerate blood vessels when NPWT applied

4 Equipment/Supplies

4.1 NPWT Component Options

4.1.1 Wound-Dressing Interface

The V.A.C.® system includes different types of foam dressings (synthetic sponge-like materials) which are placed directly on wounds.

Some alternatives:

- *Surgical Scrub Brush Sponge* (the sponge portion of the brush that is used for cleaning hands for the OR)
  - Pros:

    Comes in sterile package (no need to sterilize)
    Small size makes these easily adjusted for small wounds (such as pediatric extremity wounds)

  - Cons:
    - Relatively expensive
    - May not be available in lower-income country settings
    - Larger wounds may require multiple sponges, which may be difficult to keep together
- *Household cleaning sponge* (Fig. 1a)
  - Pros:

    Widely available in shops and stores
    Inexpensive

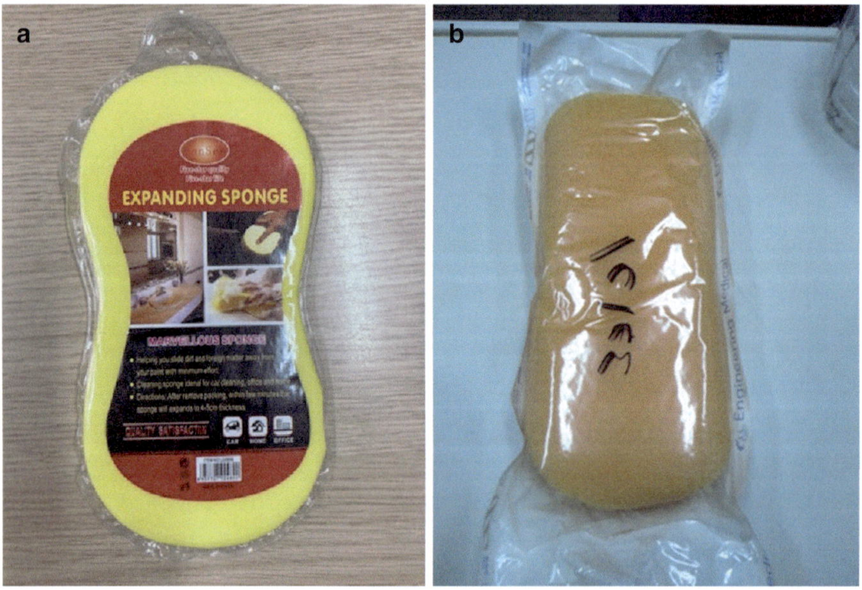

Fig. 1 (**a**) Example of household sponge. (Figure used with permission from J Lim and Dr. S. Fayik). (**b**) Sponge now autoclaved and packaged for use. (Figure used with permission from J Lim and Dr. S. Fayik)

– Cons:

Requires sterilization which can be done with standard steam autoclave used for surgical instruments (Fig. 1b)

4.2 Dressing Sealant

4.2.1 Adhesive Drapes

Alternatives to the V.A.C.® system dressing sealant include:

- Commercially available *medical-use adhesive drapes* such as OpSite (Smith & Nephew™) or Ioban™ (3M™). Some locally sourced surgical drapes are also available (Fig. 2).
- *Plastic food wrap (not pictured)*
  - A very inexpensive and widely available alternative is plastic food wrap; however, this is only amenable for use on extremity wounds (not trunk or scalp). Adhesive tape is used to secure the ends and borders around the drape and tubing.

4.2.2 Suction Tubing

- 16 or 18 French *nasogastric feeding tube (NGFT)* (Fig. 3). These work adequately as the suction tubing interfacing with the sponges. The tip is buried within the sponge (Fig. 4).

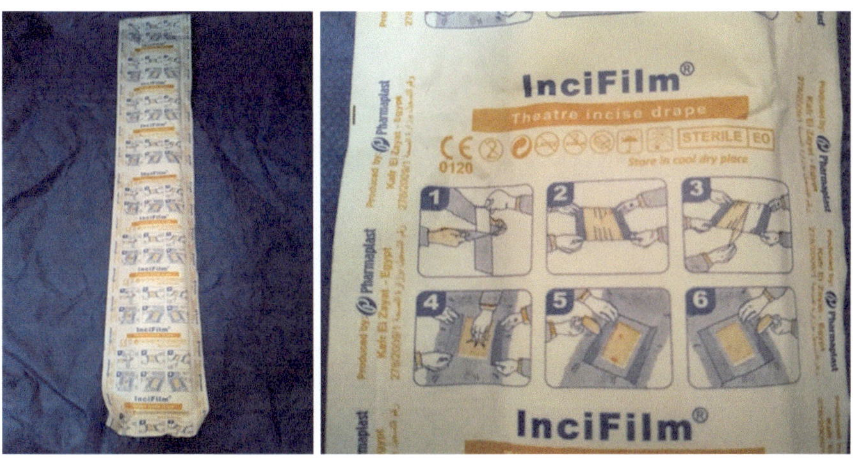

Fig. 2 Locally sourced surgical adhesive drape. (Figure used with permission from J. Lim)

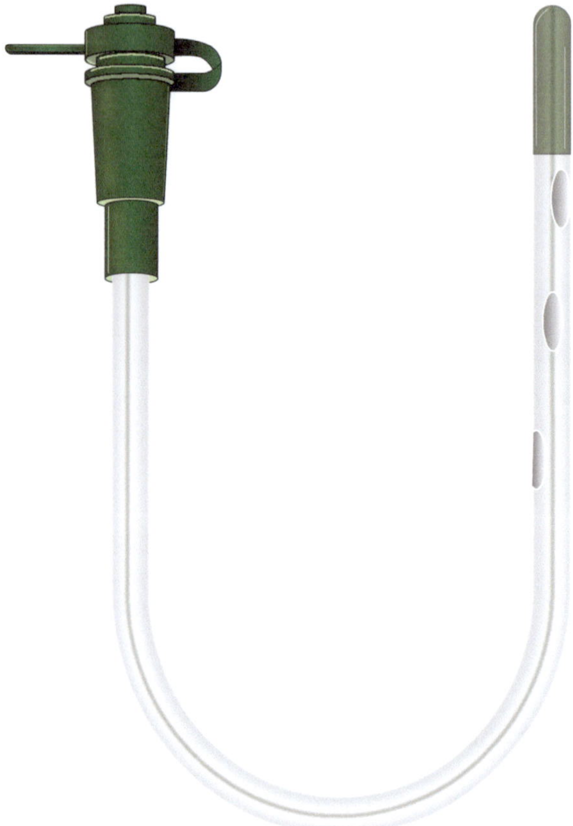

Fig. 3 Suction tube (modified NGFT with extra holes cut). (Figure used with permission from Adrian M. Slusher)

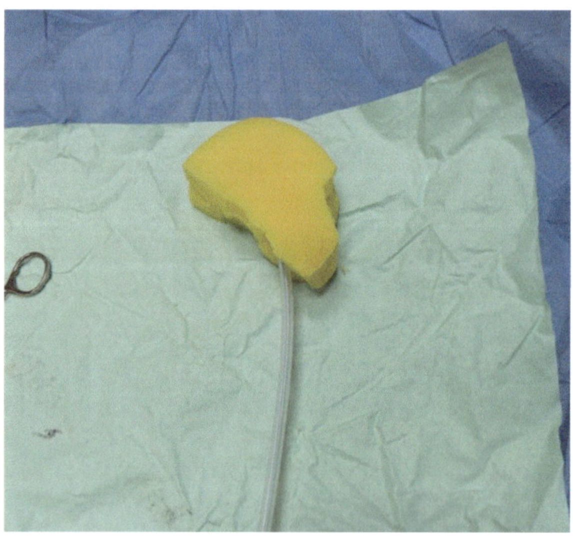

Fig. 4 NGFT buried in Sponge. (Figure used with permission from Dr. Fayik)

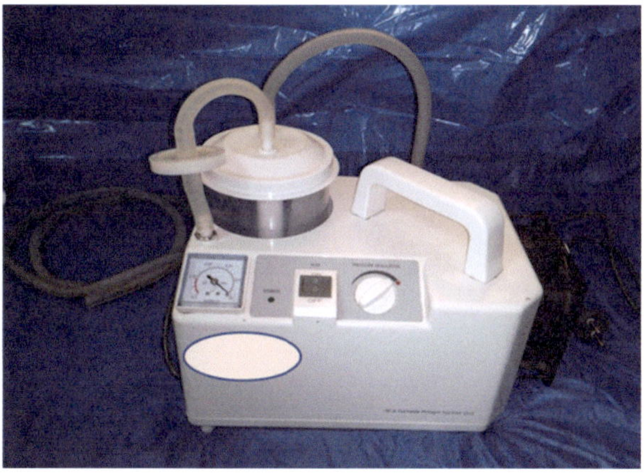

Fig. 5 Mobile suction machine. (Figure used with permission from Dr. S. Fayik)

4.2.3 Suction Device

- *Central wall suction or a mobile electric suction machine* may be used along with a standard fluid collection container (Fig. 5).

5 Technique/Instructions for Use

5.1 Wound-Dressing Interface

- The sponge should be cut precisely to the size and margins of the wound in order to avoid maceration of the surrounding skin.
- When used as a bolster for a newly applied skin graft, gauze smeared with petrolatum ointment (such as Vaseline™ petroleum jelly) should be placed on the graft before placing the sponge on top of the graft. This will help to inhibit the graft from adhering to the sponge (and coming off with the sponge when the sponge is removed).

5.2 Suction

The NGFT tip should be tunneled or buried in the sponge so as not to be occluded from the transparent drape. See Fig. 6a, b for examples of a wound before NPWT and after NPWT.

- Suction pressure should be set to 125 mmHg.
  - Continuous suction should be used since intermittent suction cycling (on and off multiple times per hour) is not feasible with wall suction or a portable suc-

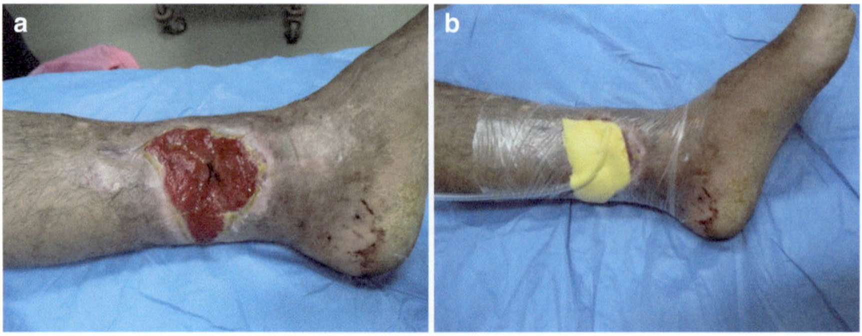

Fig. 6 (**a**) Wound before applying NPWT. (Figure used with permission from Dr. S. Fayik). (**b**) NPWT on a leg wound. (Figure used with permission from Dr. S. Fayik)

tion unit. Although much of the efficacy data with the V.A.C.® system was originally based on intermittent suction cycles, the device also has a continuous suction setting which has become the most commonly used one.

5.3 *Monitoring Suction and Seal*

If the system is functioning properly, the sponge will contract and become firm. This must be inspected frequently. If the suction and/or seal is not secure for a prolonged period of time (more than a few hours), then the occlusive dressing will effectively create an abscess environment which can cause tissue damage and sepsis.

- Nursing staff should assess the NPWT system every 4 hours.
- The surgeon should assess it twice per day on rounds (including on weekends).
- If the system is found to be malfunctioning with no resolution, the dressing and drape must be removed, and standard dressing changes instituted.

5.4 *NPWT Dressing Change Intervals*

Intervals between dressing changes should be every 3 days (no longer than every 4 days). Shorter intervals can be used based on wound characteristics and/or OR availability.

6 NPWT Endpoints

Since this is an adjunct modality for wound healing, there are no definitive endpoints. Instead, it is a matter of wound healing degree as to when to discontinue NPWT. When the wound is judged to be amenable to closure by direct suture, flap, or skin graft reconstruction or when the wound is small enough and in a favorable location for simple dressing changes to complete healing by secondary intention, NPWT can be discontinued.

7 Complications

- When NPWT is used on patients with high output wounds (such as those with enteric fistulas) or large wounds relative to the size of the patient (such as with young children), dehydration and/or electrolyte imbalances may ensue. These patients should be monitored for fluid and electrolyte imbalances and treated as indicated.
- Peri-wound skin should be protected from the wound-dressing interface. The interface is moist from the wound exudate and, when overlapping and sealed on the peri-wound skin, NPWT can cause maceration and, subsequently, tissue damage.
- Circumferential extremity NPWT dressings should be avoided due to risk of distal edema, venous congestion, and/or ischemia.

8 Case Resolution

After debridement of her wound in the OR, she had initiation of NPWT under general anesthesia. VAC changes were performed every 3 days in the OR under intravenous sedation for 2 weeks. At that point, there was sufficient granulation tissue covering the previously exposed tendons such that split-thickness skin graft closure of the wound was performed and a VAC dressing placed as the stabilizing bolster on the graft. Four days later, the VAC was removed in the OR under intravenous sedation. The graft showed a 100% take.

References

1. Invention of a vacuum-assisted wound-closure device. 2021 [cited 08/31/2021]. Available from: https://www.wakehealth.edu/About-Us/History/Firsts/Vacuum-Assisted-Wound-Closure-Device. Accessed Aug 2021.
2. V.A.C., Therapy Safety Information with V.A.C.® GRANUFOAM™ Dressing, V.A.C.® GRANUFOAM SILVER™ Dressing and V.A.C. WHITEFOAM™ Dressing application instructions. Acelity, p. 280.
3. Kim JJ, et al. Cost-effective alternative for negative-pressure wound therapy. Plast Reconstr Surg Glob Open. 2017;5(2):e1211.

Further Reading

A simplified vacuum dressing system. https://www.woundsresearch.com/article/simplified-vacuum-dressing-system.
Homemade negative pressure wound therapy: treatment of complex wounds under challenging conditions. https://pubmed.ncbi.nlm.nih.gov/25881336/.
Perez D, Exe C, Ziegler A, Bramkamp M, Von Ruden C. Modern wound care for the poor: a randomized clinical trial comparing the vacuum system with conventional saline-soaked gauze dressings. Am J Surg. 2010;199:14–20.
Simplified negative pressure wound therapy device for application in low-resource settings. https://www.ncbi.nlm.nih.gov/pmc/articles/PMC4731696/.
Vacuum-assisted closure of the open abdomen in a resource-limited setting. https://pubmed.ncbi.nlm.nih.gov/21542399/.

Burn Care in a Low-Resource Setting

Andrew W. Kiragu

Abbreviations

BSA	Body surface area
EFR	Estimated fluid resuscitation
EMS	Emergency medical services
LMICs	Low- and middle-income countries
ORS	Oral rehydration solution
TBSA	Total body surface area

1 Case Example

An 8-year-old girl presents to the hospital where you are working in Kenya. She has sustained burns to her chest and abdomen. On the day prior to presentation, she was helping her mother cook over a kerosene stove. She was carrying a pot of boiling water back into the house when she accidentally bumped into the doorframe, spilling hot water on herself, which resulted in her burns. Her mother initially took her to the local dispensary where she was given paracetamol and was advised to take her to the referral hospital where you work. Her mother was unable to get to the hospital until today because she had to borrow money from family and friends. She is very worried because large areas of the burn formed blisters and some had burst.

A. W. Kiragu (✉)
Department of Pediatrics, University of Minnesota, Minneapolis, MN, USA

Children's Hospital of Minnesota, Critical Care, Minneapolis, MN, USA

Department of Pediatrics, Division of Critical Care, Hennepin Healthcare, Minneapolis, MN, USA
e-mail: Andrew.Kiragu@childrensmn.org

T. M. Slusher et al. (eds.), *Pediatric Procedural Adaptations for Low-Resource Settings*, https://doi.org/10.1007/978-3-030-99955-1_23

On arrival, the girl is awake and crying in pain. Her burns are very painful with several blisters over her chest and abdomen. The exposed areas are moist and shiny and blanch with pressure. The medical student working with you enquires about how you should proceed with evaluation and management of this patient. While the nurse is getting vital signs and placing an IV for fluids and medication, you explain to her that classification of the child's burns is key to the evaluation and management of this patient. She also asks what you would have done in the resource-limited primary health center where there are no intravenous fluids.

2 Introduction

Burns represent a truly devastating event for children [1–5]. Worldwide, it is estimated that over 11 million people suffer burn injuries leading to more than 265,000 deaths annually [1–8]. Over 70% of burn injuries occur in low- and middle-income countries (LMICs) with the majority of these in Africa and Southeast Asia [9]. Most burns occur in the home [9]. In pediatric patients, the vast majority (61%) of burns are scald burns [10, 11]. In LMICs girls are also at increased risk of burns since in many countries they often help with cooking [9, 12]. In many low-resource settings, it is not unusual to see delays in accessing proper treatment. However, the importance of early recognition, resuscitation initiation, maintenance of euthermia, and basic wound dressings can and should be initiated at the first point of contact. Early referral to tertiary burn centers in LMICs, whenever possible, is key but unfortunately these are rare in LMICs. Building capacity in LMICs to manage burn injuries is pragmatic and morally imperative.

3 Classification of Burns

Burns are classified by their depth and the total body surface area (TBSA) involved. In addition, the etiology of the burn, location of the burn, and whether there is an inhalational component are important. It is also important to describe any associated injuries.

3.1 Burn Depth Determination

The determination of the depth of a burn injury is key to burn management. Classification is based on the layer(s) of skin involved and varies from superficial or first degree burns, that involve only the epidermis, to full-thickness burns, or third-degree burns that involve the full thickness of the skin (Figs. 1 and 2) [5, 10, 13].

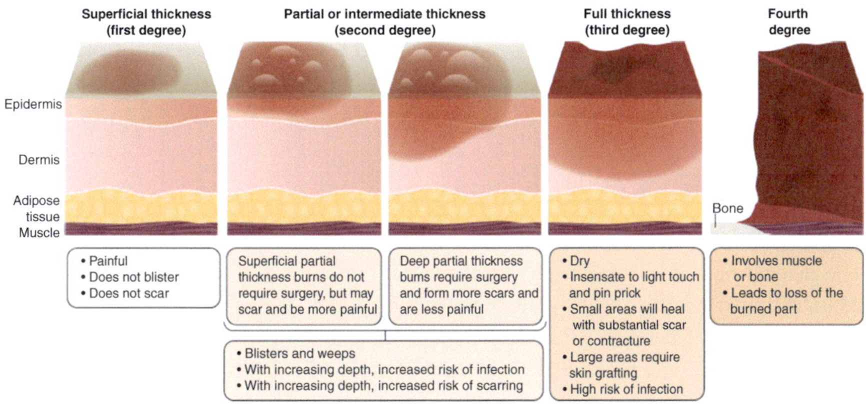

Fig. 1 Burn depth determination and characteristics. (From Jeschke et al. [12], open source [13])

Fig. 2 A child with partial thickness burns of the face, neck, and upper chest. Note the redness, blistering, and weeping nature of the wounds

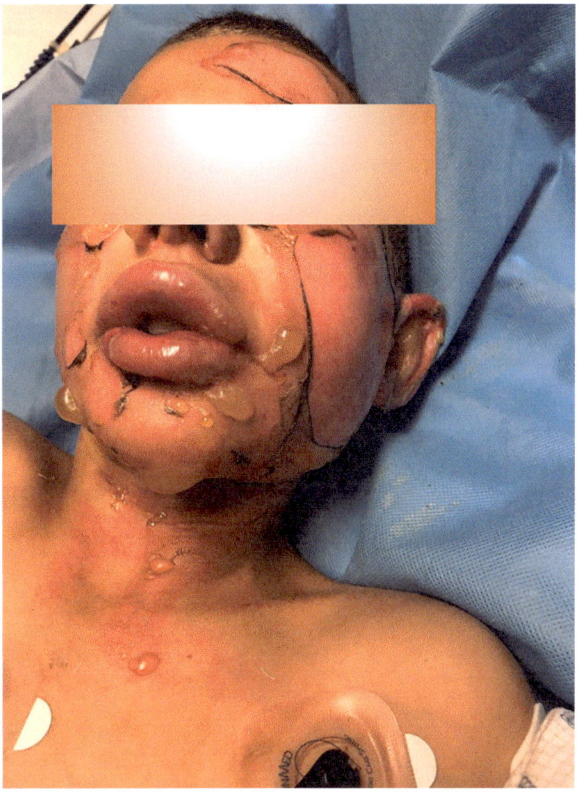

Burn depth also determines the care that will be required ranging from simple supportive skin care for superficial burns to the need for skin grafting in full-thickness burns [5, 13].

3.2 Body Surface Area Determination

The determination of total body surface area (TBSA) is key to the resuscitation of pediatric burn patients and together with burn depth, forms part of the criteria to help determine if patients will require more specialized care in a hospital that specializes in burn management [5, 13]. Only partial and full-thickness burns are used to determine TBSA. TBSA varies across age groups as illustrated in Fig. 3 [13]. The Lund-Browder Chart is used to aid in the determination of TBSA [5, 14]. Use of the Lund-Browder Chart is more accurate than the commonly used "Rule of Nines" which divides the body up into different regions, each of which represents 9% TBSA. A quick estimate is the "Rule of Palm". The area of the patient's palm, with the fingers closed, represents roughly 1% TBSA [5].

4 Case Example Continuation

Using a Lund-Browder chart, you quickly determine that this child has about 20% TBSA partial-thickness burns of her chest and abdomen. You discuss with the student the management of the burn injury, including some elements of first aid that can be used and then discuss how your patient will be managed in your hospital setting.

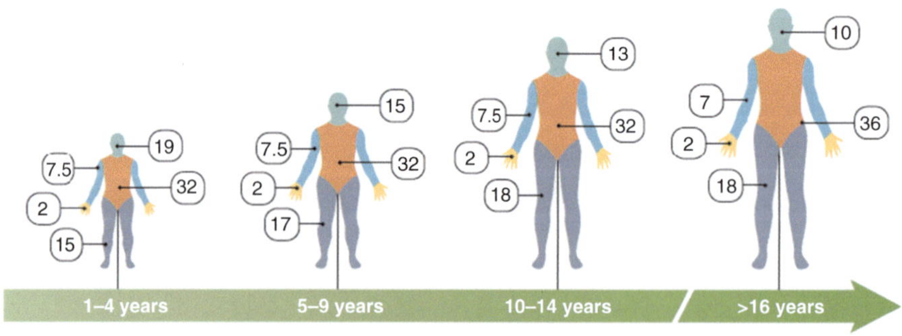

Fig. 3 The Lund-Browder chart for determining TBSA. (From Jeschke et al. [12], open source [13])

5 Burn Management: Initial Care and Evaluation

The rapid evaluation and management of pediatric patients with burn injuries is crucial. Children have an increased body surface area (BSA) to body mass ratio and even short delays in resuscitation can result in hypovolemia, longer hospital lengths of stay, acute renal failure, and increased mortality [15, 16].

5.1 *Pre-healthcare Facility*

Limitations in the availability of formal Emergency Medical Service (EMS) systems means that many children in LMICs receive the initial care for their injuries outside of the formal medical sector [5, 17, 18].

(a) The first step of first aid, as recommended by the World Health Organization (WHO), for flame burns includes stopping the burning process using the stop, drop, and roll technique to put out flames [5, 19].
(b) The next step is to place the burned area under cool running water to reduce the temperature of the burn for at least 20 min. If running water is not available and the burn area is small, place the burned area under cool water for 20 min or wrap the burned area with wet cloths and replace periodically [5].
(c) The burn should then be covered with a clean cloth [5, 17, 18].

Unfortunately, these elements of first aid are not consistently followed, and in many instances, family caregivers employ harmful practices such as the use of traditional ointments, kerosene, petroleum jelly, milk, and raw eggs [17, 18]. Community education about proper first aid for all injuries including burns is therefore key. After the administration of first aid, the burned child should be taken for evaluation at a local health facility.

5.2 *Medical Facility/Hospital Management*

As with the management of any trauma patient, the management of burn patients involves a primary and secondary survey.

1. Primary survey: Airway, Breathing, Circulation, Disability, and Exposure (with caution to avoid hypothermia) [5, 13].
    (a) Inhalational injury/airway involvement
    (b) Circulatory failure due to burn shock

2. Secondary survey:
   (a) Obtaining any necessary laboratory data and radiographic studies
   (b) Provision of tetanus prophylaxis
   (c) More definitive evaluation of the severity of the burn injury including burn TBSA extent and depth [5, 13]
   (d) Calculate the amount of fluid resuscitation required once TBSA involved is estimated [13]
3. Burn injury management-specific priorities:
   (a) Early recognition of major burns (>10–20% partial thickness and full-thickness burns)
   (b) Evaluation and management of airway involvement
   (c) Recognition of carbon monoxide and cyanide poisoning
   (d) Fluid resuscitation for management of burn shock.

6 Burn Management: Fluid Resuscitation

The recognition and early aggressive management of burn shock has been a key advancement in the management of major burn injuries and has been responsible for increased survival.

- *Smaller burns*: <10% TBSA (infants and children) or <15% TBSA (adolescents) generally can be treated with oral rehydration solution (ORS).
- *Larger burns*: >10% TBSA (infants and children) or >15% TBSA (adolescents) require prompt intravenous access and volume resuscitation [16]. Burn injuries larger than 15% TBSA often trigger the systemic inflammatory response syndrome and require intravenous fluid resuscitation to prevent burn shock and death [20].

   1. Access: Large-bore peripheral intravenous access should be obtained either percutaneously or by cut-down, preferably into unburned skin [16].
   2. Fluid resuscitation: Several pediatric-specific formulas calculate age and weight-based estimated fluid resuscitation (EFR) volumes (Table 1) [15, 16, 20]. The most used formula is the Parkland formula (Table 1), which has been adapted for pediatric use [5, 14, 15, 21].
   3. Maintenance fluids: Maintenance fluids should be given as saline with dextrose to avoid hypoglycemia [5]. The maintenance fluid rate can be calculated using the 4:2:1 rule: 4 ml/kg for the first 10 kg plus 2 ml/kg for the next 10 kg plus 1 ml/kg for each additional kg of weight [5].

A survey of burn resuscitation in Africa, revealed that parenteral fluid resuscitation protocols using Lactated Ringer's solution based upon the Parkland formula are the most utilized [19]. There was also an increased utilization of enteral hydration in the form of ORS, along with a focus on clinical endpoints such as urine output, rather than invasive monitoring in comparison to high-income countries. In certain

Table 1 Fluid resuscitation formulae

Resuscitation formula	Type of fluid infused	Volume of fluid infused in first 24 h	Rate of infusion
Parkland formula (pediatric)	Lactated ringers	4 ml/kg/%TBSA **plus** maintenance fluids	½ in first 8 h and the remaining ½ over the following 16 h
Cincinnati-Shriners	Lactated ringers+50 meq sodium bicarbonate Lactated ringers Lactated ringers+12.5 g albumin 5%	4 ml/kg/%TBSA **plus** 1500 ml/kg	First 8 h Second 8 h Third 8 h
Galveston-Shriners	Lactated ringers	5000 ml/m^2 TBSA burn plus 2000 ml/m^2 BSA	First ½ over 8 h, second ½ over 16 h

Adapted from Zuo et al. [21]

resource-poor settings, ORS is a viable option for burn resuscitation for burns less than 20% TBSA [22]. ORS consists of a simple formula containing glucose, sodium chloride, potassium chloride, and trisodium citrate [23]. For additional details on ORS see chapter "Oral Rehydration Therapy in a Low-Resource Setting". It has been used successfully for decades to treat dehydration secondary to severe diarrhea in conditions such as cholera. This intervention has saved millions of lives [23]. This highlights the possibility of rapidly mobilizing ORS following large-scale mass casualty/burn incidents and in delayed transport scenarios such as prolonged field care [23, 24].

7 Case Continuation

The calculation of our patient's fluid resuscitation needs is shown below:

Our Patient's Fluid Calculation

Our patient has 20% TBSA partial thickness burns. She weighs 35 kg.

Her initial 24-h fluid resuscitation needs would be:

4 ml × kg × %TBSA = 4 × 35 × 20 = 2800 ml of Lactated Ringers.

Half of this would be given in the first 8 h = 1400 ml/8 h = 175 ml/h.

The remaining half would be given over the following 16 h = 1400 ml/16 h = 87.5 ml/h.

In addition, she would need dextrose containing maintenance IV fluids. The rate would be: (4 ml/kg/h × 10 kg) + (2 ml/kg/h × 10 kg) + (1 ml/kg/h × 15 kg) = 75 ml/h.

Therefore, her total fluid rate in the first 8 h would be 175 ml/h + 75 ml/h = 250 ml/h and in the following 16 h would be 87.5 ml/h + 75 ml/h = 162.5 ml/h.

Your student then asks you how you should manage the patient's wounds. You explain that good wound care is essential in burn management.

8 Burn Management: Wound Care

The burn wound is an evolving wound and can worsen if conditions are suboptimal. Poor perfusion, poor nutrition, sepsis, and wound infections can delay healing and increase the need for excision and grafting [5]. Good management of the wound is essential. This involves not only appropriate dressings but prevention of infection, correct positioning, and assessment for surgery [5]. Burn dressings should provide a bacterial barrier to prevent bacteria from entering the wound or being transmitted from the wound leading to sepsis or tissue infection [25]. Burn wound care is particularly challenging in low-resource areas where adequate access to clean water is often problematic. Superficial burns do not require antibiotics or wound dressings. All deeper burns require topical antimicrobials or an absorptive occlusive dressing. Table 2 includes options for ointments and dressings.

Table 2 Burn wound care options

Wound care component	Options and alternatives
Inner layer dressing (should be non-adherent)	Silver-based dressing = ideal Paraffin gauze with petroleum jelly or Adaptic Amniotic membranes (donor screened for infections including hepatitis B & C, HIV, and syphilis infections) [27] Boiled potato peel Banana leaf
Antimicrobial ointments [22]	Silver sulfadiazine Mafenide acetate Bacitracin Honey [28, 29] (medical grade when possible) (One option, if only local honey is available, is to heat the honey on the stove to near boiling, strain if needed, allow to cool, and place in a clean jar for use with burn care for partial thickness burns) Moist exposed burn ointment (MEBO): traditional Chinese burn ointment whose primary active component is ß-sitosterol in a base of beeswax and sesame oil – added benefit of not requiring an overlying dressing [25, 26] [26, 30]
Outer layer dressing (should be thick and absorbent)	Thick gauze Wool Cotton
Adjunct	Aloe vera –for superficial or partial thickness burns [31]

8.1 Burn Wound Care Steps

1. Using aseptic technique, clean the wound. Daily cleaning with Dakin's™ solution or other antiseptic solution helps to ensure sterility of the water and is bactericidal against most bacteria in the wound [22].
2. Apply a topical antimicrobial agent.
3. Place a two-layer dressing. The inner layer of the dressing should be non-adherent, while the outer layer should be thick and absorbent [5]. Silver-based dressing and ointment should be used if available [26].
4. This should be followed by a firm bandage [5].

9 Burn Management: Pain Control and Nutrition

9.1 Pain Control and Sedation

Burn pain may be the most difficult to treat among any etiology of acute pain. Unfortunately, many of the interventions required for burn care such as dressing changes, excision and grafting, post-burn physical and occupational therapies are associated with pain which may be the same or worse than the pain of the initial burn injury [5, 10, 32]. Assessing the degree of pain is key. There are a variety of pain scales that can be utilized in children [10, 32]. A parent's presence and participation in procedures can be highly beneficial and has the added benefit of teaching parents how to do wound care [10]. Oral non-steroidal anti-inflammatory drugs and acetaminophen/paracetamol are used to treat minor burns. For hospitalized burn patients, opioids are the cornerstone of pharmacologic pain control [32]. Codeine should be avoided in pediatric patients since it is not properly metabolized in up to 30% of children. Ketamine is especially helpful in major dressing changes at the bedside, or other procedures requiring moderate sedation [32]. Ketamine controls pain, provides sedation, and amnesia. It can be given via oral, intramuscular, intranasal, or intravenous routes. One protocol using ketamine safely is described in "The Every Second Matters – Ketamine Package" and provides checklists and guidance for safely administering ketamine sedation in emergent situations" [33].

9.2 Nutrition

In LMICs, children are commonly undernourished even before they sustain the thermal injury. If they present for care days or weeks after injury, they are likely to be even more nutritionally compromised [5]. Adequate nutritional status is critical in wound healing and reduction of infection risk [5]. Nutrition should be considered as important as any medication in the management of any child with a major burn injury [5] (chapter "Malnutrition: Practical Approaches to Feeding a Severely Malnourished Child in a Low-Resource Setting").

10 Complications

Patients with burns are at high risk for many complications associated with their burns. Some common complications include

- Infection (localized or systemic)
- Fluid shifts – shock/dehydration and/or fluid overload/edema
- Malnutrition
- Electrolyte abnormalities
- Poor wound healing

11 Case Resolution

The patient was admitted for fluid resuscitation and wound care. She received a tetanus vaccination. Her burns were mostly partial-thickness burns and she would not require surgery. After her wounds were cleaned and with good pain control, her appetite improved. Her mother was taught how to dress her wounds with antibiotic ointment at home and with help from relatives was able to purchase the necessary supplies for wound care. She was discharged after 3 days and was told to return to the pediatric clinic 1–2 weeks later for evaluation. At that time her wounds were noted to be healing well. The mother also received additional counseling on keeping her children safe from burns.

References

1. Rybarczyk MM, et al. A systematic review of burn injuries in low- and middle-income countries: epidemiology in the WHO-defined African Region. Afr J Emerg Med. 2017;7(1):30–7.
2. Gali BM, Madziga AG, Naaya HU. Epidemiology of childhood burns in Maiduguri north-eastern Nigeria. Niger J Med. 2004;13(2):144–7.
3. Argenta A, Demos J. Burn management in the developing world: international volunteerism. Clin Plast Surg. 2017;44(4):875–83.
4. Thomson IK, et al. Management of paediatric burns in low- and middle-income countries: assessing capacity using the World Health Organization Surgical Assessment Tool. Int Health. 2020;12(5):499–506.
5. Falder S, Potokar T, Bendell R. Interburns essential burn care training manual. England and Wales: Interburns; 2016.
6. Aldana MC, Navarrete N. Epidemiology of a decade of pediatric fatal burns in Colombia, South America. Burns. 2015;41(7):1587–92.

7. Bailey ME, et al. Epidemiology and outcomes of burn injuries at a tertiary burn care center in Bangladesh. Burns. 2019;45(4):957–63.
8. Stokes MAR, Johnson WD. Burns in the Third World: an unmet need. Ann Burns Fire Disasters. 2017;30(4):243–6.
9. Gandhi M, et al. Management of pain in children with burns. Int J Pediatr. 2010;2010:1–9. https://doi.org/10.1155/2010/825657.
10. Tripathee S, Basnet SJ. Epidemiology of burn injuries in Nepal: a systemic review. Burns Trauma. 2017;5:10.
11. Banerjee S, Shumba C. A systematic review of epidemiological patterns and proposed interventions to address pediatric burns in Nigeria. Afr Health Sci. 2020;20(2):991–9.
12. Jeschke MG, et al. Burn injury. Nat Rev Dis Primers. 2020;6(1):11.
13. Shah AR, Liao LF. Pediatric burn care: unique considerations in management. Clin Plast Surg. 2017;44(3):603–10.
14. Partain KP, Fabia R, Thakkar RK. Pediatric burn care: new techniques and outcomes. Curr Opin Pediatr. 2020;32(3):405–10.
15. Arbuthnot MK, Garcia AV. Early resuscitation and management of severe pediatric burns. Semin Pediatr Surg. 2019;28(1):73–8.
16. Gyedu A, et al. Pediatric first aid practices in Ghana: a population-based survey. World J Surg. 2015;39(8):1859–66.
17. Seow SN, et al. The practice of first aid for burn injuries among the population of East Coast of Peninsular Malaysia for 2012–2016. J Burn Care Res. 2020;41(4):905–7.
18. Jeng J, Gibran N, Peck M. Burn care in disaster and other austere settings. Surg Clin N Am. 2014;94(4):893–907.
19. Rode H, et al. Burn resuscitation on the African continent. Burns. 2014;40(7):1283–91.
20. Zuo KJ, Medina A, Tredget EE. Important developments in burn care. PlastReconstr Surg. 2017;139(1):120e–38e.
21. Wasiak J, et al. Dressings for superficial and partial thickness burns. Cochrane Database Syst Rev. 2013;3:CD002106.
22. Gomez BI, et al. Enteral resuscitation with oral rehydration solution to reduce acute kidney injury in burn victims: evidence from a porcine model. PLoS One. 2018;13(5):e0195615.
23. Michell MW, et al. Enteral resuscitation of burn shock using World Health Organization oral rehydration solution: a potential solution for mass casualty care. J Burn Care Res. 2006;27(6):819–25.
24. Romanowski KS, Palmieri TL. Pediatric burn resuscitation: past, present, and future. Burns Trauma. 2017;5:26.
25. Charles AG, Gallaher J, Cairns BA. Burn care in low- and middle-income countries. Clin Plast Surg. 2017;44(3):479–83.
26. Mabvuure NT, et al. The use of moist exposed burn ointment (MEBO) for the treatment of burn wounds: a systematic review. J Plast Surg Hand Surg. 2020;54(6):337–43.
27. Eskandarlou M, et al. The healing effect of amniotic membrane in burn patients. World J Plast Surg. 2016;5(1):39–44.
28. Okeniyi JAO, et al. Healing of burns in children: which is the better agent, honey or silver sulphadiazine? Niger J Paediatr. 2006;32:7–11.
29. Aziz Z, Abdul Rasool Hassan B. The effects of honey compared to silver sulfadiazine for the treatment of burns: a systematic review of randomized controlled trials. Burns. 2017;43(1):50–7.
30. Maenthaisong R, et al. The efficacy of aloe vera used for burn wound healing: a systematic review. Burns. 2007;33(6):713–8.
31. Griggs C, et al. Sedation and pain management in burn patients. Clin Plast Surg. 2017;44(3):535–40.
32. Palmieri TL. Pediatric burn resuscitation. Crit Care Clin. 2016;32(4):547–59.
33. Schwartz KR, et al. An innovative safe anesthesia and analgesia package for emergency pediatric procedures and surgeries when no anesthetist is available. Int J Emerg Med. 2016;9(1):16.

Unique Considerations for Simulation Use in a Low-Resource Setting

Colleen Fant, Kristin Van Genderen, Gatwiri Murithi, and Michael B. Pitt

Abbreviations

HBB	Helping Babies Breathe
HIC	High-Income Countries
LMIC	Low- and middle-income countries
PEARLS	Promoting Excellence and Reflective Learning in Simulation
RLS	Resource-limited settings
SBME	Simulation-Based Medical Education
SUGAR	Simulation Use for Global Away Rotations

1 Introduction

Simulation-Based Medical Education (SBME) is a novel educational tool in LMICs that can be integrated into medical training programs to prepare trainees for real-life challenges. Simulation helps generalists and providers at different levels of training

C. Fant · K. Van Genderen
Feinberg School of Medicine, Northwestern University, Chicago, IL, USA
e-mail: Cfant@luriechildrens.org; kvangenderen@luriechildrens.org

G. Murithi
Center for Public Health and Development, Center for Experiential Learning, Safe Anesthesia and Surgery Advocate Project Manager, HRH Specialist, Kisumu, Kenya
e-mail: gatwiri.murithi@cphdev.org

M. B. Pitt (✉)
Department of Pediatrics, Division of Hospital Medicine, University of Minnesota, Minneapolis, MN, USA
e-mail: mbpitt@umn.edu

T. M. Slusher et al. (eds.), *Pediatric Procedural Adaptations for Low-Resource Settings*, https://doi.org/10.1007/978-3-030-99955-1_24

learn medical skills not traditionally part of their training. One significant value of SBME is to prepare students for crisis resource management leading to reduction in errors, increase in patient safety, and improve resource allocation [1]. As a training tool, the combination of didactic teaching and repeated simulation sessions prepare health workers to work effectively and handle emergencies [2, 3]. Simulation – with or without procedural practice – can be used to address some of the nuanced emotional and practical preparation needs for work in resource-limited settings (RLS).

Thus far, this textbook has focused on procedural modifications for use in resource-limited settings. In this chapter, we shift focus to highlight unique considerations where these procedural modifications can be incorporated into simulation experiences for learners. We describe simulation for preparation for work in RLS settings and provide some practical tools for how to conduct simulations o-site with partners in resource-limited environments.

2 Simulation for Preparing to Work in Resource-Limited Settings

Pre-departure training for work in global health settings is a well-established best practice [4, 5]. Simulation can be a useful tool to support this preparation by "pre-creating" some of the practical and emotional challenges that are common when working in RLS [5–9]. Cases can be designed to expand educational domains including *knowledge* [8, 10] (e.g., exposure to real-time management of rarely encountered conditions such as cerebral malaria), *attitudes* [10, 11] (e.g., managing the emotions often encountered when working in resource-limited settings such as frustration at not being able to manage a case the same way as one would in their home institution), and *skills* [7] (e.g., incorporating the procedural modifications as laid out in this textbook).

2.1 SUGARPREP Curriculum

In 2013, members of the multi-institution Midwest Consortium of Global Child Health Educators [12] developed a simulation curriculum called Simulation Use for Global Away Rotations (SUGAR) [10]. In SUGAR cases, the facilitator allows time for participants to problem solve and navigate through the emotional hurdles of the case, and then creates a psychologically safe space for learners to debrief these emotions and address knowledge gaps. There are over a dozen cases available to use on www.sugarprep.org as well as training videos for facilitators.

In addition to the SUGAR cases, the Midwest Consortium of Global Child Health Educators developed simulation cases to pair with several of the procedural adaptations described in this textbook. For example, one case describes a 6-year-old in shock who requires an intraosseous line, and the learners practice the case with the procedural modification of using a modified large-bore needle instead as described in chapter "Intraosseous Line Placement for Medical Therapy in a Low-Resource Setting". In another, a patient with respiratory failure necessitates the use of modified oxygen delivery devices and chest tube drainage as described in chapter "Modified Chest Drainage System for Use in a Low-Resource Settings". These case pairings, which also include tailored debriefing scripts, allow learners to practice the new skill modifications in a clinically relevant simulated environment. Similarly, these cases can be used with learners in resource-limited settings at a host institution.

3 Simulation Training in Resource-Limited Settings

One of the significant challenges facing healthcare systems in LMICs is an inadequately trained workforce and a lack of specialty training for providers. Simulation training is well-suited to address this issue, with a variety of ways to increase training and capacity building within resource-limited or resource-variable settings. Simulation training allows providers to gain skill and clinical confidence in areas of medicine that may not have been available in their training.

In particular, simulation-based training in Africa is still in its infancy but is rapidly expanding. There is a paucity of data available on the work being done but countries like South Africa, Kenya, Rwanda, Ethiopia, Tanzania, and Uganda have institutions with dedicated simulation centers. Different forms of low fidelity simulation are also widely available and are used to train health workers on basic skills including first aid, Basic Life Support (BLS), and Advanced Cardiac Life Support (ACLS) among other simulation programs. Partnerships for SBME between academic centers in LMICs and HICs allow for more resources and access to expanded subspecialty training. This educational partnership model has been successfully implemented in a variety of different iterations with a variety of trainers and learners from both LMICs and HICs (Table 1).

Table 1 Simulation setup for trainers and learners

	Trainer in high-income countries	Trainer in low- and middle-income countries
Learner in high-income countries	Example: Simulation training in US medical education Example: SUGAR pre-departure cases for HIC learners preparing for global health rotations	A potential area for future work (especially in pre-departure training) Example: Visiting trainees and faculty from LMIC running simulation cases for HIC partner trainees on a country-specific case as part of bidirectional partnership
Learners in low- and middle-income countries	Example: Lurie Children's faculty from Chicago, IL, USA traveling to Bugando medical Center in Mwanza, Tanzania to run simulation cases on pediatric emergencies for clinical staff	Example: The JOOTRH simulation lab running cases for hospital staff on COVID-19

4 Case Example

Simulation in Western Kenya: The Center for Experiential Learning at Jaramogi Oginga Odinga Teaching and Referral Hospital (JOOTRH) was established in 2016 to support the training of nurse anesthetists who use the hospital as their clinical training site. It is currently managed by the Center for Public Health and Development, a local NGO that received funding to build capacity for anesthesia training in Kenya. It is equipped with a mix of low fidelity and high-fidelity mannequins (SimMan®, SimMom®, and SimBaby®). In addition to the simulation equipment the space is equipped with medical equipment including an anesthesia machine, ventilator, and defibrillator allowing for a range of simulation scenarios including surgical/anesthesia care, critical and emergency care.

To build faculty for this center, the funding available was used to send 6 Kenyans to Vanderbilt University Medical Center for an 8-week training program. Four of this six-member team were health workers from Western Kenya; one gynecologist/obstetrician, one anesthesiologist, and two non-physician anesthetists (one nurse and a clinical officer). The four formed the foundational faculty for training programs offered at the center. The initial programs focused on obstetric care since cesarean sections and other obstetric surgeries were the most common surgeries done in Kenya. In addition to support for training nurse anesthetists, the center is used for continuing medical education by external providers training on a range of short courses including ACLS, Basic Emergency Course, and Introduction to Critical Care.

Since inception, the center has hosted a range of trainees including pre-service (nurse anesthesia students) and in-service health workers. Learners are exposed to scenarios that build both technical and non-technical skills at an individual and team level. Real-time debrief sessions prepare learners to engage in individual and collaborative reflection. This is done by giving them the opportunity to review scenarios, break down their decision making and discuss areas for improvement. The center has trained more than 800 individual health workers from the Western Kenya Region. Ongoing training projects have been implemented in the care of the patients with the novel coronavirus and training in pediatric emergencies.

5 Simulation Partnerships

Given that simulation is yet to be widely utilized in LMICs, it is important for leaders in SBME to engage with local stakeholders who can champion the adoption of this mode of training. One strategy to ensure sustainability is partnership with local academic training institutions. Training of faculty using a train-the-trainer model is critical to promote and spread the use of SBME in medical education programs. The simulation faculty serve as champions and give accurate feedback on the impact this mode of training has on learning outcomes. In a data-driven world, it is critical to

Table 2 Key components of a simulation training partnership

Key components to a simulation training partnership
Pairing of academic institutions (if possible) in both sites with existing engagement in medical education
Identification of local champions for simulation
Identify partnership goals early and explicitly
Acknowledgment of limitations at each institution
Collaboratively build goals, learning objectives, and case topics with rigorous medical education pedagogy
Collaborative simulation case development
Emphasis on operating within local structures
Early implementation of evaluation frameworks to identify barriers and measure outcomes

set up a robust evaluation framework to allow the partner institution to measure progress and identify barriers to success during the implementation of the simulation project. (Table 2).

6 Location, Technology, and Equipment

Two important considerations prior to implementing any simulation case are (1) the location where your simulation will take place and (2) your access to resources in that space. Will you conduct your case in a dedicated simulation lab such as The Center for Experiential Learning at Jaramogi Oginga Odinga Teaching and Referral Hospital, in a conference or classroom space, or in-situ (i.e., location of clinical care)? What physical and human resources are available in your space? Below we discuss several options ranging from low- to high-fidelity simulators as well as options for running simulations in different settings. It is imperative that simulation prepare learners to successfully practice in their own environment so technology should reflect available resources. A detailed pre-brief should include orienting learners to the simulator including its capabilities and limitations as well as the simulation environment, roles, and resources.

The Laerdal NeoNatalie Newborn Simulator [13] is a low-fidelity simulator that was developed for use in RLS with the Helping Babies Breathe [14] training program. The simulator can be filled with air, water, or rice and is available with light or dark skin tone. NeoNatalie demonstrates chest rise with effective bag mask ventilation technique and simulates umbilical pulse and spontaneous breathing using separate squeeze bulbs attached to the simulator. Laerdal offers several additional products, including the PreemieNatalie Preterm Simulator and MamaNatalie Birth Simulator designed for simulation of normal maternal and pediatric delivery and postpartum care as well as potential complications. Laerdal Global Health offers simulators at not-for-profit prices to 95 countries with neonatal and/or maternal mortality greater than the Sustainable Development Goals targets [15].

Low-fidelity simulators such as NeoNatalie can be combined with electronic applications, for example, SimMon (a downloadable phone app), to provide a remote-controlled simulated patient monitor allowing facilitators to display and adjust continuous vital signs including heart rate, oxygen saturation, and blood pressure. SimMon is a low-cost application that requires a pair of android or iOS devices to use and can be operated without internet access using Bluetooth technology [16]. Using SimMon is significantly more affordable than traditional simulation monitoring systems. Both the low-fidelity mannequins and vital sign display technology have the added benefit of being easily moveable and can be used in a simulation lab, a classroom, or in situ.

While high-fidelity simulators offer myriad capabilities, it is critical to consider if these reflect the resources that are available in the clinical setting being simulated. For example, access to continuous vital sign monitoring may be limited or only available to patients in the intensive care unit and utilizing this technology in simulation may misrepresent the clinical reality – so it would be discouraged in simulation practice [9].

The primary role of a simulator or mannequin simulation is to provide a central focus – i.e., the patient – for the learner to engage. Using an explicit pre-brief, almost anything can be used to represent "the patient." Simulation cases have been successfully run with items such as a bag of rice or a doll taking the role of the patient when a high- or low-fidelity simulator is not available (Figs. 1 and 2). An embedded actor playing the role of a nurse or patient caregiver can also easily communicate physical exam findings and provide learner feedback using a low-fidelity simulator.

An ideal way to conduct a simulation with limited resources is to run the case in-situ (in the clinical setting), such that the learner is truly limited by the available resources and will use exactly what is clinically available with care taken not to open any clean products. Running the simulation in situ also serves to highlight any process challenges that arise for the learner as well as engage multidisciplinary team members.

If the facilitator chooses to run a case in a classroom or lab without resources, there are multitude creative solutions to mimic the clinical setting. With proper pre-brief and the use of an embedded actor, anything from a rock to a box can mimic a glucometer or pulse oximeter, face masks can be made from recycled plastic bottles or cloth, and labeled tubes and bags can play the role of medications. Having the embedded actor treat these items as their counterpart elicits buy-in from the learners.

There are several ways to replace patient monitoring tools if they are not available: vital signs can be shared ad-hoc by the embedded actor when the learner places the rock or box near the finger of the mannequin – mimicking the way intermittent vital signs are normally obtained. In contrast, if continuous monitoring is available, a chalk board or board with attached paper or sticky notes can be used and updated throughout the case to represent a clinical monitor.

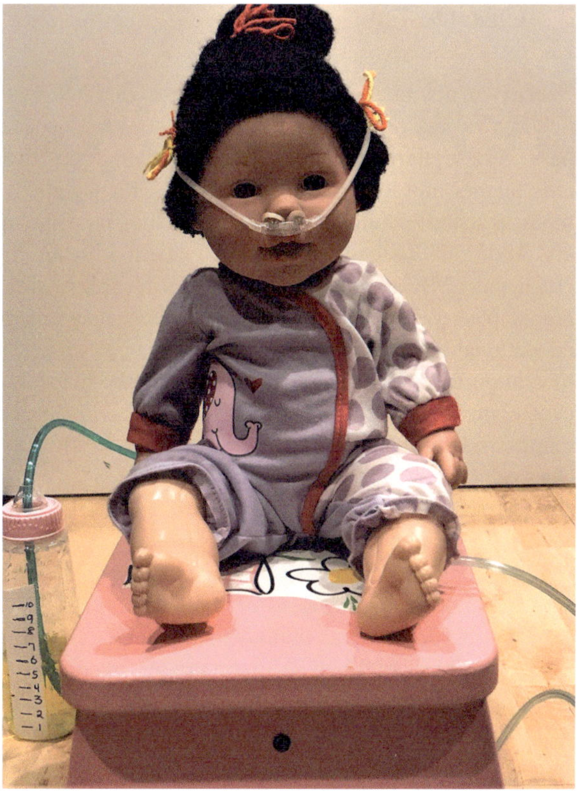

Fig. 1 Using a baby doll as a mannequin

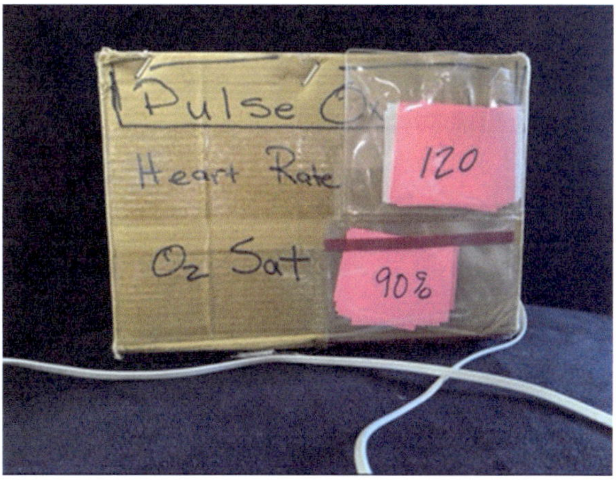

Fig. 2 Cardboard with changeable sticky notes as a monitor

7 Case Design

There is an abundance of simulation cases in the literature and that are used in practice in a variety of settings. One of the keys for a successful simulation is to take a basic case scenario or clinical condition and adjust the case flow based on the specific learner and learning objectives. The management expectations for learners in medical school would be different than those for nursing staff or practicing providers. Additionally, the medical management and care logistics likely differ between HICs and LMICs due to available resources. It is imperative that simulation cases are adapted to learners to meet them where they are with the goal to take them an educational step forward. To achieve this goal when adapting HIC cases for implementation in LMICs, strict attention must be made to the relevancy of simulation case content, i.e., if a specific medication is not a local option, it should not be emphasized in the case. Having clear learning objectives specific to local learners can keep case content appropriate.

When adapting a case that is in use in a HIC, it is imperative that local leadership, knowledge, and capabilities are directly addressed with any modifications. Interventions such as invasive procedures, specific medications, and specialty consult may not be available in an LMIC. Simulations should emphasize the best, evidence-based medical management that is available in the setting the learner intends to practice. When debriefing cases, attention can also be given to additional evidence-based interventions that may not currently be available at a specific site but would be important for learners in their future practice.

8 Case Facilitation

Facilitating a simulation case is split into three parts: the Pre-Brief, the Case Facilitation, and the Debrief (Table 3).

8.1 Pre-brief

The pre-brief occurs prior to the simulation case and serves to orient the learner to a potentially novel educational modality. Traditional medical education in many LMICs often emphasizes didactic learning and institutional hierarchy so there may be an expected learner adjustment phase, as with learners anywhere, when first exposed to SBME.

Table 3 PEARLS debriefing script [10]

<table>
<tr><td colspan="3">Setting the scene (may also occur before the first scenario debriefing, may abbreviate or omit for subsequent debriefings): "I'll spend about XX minutes debriefing the case with you. First, I'll be interested to hear from you how you are feeling now that the case is over; second, I'd like someone to describe what the case was about to make sure we are all on the same page. Then, we'll explore the aspects of the case that worked well for you and those you. Would manage differently and why. I'll be keen to hear what was going through your mind at various points in time. We'll end by summarizing some take-home points and how to apply them in your clinical practice"</td></tr>
<tr><td colspan="3">Reaction
"How are you feeling?"
Potential follow-up question:
"Other reactions?" or "how are the rest of you feeling?"</td></tr>
<tr><td colspan="3">Description
"Can someone summarize the case from a medical point of view so that we are all on the same page?"; "from your perspective, what were the main issues you had to deal with?"
Potential follow-up questions:
"What happened next?"; what things did you do for the patient?"</td></tr>
<tr><td colspan="3">Analysis
Signal the transition to the analysis of the case and frame the discussion:
"Now that we are clear about what happened let's talk more about the case. I think that there were aspects you managed effectively and others that seemed more challenging. I would like to explore each of these with you."</td></tr>
<tr><td>Learner self-assessment (e.g. plus-delta)
"What aspects of the case do you think you managed well and why?"<br>"What aspects of the case would you want to change and why?"
Close performance gaps selectively using directive feedback and teaching or focused facilitation</td><td>Directive feedback and teaching
Provide the relevant knowledge or tips to perform the action correctly.
"I noticed you (behavior). Next time, you may want to… [suggested behavior]… because [provide rationale]."</td><td>Focused facilitation (e.g., alternatives-pros and cons; self-guided team correction; advocacy-inquiry)
Specifically state what you would like to talk about ("I would like to spend a few minutes talking about XXX."
Elicit underlying rationale for actions: See SDC 2, http://links.lww.com/SIH/A175 for advocacy-inquiry approach</td></tr>
<tr><td colspan="3">Are there any outstanding issues before we start to close?</td></tr>
<tr><td colspan="3">Application summary
Learner guided: "I like to close the debriefing by having each you state one-two take-aways that will help you in the future."
Educator guided: "In summary the key learning points from this case were…"
Simulation in Healthcare</td></tr>
</table>

8.2 Case Facilitation

During the Case Facilitation, learners less familiar with simulation as an educational tool may require additional prompting to engage with the "patient" and to seek information from interactions with the simulator. Having an embedded actor play the role of a nurse, assistant, or other medical provider – as is contextually appropriate – can be useful to communicate information without breaking the realism of the case. This is preferable to a call and response approach where a learner directly solicits information from a facilitator rather than the "patient."

8.3 Debriefing

Focused and deliberate debriefing is critical to achieving learning objectives with SBME. The Promoting Excellence and Reflective Learning in Simulation (PEARLS) framework [10] has been successfully implemented at JOOTRH with faculty training as well as in other settings [17]. Based on the experience at JOOTRH, the content and steps of PEARLS translate easily to this context. The major adaptation was to provide an example debrief for planned debriefers to watch early in the training process. With this simple addition, faculty at JOOTRH learned and have successfully implemented the PEARLS debriefing framework with their learners (Tables 3 and 4).

Table 4 Key adaptations for designing and facilitating simulation in resource-limited settings

	Key adaptations for simulation in resource-limited settings	Virtual considerations
Setting the stage	Consider your location: Simulation lab, conference/classroom space, in-situ (hospital ward or clinic) Simulator type (high- vs low-fidelity, can substitute a doll or bag of rice with clear instructions on how to use in your pre-brief) Supplies should reflect resources available in the clinical environment where your learners practice (i.e., no monitors if these are only available in the ICU) Be creative and take care not to waste clean supplies, rely on embedded providers to guide learners	Ensure reliable internet access Familiarize yourself with the videoconferencing platform you will be using for the case and available features Consider where facilitators, learners, and simulators will be located and how they will interact

Table 4 (continued)

	Key adaptations for simulation in resource-limited settings	Virtual considerations
Case selection	Partner with local medical educators and clinicians to develop cases that address learning objectives that meet your learners' specific needs Tailor to training level and professional role Consult local hospital/clinic, national, and WHO guidelines to ensure management reflects local best, evidence-based practices	Consider if learning objectives can be met using the technology available (i.e., procedure skill practice will require learners to access equipment for practice from home or on-site)
Pre-brief	Additional exposition on the role of simulation, particularly with participants with limited simulation exposure Establish psychological safety Orient learner to any equipment and its role Encourage suspension of disbelief Clarify the role of any embedded provider Remind the learner that they must interact with the simulator and plan to mimic any actions they would do to a patient If the learners have not previously done simulation, remind them that making mistakes is OKAY and provides an opportunity for learning	Manage learner expectations and set the stage prior to the session Give explicit instructions on how learners should manage microphone, camera, chat feature, and set up their screens Emphasize suspension of disbelief and encourage learners to minimize distractions Acknowledge linear flow and limited ability of learners to multitask in the virtual environment, awkwardness of virtual interaction Let learners know if you plan to record the case and obtain consent before doing so
Simulation case facilitation	Consider where learners may get stuck in your case and develop rescue statements to help them navigate through the case successfully Gently remind learners (if needed) to stay engaged in the case and act as though caring for a real patient Use an embedded actor or facilitator playing a locally relevant role to guide learners and provide suggestions as needed	Turn off your video and sound briefly and restart to help learners transition to the start of the case, mimicking entering the patient room Use this break as an opportunity to have learners divide up roles amongst themselves Use a digital pause to transition again at the end of the case to the debrief

(continued)

Table 4 (continued)

	Key adaptations for simulation in resource-limited settings	Virtual considerations
Debrief	The debriefer should create a positive, collegial, and locally appropriate environment for learners to discuss clinical performance Co-debrief with faculty with significant experience practicing in the clinical environment you are simulating (if you do not) Explicitly elicit initial emotional reactions first Encourage learners not to focus only on errors and highlight positive performance Specific reference should be made to utilization of best practices and available resources within the specific RLS (i.e., referencing guidelines you used in developing your case) If learners have experiences from areas with more resources, encourage peer to peer teaching of practices (i.e., if bubble CPAP is not available, but a learner knows of this, have them discuss this with their peers)	Silence can feel longer in the virtual environment than in-person. Be patient and allow learners time to reflect and respond to your prompts Some learners may be more comfortable sharing their thoughts in the chat vs coming off mute
Training local simulation educators	Provide a video or in-person example of what a debriefing session and simulation case looks like and have your future debriefers experience being debriefed prior to working with their trainees When training local or novice debriefers, experienced debriefer can provide mentored feedback by directly observing sessions	Practice your virtual simulation session multiple times to help troubleshoot potential issues and gain comfort with your virtual platform

9 Virtual Simulation Adaptations

Telesimulation is a novel tool which can increase access to simulation-based education in RLS. Telesimulation has been described as an effective technique to teach procedural skills, including intraosseous insertion and chest tube placement, as well as neonatal resuscitation [18–21]. There are multiple models for how to implement telesimulation for teaching procedural skills (Fig. 3) utilizing task trainers on-site at both participating institutions with video conferencing software and equipment allowing trainers to demonstrate procedures and coach learners as they practice using the same or similar equipment [18]. Trainers may also consider distributing equipment (such as NeoNatalie kits for teaching neonatal resuscitation) to

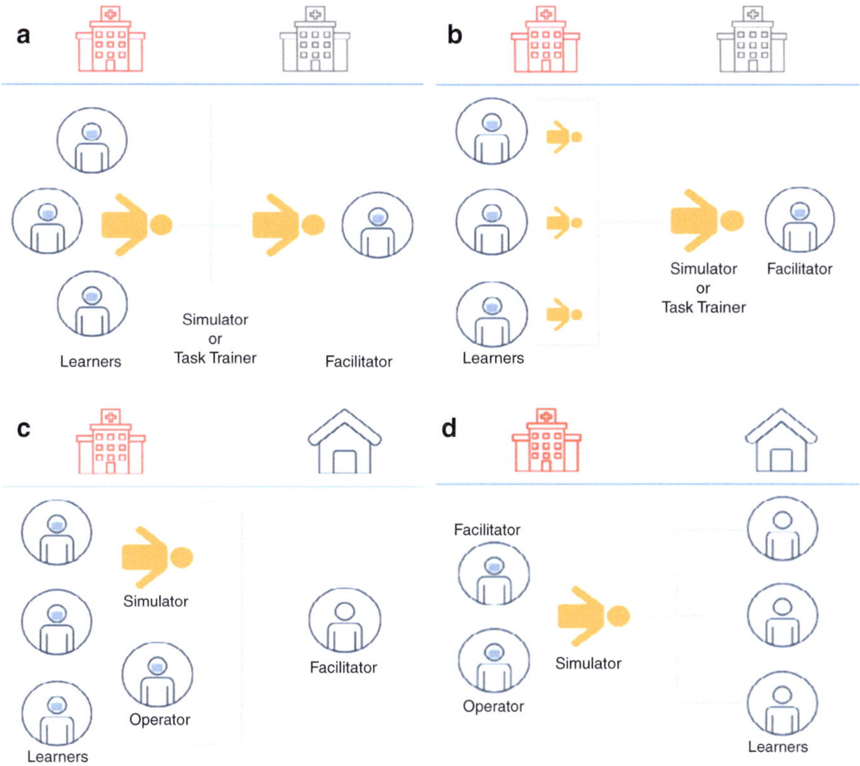

Fig. 3 (**a**) Virtual simulation models. Learners and a facilitator at remote sites utilize the same or similar simulator or task trainer and connect using video conferencing technology for procedural skills training, such as described by Garland et al. and Mikrogianakis et al. [18]. (**b**) Virtual simulation models. Learners at separate sites each with a simulator, task trainer, or procedural supplies connect to a facilitator at a remote site who demonstrates procedural skills and provides feedback to learners as they practice using video conferencing technology. (**c**) Virtual simulation models. Learners practice procedural skills or case on a simulator on-site with guidance from a remote facilitator. An operator or embedded confederate may be present on-site to assist learners, set up equipment and connection, and manage technical issues as in Donohue et al. [19] The facilitator may run the simulator remotely, or the operator on-site may control the simulator. (**d**) Virtual simulation models. The facilitator and operator are present with the simulation for the case or procedural skills. Learners are remote and connected virtually to observe and verbally guide the case

individual learners participating in simulation from multiple different locations. Some of the procedural skills described in this book, such as creating a spacer for a metered dose inhaler (MDI), may be taught with telesimulation using equipment participants may have already at their location and can gather with advance notice prior to the training session. Alternatively, learners may engage with a simulator that is remotely controlled by a facilitator to practice procedural skills and receive feedback [19].

Similarly, simulation cases themselves can be facilitated virtually with facilitator and learners separate (Fig. 3). If the simulator is with the facilitator, the virtual learners would be expected to explicitly state what physical exam maneuvers and diagnostic or therapeutic interventions they would perform, with either the facilitator or an embedded actor interacting with the patient – or if the simulator is with the learners, the facilitator must seek clarification for the learners' actions and provide the feedback verbally.

The greatest limitation to implementing telesimulation is its dependence on a reliable internet connection. However, Mikrogianakis et al. [18] overcame this barrier by using telesimulation to train a core group of clinicians in interosseous needle insertion who could then disseminate these skills to clinicians practicing in remote areas without internet access using a train the trainer model.

More detail regarding virtual education including expansion of many of the topics covered in this chapter can be found on the VE Pack website [22].

10 Conclusion

Simulation, which can incorporate some of the procedural modifications discussed elsewhere in this text, can be a valuable educational tool for use in resource-variable settings. While best practices in facilitating simulation such as pre-briefing, developing psychological safety, and structured debriefing are valuable regardless of where the simulation takes place, addressing some of the nuances of working in settings with limited resources in the design and facilitation is essential in creating a meaningful learning experience.

References

1. Datta R, Upadhyay K, Jaideep C. Simulation and its role in medical education. Med J Armed Forces India. 2012;68(2):167–72.
2. Balki M, et al. Effectiveness of using high-fidelity simulation to teach the management of general anesthesia for cesarean delivery. Can J Anaesth. 2014;61(10):922–34.
3. Ruesseler M, et al. Simulation training improves ability to manage medical emergencies. Emerg Med J. 2010;27(10):734–8.
4. Crump JA, Sugarman J, T. Working Group on Ethics Guidelines for Global Health. Ethics and best practice guidelines for training experiences in global health. Am J Trop Med Hyg. 2010;83(6):1178–82.
5. St Clair NE, et al. Global health: preparation for working in resource-limited settings. Pediatrics. 2017;140(5):1–16.
6. Butteris SM, et al. Simulation use for global away rotations (SUGAR): preparing residents for emotional challenges abroad--a multicenter study. Acad Pediatr. 2014;14(5):533–41.
7. Pitt MB, Gladding SP, Butteris SM. Using simulation for global health preparation. Pediatrics. 2016;137(5):1–4.
8. Schwartz KR, Prentiss KA. Simulation in pre-departure training for residents planning clinical work in a low-income country. West J Emerg Med. 2015;16(7):1166–72.
9. Pitt MB, et al. Using simulation in Global Health: considerations for design and implementation. Simul Healthc. 2017;12(3):177–81.

10. Eppich W, Cheng A. Promoting excellence and reflective learning in simulation (PEARLS): development and rationale for a blended approach to health care simulation debriefing. Simul Healthc. 2015;10(2):106–15.
11. Rosenman JR, et al. Global health simulation during residency. Glob Pediatr Health. 2016;3:2333794X16663545.
12. St Clair NE, Fischer PR, Hagen SA, Kuzminski J, Al-Nimr A, Pitt MB, Schubert C, Umphrey LA-M, Warrick S, Conway JH. Midwest consortium of global child health educators: local collaboration to strengthen global education. Ann Glob Health. 2014;80(3):178.
13. NeoNatalie. Available from: laerdal.com/us/products/simulation-training/obstetrics-pediatrics/neonatalie. Accessed April 27, 2022.
14. Helping Babies Breathe. American Academy of Pediatrics. Available from: https://www.aap.org/en/aap-global/helping-babies-survive/our-programs/helping-babies-breathe/. Accessed April 27, 2022.
15. Laerdal Global Health. Available from: https://laerdalglobalhealth.com/.
16. SimMon. Castle+Andersen ApS. 2018 [cited 2021 February 1, 2021]; Available from: Laerdal Medical.
17. Robinson T, et al. Sim for life: foundations-a simulation educator training course to improve debriefing quality in a low resource setting: a pilot study. Simul Healthc. 2020;15(5):326–34.
18. Mikrogianakis A, et al. Telesimulation: an innovative and effective tool for teaching novel intraosseous insertion techniques in developing countries. Acad Emerg Med. 2011;18(4):420–7.
19. Donohue LT, Hoffman KR, Marcin JP. Use of telemedicine to improve neonatal resuscitation. Children (Basel). 2019;6(4):1–11.
20. Garland C, et al. The application of low-fidelity chest tube insertion using remote Telesimulation in training healthcare professionals. Cureus. 2019;11(12):e6273.
21. Hayden EM, et al. Mannequin-based Telesimulation: increasing access to simulation-based education. Acad Emerg Med. 2018;25(2):144–7.
22. Lam SK, CC, Fant C, Umphrey L, Bensman R, An C, Arteaga G, Ben Abdallah M, Bjorklund A, Bothe D, Dalal Hardman P, Greene B, Gundacker C, Hoekstra N, Houser L, Jasthi D, Khron K, Lauden S, Leuche V, Mikkelsen M, Mitchell J, Moskalawicz R, Mumuney S, Perera S, Rule A, Runsewe O, Santoso Clark S, Slusher T, Van Genderen K, Weinstein I on behalf of the Midwest Consortium of Global Child Health Educators. VE-PACK: Virtual Education Partnership and Curricular Kit. 2021 Curriculum launched July 30, 2021; Available from: https://sugarprep.org/ve-pack.

Practice and Implementation of Procedural Adaptations in a Low-Resource Setting

Ashley R. Bjorklund, Stephanie M. Lauden, and Tina M. Slusher

Abbreviations

AAP	American Academy of Pediatrics
CPAP	Continuous Positive Airway Pressure
EBT	Exchange blood transfusion
GHEC	Global Health Education Course
HBB	Helping Babies Breathe
IO	Intraosseous
ISEC	Interdisciplinary Simulation Education Center at Hennepin Healthcare
IV	Intravenous drops
MDI	Metered Dose Inhaler
PAS	Pediatric Academic Society
SUGAR PEARLS	Simulation Use for Global Away Rotations – Procedural Education for Adaptations to Resource-Limited Settings
UVC	Umbilical venous catheter
VE-PACK	Virtual Education Partnership and Curricular Kit

A. R. Bjorklund (✉) · T. M. Slusher
Department of Pediatrics, Division of Critical Care, Global Pediatric Program, University of Minnesota, Minneapolis, MN, USA

Department of Pediatrics, Division of Critical Care, Hennepin Healthcare, Minneapolis, MN, USA
e-mail: bals0064@umn.edu

S. M. Lauden
Department of Pediatrics, Division of Hospital Medicine, University of Colorado, Denver, CO, USA
e-mail: stephanie.lauden@childrenscolorado.org

T. M. Slusher et al. (eds.), *Pediatric Procedural Adaptations for Low-Resource Settings*, https://doi.org/10.1007/978-3-030-99955-1_25

1 Self-Study and Available Resources

Any healthcare provider intending to incorporate the procedural adaptations and modifications described in this book requires dedicated training and supervision before implementing these skills in a clinical setting. There are a variety of resources that can be utilized to review these procedures to ensure adequate understanding of the steps. Knowing your resources is half the battle! A portion of that training can come from self-study resources such as this book, the free online training resource SUGAR PEARLS (Simulation Use for Global Away Rotations – Procedural Education for Adaptations to Resource-Limited Settings), and other resources for practice in low-resource settings.

Below are links and descriptions of some of the well-known resources that providers in the United States utilize. One thing that is wonderful about the community of global health providers is the willingness to share ideas and support each other in providing evidence-based, safe, and appropriate care for children throughout the world.

- PEARLS on Sugar Prep website:
  - https://sugarprep.org/pearls/
- Helping Babies Breathe (HBB) website:
  - https://laerdalglobalhealth.com/partnerships-and-programs/helping-babies-breathe/
- Global Pediatrics Education Series (GPEDS) (available for purchase through the University of Minnesota Global Pediatrics Program)
  - z.umn.edu/GPEDS
- Global Health Education Course (GHEC):
  - https://shop.aap.org/2021-global-health-education-course-virtual-only/
- Open Pediatrics Website:
  - https://www.openpediatrics.org

2 Importance of Hands-On Training and Supervision

However, hands-on training and opportunities to practice learned skills in a proctored setting are essential before attempting to utilize these procedural adaptations in any clinical setting. As emphasized throughout this book, procedural modifications and adaptations should only be completed by clinicians already trained and licensed to perform them. Thus, trainees or clinicians who have not previously performed a procedure must receive dedicated teaching and supervision from an experienced clinician. That teacher often is the clinician from the low-resource setting.

Over the last several decades, we have utilized a variety of formats to provide both instruction and opportunities to practice procedural adaptations and the construction of modified devices. In-person "procedural workshops" have been a highly successful model. These workshops utilize low-cost models and re-useable supplies in a number of stations, allowing hands-on instruction, practice, and review of the procedure or device. Generally, we have found that dividing learners into small groups (6–8 learners: 1 instructor maximum) creates the most ideal learning environment. We have led "procedural workshops" at multiple conferences, including the Pediatric Academic Society (PAS) annual meeting and the American Academy of Pediatrics (AAP) National Convention, as well as various global health courses both nationally and internationally.

Workshop Format: Here is an example of the format for one session.

Preparation for the workshop: Gather supplies and sort into "station boxes" with individual bags or packets for each participant who will be rotating through this station. Ideally, each participant should have their own supplies, so they can practice the skillset.

Supply list: Table 1 provides an example supply list for a procedural workshop. For in-person workshops, supplies are typically provided by the instructors/facilitators. For virtual workshops, some supplies are provided by the instructor and mailed ahead of time to the participants and some supplies are provided by the student. See VE-PACK website for more details – https://sugarprep.org [1].

Total participants: 36.

Total station facilitators: 6.

Time keeper: Helpful to have an extra person that can be a runner for supplies, and monitor time participants spend at each station.

Workshop timeline – 2.5 hours

- 15–20 min: Introduction (whole group) – Basic concepts/ethics as described in chap. 1. Discuss station rotations and format for the workshop.
  - Divide into 6 small groups to rotate between stations
- 120 min (15 min at each station with 5 minutes to switch/set up between)

6 Stations: Instructor demo with learners following along step by step with their own supplies.

- Station 1:
  - Skill: Place an umbilical venous catheter (UVC)
- Station 2:
  - Skill: Perform an exchange blood transfusion (EBT)
- Station 3:
  - Skill 1: Make a water bottle spacer for a metered dose inhaler (MDI)
  - Skill 2: Insert an intraosseous (IO) needle with a locally produced needle

Table 1 Sample supplies list for virtual

Station		Faculty/ facilitator supplies	Student supplies (from facilitators)	Student supplies (student brings)
Bubble CPAP				
	Oxygen tubing	X	X	
	Nasal cannula adult or pediatric	X	X	
	Ruler	X		X
	Marker/pen	X		X
	Super glue	X		X
	Tape roll	X	X	
	Water bottle	X		X
	Ear plugs	X	X	
	Nail (or toothpick)			
	Scissors (small sharp)	X		X
	Baby hat	X		
	Safety pin	X		
UVC/ EBT				
	Baby bottles with cord	X	X	
	6F NG tube	X	X	
	String	X	X	
	10 mL syringe	X	X	
IO				
	Spinal needles	X		
	Commercial IO	X		
	List/picture of possible placement sites	X		
	IV 18G with caps		X	
	Scissors			X
	10 or 20 mL syringe	X	X	
	Tape roll	X	X	
	Gauze	X		
	Bones (chicken leg)	X		X
Drips				
	Paper	X		X
	Pens	X		X
	Wipe board	X		
	Buretrol™	X		
	Microdrip Buretrol™	X		
	Fluid bag	X		
	IV pole	X		
	Worksheet with example problems		X	

Course courtesy of VE-PACK

- Station 4:
  - Skill: Construct a low-cost bubble continuous positive airway pressure (BCPAP) Circuit
- Station 5:
  - Skill: Make a chest drainage system
- Station 6:
  - Skill: Calculate intravenous fluid drip count without an infusion pump

10–15 min: Conclusion and final questions (whole group).

3 Low-Cost Model Examples

In other simulations, such as those focused on procedural skills, it is helpful to have low-cost models. Commercially, models such as the Helping Babies Breath mannequin or commercial IO practice bones can be purchased for a relatively low cost. Alternatively, we have found that clean chicken bones work well for teaching intraosseous needle insertion, pig ribs work well for teaching chest tube insertion, and a baby bottle umbilical cord model (described below) works well for teaching UVC placement (Table 2).

Umbilical cord model – This model can be used to teach umbilical venous line placement. Select either a commercial cord or a locally produced cord (Fig. 1). Add red food color to water for "blood" and fill a baby bottle with the red water. Consider putting a small rim of tape at the bottom of the bottle nipple to simulate skin (Fig. 2).

Intra-osseous model can be commercial IO model, chicken bone model (Fig. 3), or locally produced IO model (Table 2 and Fig. 4).

4 Implementation in the Clinical Setting

It is important that each procedural adaptation be reviewed carefully within the context it is to be used in. If further adaptation is warranted that should be studied carefully for safety and efficacy if it deviates significantly from that described in these chapters or currently used in your setting.

The term "low-resource" applies to a wide range of technology and equipment. For instance, continuous positive airway pressure (CPAP) using a modified nasal canula, a water bottle attached to a flow meter, and no blended oxygen may be appropriate in settings where nothing is available beyond a simple nasal cannula and transport to a higher level of care is not feasible. This level of support would not be appropriate for a setting where commercial bubble CPAP with built-in blenders are available, unless this unit's demand for commercial CPAP exceeded their supply.

Table 2 Making locally produced models

Model	Ingredients[a]/Supplies	Instructions
"Skin/tissue" material[b]	Glass mixing bowl Wisk 5 c (1200 mL) distilled water 3.5 c (800 mL) glycerin 1.2 c (280 mL) powdered gelatin 6 tsp. sugar-free psyllium containing powdered dietary fiber supplement	Mix all ingredients together in glass bowl Microwave until boiling Pour into mold being careful not to burn yourself Refrigerate (can keep extra in the refrigerator until another model needed)
Umbilical cord	Tubing about the size of an umbilical cord (ex. Teleflexg® Pleur-Evac™ tubing) 8 Fr suction catheter (2) 10 Fr suction catheter (1)	Tape the three suction tubes together and twist Thread the suction tubing into the "umbilical cord" tubing Place the tubing in the pink basin so that both ends are at the same height Pour the locally produced "skin" in the "umbilical cord" tubing, while not getting any in the suction tubing. After cord "hardens" test to make sure the 10 French tube "UVC" remains patent (Fig. 2b)
Intraosseous model	Hollow doll leg (or other mold) 10 ml syringe	Pour the locally produced "skin" into the mold/ hollow leg If desired, place a 10 ml syringe in the middle of the mold – which can act either as handle (Fig. 3) or can serve as a way to put colored water into the leg to simulate bone marrow

[a] Depending on the quantity needed the above recipe can be cut down, i.e., for the UVC model cutting ingredients to 1/10th is enough to make at least 20 "cords"

[b] We would like to acknowledge Troy E. Reihsen, for his creation of the recipe and formulation of materials used for this application

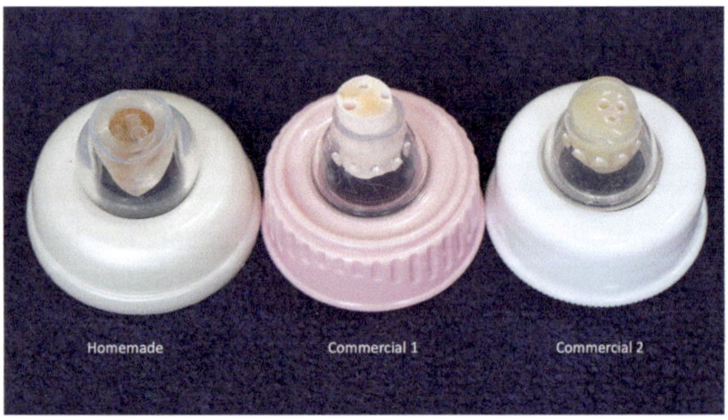

Fig. 1 Examples of locally produced and commercially available umbilical cord models

And of course, if even higher levels of support such as BiPAP and invasive ventilation are indicated and available in a unit staffed for these devices then of course these should be used. The same could be said about counting intravenous (IV) drops, mixing intravenous fluids, inserting umbilical catheters, doing exchange blood transfusions, and most of the procedures discussed in this book. *When possible, we should provide the best level of care available in order to meet the patient's needs.*

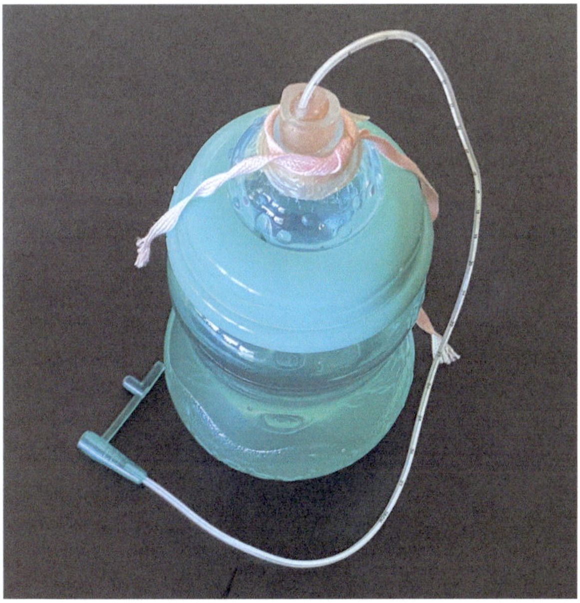

Fig. 2 Umbilical cord model (locally produced) in baby bottle with cord tie and feeding tube for simulations

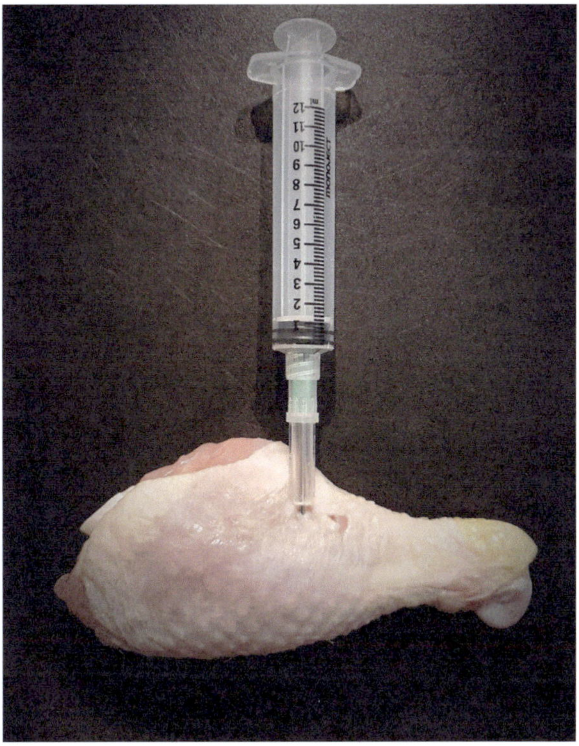

Fig. 3 Chicken bone. (Courtesy of https://sugarprep.org)

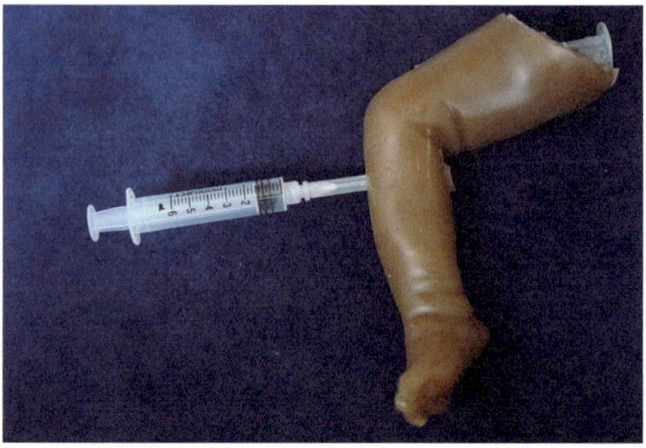

Fig. 4 Intraosseous model. (Courtesy of Mr. Russ Siekman and the Interdisciplinary Simulation Education Center (ISEC))

If there are restrictions from any regulatory board or other agency in the country on using any of these adaptations, they should not be used in that country. If in doubt, confirm with the in-country clinician and the appropriate regulatory board(s) before using the adaptation. Some adaptations may require an in-country study even if used and approved in other countries.

5 Concluding Thoughts

Above all, we are called to do no harm. We must be aware of our limitations, but also think creatively to improve the quality of life for children regardless of their origin. We hope that the suggested modifications and adaptations presented in this book empower existing clinicians working in low-resource settings with the skills to provide high-quality care. We also hope that this collection of adaptations serves, as both a framework and inspiration for further advancements. These advancements will only occur in the context of ongoing sustainable collaborations and partnerships between high and low-income countries. We have much to learn from one another.

Reference

1. Lam SK, CC, Fant C, Umphrey L, Bensman R, An C, Arteaga G, Ben Abdallah M, Bjorklund A, Bothe D, Dalal Hardman P, Greene B, Gundacker C, Hoekstra N, Houser L, Jasthi D, Khron K, Lauden S, Leuche V, Mikkelsen M, Mitchell J, Moskalawicz R, Mumuney S, Perera S, Rule A, Runsewe O, Santoso Clark S, Slusher T, Van Genderen K, Weinstein I on behalf of the Midwest Consortium of Global Child Health Educators. VE-PACK: virtual education partnership and curricular kit. 2021 Curriculum launched July 30, 2021; Available from: https://sugarprep.org/ve-pack.

Index

T. M. Slusher et al. (eds.), *Pediatric Procedural Adaptations for Low-Resource Settings*, https://doi.org/10.1007/978-3-030-99955-1

MIX
Papier aus verantwortungsvollen Quellen
Paper from responsible sources
FSC® C105338

If you have any concerns about our products,
you can contact us on
ProductSafety@springernature.com

In case Publisher is established outside the EU,
the EU authorized representative is:
Springer Nature Customer Service Center GmbH
Europaplatz 3, 69115 Heidelberg, Germany

Printed by Libri Plureos GmbH
in Hamburg, Germany